Aesthetic Facial Anatomy Essentials for Injections

Aesthetic Facial Anatomy Essentials for Injections is the first title of a series to be published in partnership with *PRIME Journal* and the World Society of Interdisciplinary Aesthetic & Anti-Aging Medicine (WOSIAM).

PRiME

PRIME Journal is the leading authority on aesthetic and anti-aging medicine, providing industry news, insightful analysis, and key data, as well as the most high-quality research articles in the market. It's because of this that *PRIME* attracts leading authors who provide authoritative analysis on the issues that matter most to the industry. The aesthetic and anti-aging industry is a global one and deserves a dedicated international publication—a voice that will not only communicate, but educate, motivate, and inspire you with the latest, most applicable and usable information you need to do your work smarter, better, and more effectively. This is *PRIME*'s mission.

PRIME's editorial, sales, marketing, and management staff have created the leading international aesthetic and anti-aging publication, one that provides every aesthetic medical professional and supplier with a more effective communication forum to discuss, understand, implement, and apply the latest applications and technologies shaping the present and future development of the industry. Published both in print and online, *PRIME* is an essential tool for physicians, surgeons, dermatologists, and practitioners alike.

If you have not already subscribed to *PRIME*, visit the website today at www.prime-journal.com to guarantee each issue of the journal is delivered to your work or home.

WOSIAM

WORLD SOCIETY OF INTERDISCIPLINARY AESTHETIC & ANTI-AGING MEDICINE

The World Society of Interdisciplinary Aesthetic & Anti-Aging Medicine was created with a strong belief that good practice in aesthetic and anti-aging medicine must be comprehensively addressed. To achieve this, its mission is to disseminate knowledge in medical aesthetics and anti-aging medicine, as well as to federate scientific associations with shared values.

The WOSIAM is a nonprofit organization based in Paris, and membership is available to anyone who has participated in any event co-organized by the WOSIAM. Benefits of joining the WOSIAM include:

- WOSIAM membership certificate
- Special discounted rates on many international conferences
- Access to online educational video content
- Discounted rates on scientific books and peer-reviewed journals
- Priority to submit your article in *PRIME Journal*
- Priority to apply to be a speaker at a WOSIAM-affiliated congress and/or educational training course worldwide
- Listing in the WOSIAM's directory of aesthetic and/or anti-aging professionals
- Receive the WOSIAM newsletter with updates on the market products, scientific articles, and events

The WOSIAM board of directors includes Dario Bertossi, editor of *Aesthetic Facial Anatomy Essentials for Injections*, as well as other core specialists with the ambition to advance aesthetic and anti-aging medicine by creating high-quality programs at leading educational events.

The WOSIAM also hosts the annual Anti-Aging & Beauty Trophy awards, which gives recognition to the companies and physicians striving to make breakthrough innovations in the field of aesthetics and anti-aging. For more information on the awards or how to enter, visit the website at https://wosiam.org.

Aesthetic Facial Anatomy Essentials for Injections

Edited by

Ali Pirayesh, MD, FCC (Plast)
Plastic, Reconstructive and Aesthetic Surgeon
Founder, Amsterdam Plastic Surgery Clinic, the Netherlands
Consultant, Burns and Tissue Regeneration Unit
University Hospital, Gent, Belgium
Research Consultant, University College Hospital, London, UK

Dario Bertossi, MD
Associate Professor of Maxillofacial Surgery
Specialist in Maxillofacial Surgery, Otolaryngology
Facial Plastic Surgeon
Department of Surgery, Dentistry, Pediatrics and Gynaecology
Chief of Maxillofacial Plastic Surgery Unit
University of Verona, Verona, Italy
Professor of Practice, University of London
Centre for Integrated Medical and Translational Research, London, UK

Izolda Heydenrych, MD
Dermatologist, Founder and Director, Cape Town Cosmetic Dermatology Centre
Consultant, Division of Dermatology, Faculty of Health Sciences
University of Stellenbosch, Stellenbosch, South Africa

With Forewords from Mauricio de Maio, Pierfrancesco Nocini, and Foad Nahai

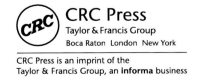

CRC Press
Taylor & Francis Group
Boca Raton London New York

CRC Press is an imprint of the
Taylor & Francis Group, an **informa** business

CRC Press
Taylor & Francis Group
6000 Broken Sound Parkway NW, Suite 300
Boca Raton, FL 33487-2742

Printed on acid-free paper

International Standard Book Number-13: 978-1-138-50571-1 (Paperback; pack/eBook)
978-1-138-50572-8 (Hardback)

Artwork and illustrations have been done by Alessandro Meggio of 3Dshift srls

Library of Congress Control Number: 2020930259

Visit the Taylor & Francis Web site at
http://www.taylorandfrancis.com

and the CRC Press Web site at
http://www.crcpress.com

CONTENTS

PREFACE

Anatomy has long been the compass guiding clinicians through the astounding complexity of the human body.

Many textbooks of anatomy display the vital structures and their anatomical relationships in order to guide medical students and physicians, thus enabling them to learn and execute medical treatments.

We encountered a void in the plethora of anatomical scripts where both essential clinical anatomy and an aesthetic eye for beautification and rejuvenation need to merge. Only a paucity of mostly single-author texts exist on the essential anatomy for aesthetic medicine.

The global conference platform of Euromedicom and its network provided us with unparalleled access to the greatest minds in surgical and medical aesthetics who enjoy passing on their passion, tips and tricks in this ever expanding field.

This book by the Aesthetic Facial Anatomy group is a multi-author, cross-specialty consensus on the essential knowledge of clinically relevant anatomy and injection guidelines mandatory for safe, effective and aesthetically pleasing application of aesthetic medicine, and is encouraged to be regularly updated online by the many authors.

The men and women who allowed us to explore their anatomical structures after their passing in order for us to pass on this knowledge to our peers are the true hero educators which we should honour. It has been a privilege to work on this ongoing project.

Ali Pirayesh, Dario Bertossi, and Izolda Heydenrych

FOREWORDS

"We shall not cease from exploration
And the end of all our exploring
Will be to arrive where we started
And know the place for the first time..."

—from TS Eliot, "Little Gidding", *Four Quartets*, with permission from Faber & Faber Ltd.

The ancient art of anatomy, which has long fascinated the human mind, has in recent years been considerably expanded by the field of aesthetic medicine. This book beautifully demonstrates the fascinating detail beneath the surface of our everyday work and should form an invaluable practical resource for those passionate about the field of medicine.

This initiative is aimed at elevating both procedural safety and clinical excellence.

I am proud to be part of it.

Mauricio de Maio, MD

During my 40 years of practice, I have trained many residents, some of them who are now masters in the field of facial aesthetics, where they are witnesses of the impressive growth this field has undergone during the last few decades. As a teacher, my role has always been to accurately evaluate the international scientific production. As I received the first draft of this comprehensive book, I realized that its impact on the medical aesthetic field will be great as it will provide the reader a solid scientific knowledge and a practical tool for beginners as well as for the advanced injectors.

I wish for all readers to understand the deepest meaning of this work. If culture and learning are made to light up our minds before our hands, the result has been achieved.

Pierfrancesco Nocini, MD

Fillers and toxins have proven to be affordable and safe treatments for the aging face. Injectables continue to gain popularity and are by far the most sought after cosmetic treatments worldwide. With this increase in demand and popularity, there arises the need for appropriate training; a need to assure safety as well as efficacy of results.

I congratulate the editors Dr Pirayesh, Dr. Bertossi and Dr. Heydenrych for bringing together such an illustrious group of thought leaders to share their knowledge and expertise in this book which is designed to improve results and enhance safety.

The most feared and devastating complication of injectables is intra-arterial injection of fillers leading to tissue necrosis and vision loss. The chapters organized by facial regions accurately describe the anatomy in minute detail, with beautiful medical illustrations and immaculately clear cadaver dissections which highlight the location and course of blood vessels at risk. The risk to blood vessels in each location is outlined and safe injection techniques are recommended that reduce risk.

This book will be invaluable not only to the novice eager to perfect their injection technique but also to those of us who have had years of experience. As someone with a long career as a surgical educator and proponent of patient safety, I plan to put this book in the hands of all our trainees.

Foad Nahai, MD FACS FRCS (Hon)

CONTRIBUTORS

Shino Bay Aguilera
Dermatologist
Assistant Professor of Dermatology
Shino Bay Cosmetic Dermatology
and Laser Institute
and
Dermatology Department
NOVA Southeastern University
Fort Lauderdale, Florida, USA

Khalid Alawadi
Consultant Plastic and Hand Surgeon
Department of Hand and Reconstructive
Microsurgery
Rashid Hospital
Dubai Health Authority
Dubai, United Arab Emirates

Chytra V. Anand
Chief Cosmetic Dermatologist
Kosmoderma Clinics
Bangalore, India

Fazıl Apaydın
ENT Surgeon
Department of Otorhinolaryngology
Ege University
Izmir, Turkey

Raul Banegas
Plastic Surgeon
Director of Centro Arenales
Medical Center
Buenos Aires, Argentina

Emanuele Bartoletti
Plastic Surgeon
Studio Bartoletti-Cavalieri
Fatebenefratelli Hospital
Rome, Italy

Laura Bertolasi
Department of Neurosciences
Unit of Neurology AOUI
Verona, Italy

Thierry Besins
Plastic Surgeon
Private Clinic
Nice, France

Luis Fernando Botero
Plastic Surgeon
Clinica Quirofanos El Tesoro
Medellín, Colombia

Chiara Botti
Plastic Surgeon
Villa Bella Clinic
Salo, Italy

Giovanni Botti
Plastic Surgeon
Villa Bella Clinic
Salo, Italy

Koenraad De Boulle
Dermatologist
Aalst Dermatology Clinic
Aalst, Belgium

André Braz
Dermatologist
Private Practice
Rio de Janeiro and São Paulo, Brazil

Alastair Carruthers
Dermatologist
Clinical Professor of Dermatology
University of British Columbia
and
Private Practice
The Carruthers Clinic
Vancouver, British Columbia, Canada

Maurizio Cavallini
Plastic Surgeon
Unit of Plastic Surgery and Dermatology
CDI Hospital
Milan, Italy

Steven R. Cohen
Plastic Surgeon
Clinical Professor of Plastic Surgery
University of California, San Diego and Private Practice
FACES+
La Jolla, California, USA

Sebastian Cotofana
Associate Professor of Anatomy
Department of Clinical Anatomy
Mayo Clinic
Rochester, Minnesota, USA

Steven Dayan
Facial Plastic Surgeon
Clinical Assistant Professor
University of Illinois
Chicago, Illinois, USA

Henry Delmar
Plastic Surgeon
Clinique Del Mar
Antibes, France

Wolfgang G. Philipp-Dormston
Dermatologist
Medical Director, Department for Dermatology, Dermatosurgery and Allergology
Clinic Links vom Rhein
Cologne, Germany

Paul van der Eerden
ENT/Facial Plastic Surgeon
Lange Land Hospital
Zoetermeer, the Netherlands

Steven Fagien
Oculoplastic Surgeon
Aesthetic Eyelid Plastic Surgery
Private Practice
Boca Raton, Florida, USA

Fernando Felice
Associate Professor in Anatomy
University of Buenos Aires
Aesthetic Plastic Surgeon, Private Practice
Buenos Aires, Argentina

Jay Galvez
Facial Plastic Surgeon
Galvez Clinics
Makati City, the Philippines

Jennifer Gaona
Plastic and Reconstructive Surgeon
Founder of Keraderm and INTI Foundation
Private Practice
Bogota, Colombia

Giorgio Giampaoli
Resident in Maxillofacial Surgery
Maxillofacial Surgery Department
University of Verona
Verona, Italy

Kate Goldie
Aesthetic Physician
Medical Director, European Medical Aesthetics Ltd
London, UK

Uliana Gout
Aesthetic Physician
London Aesthetic Medicine Clinic and Academy
London, UK

Alessandro Gualdi
Plastic Surgeon
Clinical Professor
Vita-Salute San Raffaele University
Milano, Italy

Ekaterina Gutop
Dermatologist
Actual Clinic
Yaroslavl, Russia

Per Heden
Plastic Surgeon
Associate Professor in Plastic Surgery
Karolinska Institute
Stockholm, Sweden

Benoit Hendrickx
Plastic Surgeon
Associate Professor
University Hospital Brussels
Brussels, Belgium

Haideh Hirmand
Plastic Surgeon
Clinical Assistant Professor of Surgery
Cornell-Weill Medical College
New York-Presbyterian Hospital
New York City, New York, USA

Rene van der Hulst
Head and Professor of Plastic Surgery
Maastricht University Medical Center
Maastricht, the Netherlands

Shannon Humphrey
Clinical Assistant Professor
Department of Dermatology and Skin Science
University of British Columbia
Vancouver, Canada

Fabio Ingallina
Plastic Surgeon
Private Practice
Catania, Italy

Mohammad Ali Jawad
Plastic, Reconstructive and Burn Surgeon
R5 Aesthetic and Healthcare
Karachi, Pakistan

Krishan Mohan Kapoor
Consultant Plastic Surgeon
Plastic and Cosmetic Surgery
Fortis Hospital
Mohali, India

and

Honorary Senior Clinical Lecturer
University of London
London, UK

Philippe Kestemont
Facial Plastic Surgeon
Saint George
Aesthetic Medicine Clinic
Nice, France

Paraskevas Kontoes
Plastic Surgeon
DrK Medical Group
Athens, Greece

Berend van der Lei
Plastic, Reconstructive and Aesthetic Surgeon
Professor, Aesthetic Plastic Surgery
Department of Plastic Surgery
University Medical Centre Groningen
Bey Bergman Clinics
Groningen, the Netherlands

Shirong Li
Professor of Plastic Surgery
Department of Plastic Surgery
Third Military Hospital
Chongking, China

Steven Liew
Plastic Surgeon
Medical Director Shape Clinic
Darlinghurst, Australia

Philippe Magistretti
Consultant Radiologist and Aesthetic Physician
The Summit Clinic
Crans Montana, Switzerland

Mauricio de Maio
Plastic Surgeon
MD Codes™ Institute
São Paulo, Brazil

Natalia Manturova
Plastic Surgeon
Head, Department of Plastic and Reconstructive Surgery
Cosmetology and Cell Technologies
Russian National Research Medical University
Moscow, Russia

Alberto Marchetti
Plastic Surgeon
San Francesco Clinic
Verona, Italy

John J. Martin
Oculoplastic Surgeon
Oculo-facial Plastic Surgery
Miami, Florida, USA

Leonard Miller
Plastic Surgeon
Founder, Boston Center for Facial Rejuvenation
Brookline, Massachusetts, USA

Randy B. Miller
Plastic Surgeon
Miller Plastic Surgery
Miami, Florida, USA

Stan Monstrey
Professor in Plastic Surgery
Plastic Surgery, Burns and Tissue Regeneration Unit
Gent University Hospital
Gent, Belgium

Colin M. Morrison
Consultant Plastic Surgeon
St. Vincent's University Hospital
Dublin, Ireland

Ash Mosahebi
Professor of Plastic Surgery
Royal Free Hospitals and University College Hospital
London, UK

Paul S. Nassif
Facial Plastic and Reconstructive Surgery
Assistant Clinical Professor
Department of Otolaryngology – Head and Neck Surgery
Division of Facial Plastic and Reconstructive Surgery
University of Southern California Keck School of Medicine
Los Angeles, California, USA

Marc Nelissen
Plastic Surgeon
Global Care Clinic
Heusden-Zolder, Belgium

Riccardo Nocini
ENT Surgery
Department of Otolaryngology
Department of Surgical Sciences, Dentistry, Gynecology and Pediatrics
University of Verona
Verona, Italy

Anna Marie C Olsen
Dermatologist
Private Practice
London, UK

Tim Papadopoulos
Plastic Surgeon
Private Practice
Sydney, Australia

Michele Pascali
Plastic Surgeon
Plastic Surgery Academy Roma
Rome, Italy

Tatjana Pavicic
Dermatologist
Private Practice for Dermatology and Aesthetics
Munich, Germany

Eqram Rahman
General Surgeon
Associate Professor
Division of Surgery and Interventional Science
University College London
London, UK

Jinda Rojanamatin
Dermatologist
Head of Dermatosurgery and Laser Department
Institute of Dermatology
Bangkok, Thailand

Hervé Raspaldo
Facial Plastic Surgeon
Chef de Clinique des Universités
Face Clinic Genève
Geneva, Switzerland

Enrico Robotti
Plastic Surgeon
Chief, Department of Plastic Surgery
Papa Giovanni XXIII Hospital
Bergamo, Italy

Yves Saban
Facial Plastic Surgeon
Private Practice
Nice, France

Neil Sadick
Dermatologist
Sadick Dermatology
New York City, New York, USA

Massimo Signorini
Plastic Surgeon
Studio Medico Skin House
Milano, Italy

Jianxing Song
Professor of Plastic and Reconstructive Surgery
Changhai Hospital, Second Military Medical University
Shanghai, China

Alwyn Ray D'Souza
Plastic Surgery
London Bridge Hospital
London, UK

Ruth Tevlin
Department of Surgery
Stanford University School of Medicine
Stanford, California, USA

Gloria Trocchi
Specialist in Internal Medicine
Aesthetic Medicine Department
Fatebenefratelli Hospital
Rome, Italy

Ines Verner
Dermatologist
Department of Dermatology and Regenerative Medicine
Verner Clinic
Tel Aviv, Israel

Daria Voropai
Aesthetic Physician
AEGIS London
London, UK

Heidi A. Waldorf
Dermatologist
Waldorf Dermatology Aesthetics
Nanuet, New York, USA

and

Associate Clinical Professor
Department of Dermatology
Icahn School of Medicine of Mount Sinai
New York City, New York, USA

Vitaly Zholtikov
Plastic Surgeon
Private Practice "Atribeaute Clinic"
Saint Petersburg, Russia

A AESTHETIC REGIONS OF THE FACE

Alessandro Gualdi, Michele Pascali, Heidi A. Waldorf, Rene van der Hulst, Philippe Magistretti, and Dario Bertossi

FOREHEAD

The superior forehead margin lies at the hairline, whilst the lateral border is formed by the temporal crest where the frontalis and temporalis muscles fuse. The glabella, frontonasal groove (central), and the eyebrows overlying the supraorbital ridges form the inferior boundary (Figure A.1). The forehead does not demonstrate overt ethnic variations, but is usually shorter in South American and Asian patients whilst Caucasians and Africans have a higher, yet variable forehead height.

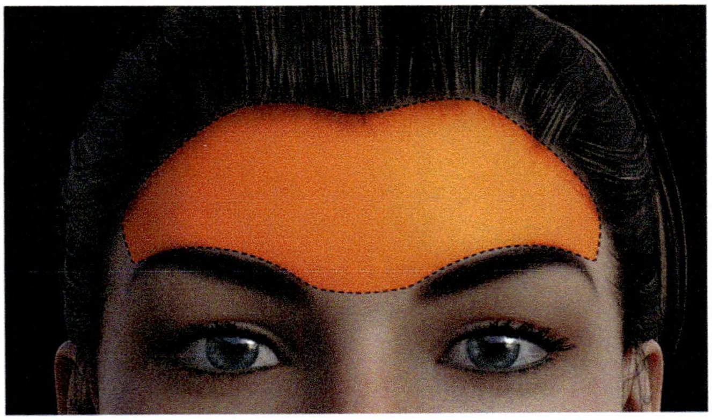

Figure A.1 The frontal area.

During the aging process, the forehead surface increases due to progressive hairline recession and widening of the orbital rims, with subsequent descent of the eyebrows. The lateral forehead aspect remains relatively unchanged.

Insightful understanding of the forehead and glabella is of great clinical importance. The frontalis is a very superficial muscle which may demonstrate several anatomical variants which need be taken into account for effective treatment with neuromodulators. The corrugator, one of the most important targets for neuromodulator treatment, lies at the medial orbital rim. Its medial origin is deep on bone, after which it courses superolaterally to insert into the skin over the lateral brow. Here it fuses with inferior frontalis fibers. Procerus is a vertical, medial muscle lying deep at the radix of the nose. The supratrochlear and supraorbital vessels are the major vessels in this area. They are delineated by overlying creases, and knowledge of their anatomical depth is of paramount importance as communications between internal and external carotid circulations pose a high risk for blindness after inadvertent intravascular filler injection. Nerves and vessels generally follow an adjacent course.

It is important to note that a deep branch of the supraorbital nerve runs approximately 1 cm medial to the temporal crest. To minimize pain or nerve damage, it is advisable to avoid injecting this region with sharp needles.

TEMPORAL REGION

The temporal region is a well-defined region extending from the temporal crest to the zygomatic arch (Figure A.2). The orbital margin forms the anterior and hairline the posterior limit. There is little ethnic variation in the extent of the temporal region, but in African skulls, the temporal bone is very thick, making temporal hollowing uncommon. The temporal area contributes to the aging process due to widening of the lateral orbital margin and concomitant underlying bone resorption, thus causing a hollowed, aged or diseased appearance. The temporal artery courses from deep to superficial through the temporal fossa. It passes close to the ear, near the root of the helix, before running in the temporoparietal fascia to pass approximately 2 cm lateral to the brow. It may anastomose with the supratrochlear and supraorbital vessels, thus comprising another danger zone for potential blindness after inadvertent filler injection.

The temporal area contains important veins, the most important and dangerous of which is the middle temporal vein. This is a very large vein draining retrogradely to the jugular vein and inadvertent injection may cause embolism and death. The middle temporal vein anastomoses with the sentinel vein. Injections should be either very deep or very superficial, and done with knowledge of the course of the middle temporal vein, which runs 1–2 cm above the zygomatic arch.

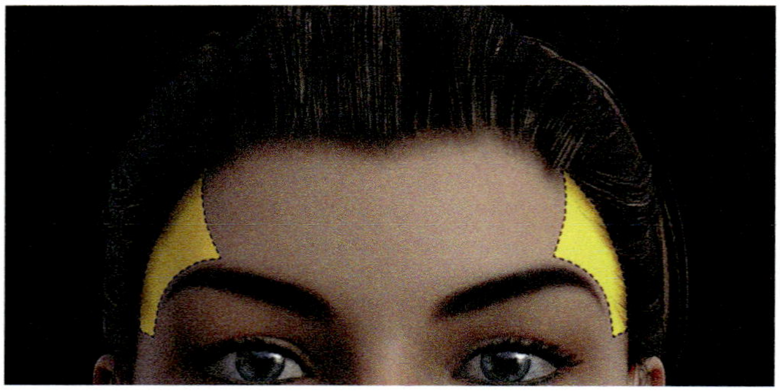

Figure A.2 The temporal area.

EYE AND PERIORBITAL REGION

The periorbital region extends from beneath the eyebrow to the zygomatico-malar ligament, and lies between the nasojugal sulcus and lateral aspect of the orbicularis retaining ligament (Figure A.3).

The periorbital region is the area demonstrating the most pronounced age and ethnic variation. In African skulls, the orbits are wider and more rectangular, and demonstrate earlier onset of bone resorption. The scant subcutaneous fat and protruded superior orbital margin causes a hollow-eyed look due to significant retraction of the periorbital tissues. Although the bone structure in Asian patients is similar to Caucasians, the tendon structure differs and the upper eyelid forms an epicanthic fold.

During the aging process, underlying bone resorption leads to progressive widening of the orbit. The

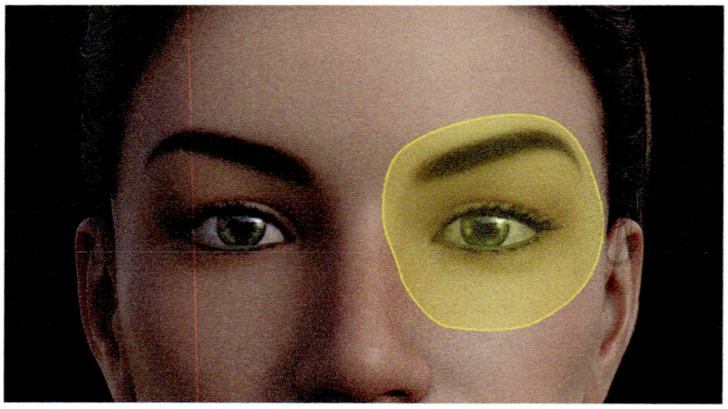

Figure A.3 The periorbital area.

eyebrows descend, and eyelid skin laxity may cause blepharochalasis and ptosis, thus impairing vision. The site for the neuromodulator injection is usually in the lateral preseptal orbicularis oculi muscle where there is no vascular danger zone. The use of neuromodulators in the upper eyelid is not recommended, because of the high risk of upper eyelid ptosis. The upper lid is a highly dangerous zone for filler injections as connections between the supratrochlear, medial palpebral and ophthalmic arteries may lead to blindness after inadvertent intravascular filler placement. It is thus imperative to have insightful anatomy knowledge and to use a cannula when treating the A-frame deformity of the upper eyelid.

NOSE

The nose is ethnically distinct, with variable bone structure and cartilage development.

It extends from the radix superiorly, to the nostrils and the columella inferiorly, and naso-jugal grooves laterally (Figure A.4).

The nose represents a vascular danger area. Above the modiolus, the facial artery superficializes and branches in two.

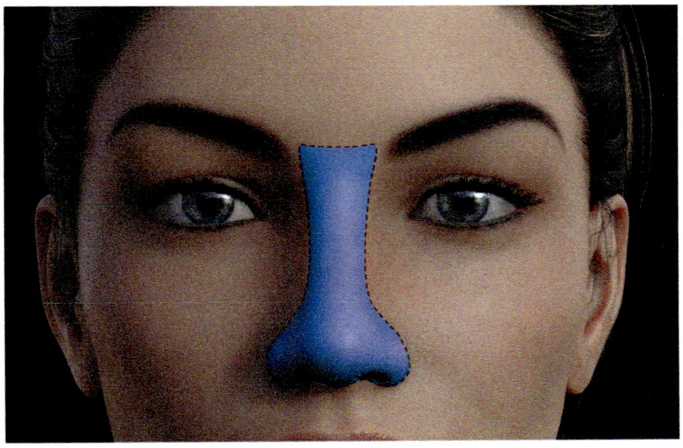

Figure A.4 The nasal area.

The deep subcutaneous branch divides close to the alar nasal sulcus to form the lateral nasal and angular arteries. In Africans, short noses with large nostrils and tips are characteristic. The central maxilla is well developed and protrudes anteriorly. The nasal dorsum is usually flat and the radix is located slightly above the intercanthal line. Asian patients have a flat nose, low radix and underrepresented dorsum. The nostrils are thin, and the tip is usually very short and rounded. With aging, the nasal cartilage enlarges and the nasal bone cavity widens. The cartilage becomes thinner and the tip falls downward. Although the bony dorsum does not change in older patients, it may become thinner, with a "sharper" edge. The lateral nasal vessels run above the alar groove to provide vascularization to the tip of the nose, together with an artery coming from the superior labial artery and passing through the columella. The tip is highly vascularized, especially in the superficial plane.

The radix of the nose is also a dangerous area due to the arborization of vessels. It is important to inject on the periosteum to avoid embolization or compression of especially the dorsal branch of the supratrochlear artery. Close to the radix, just below the medial canthus, the angular and facial veins anastomose before draining into the cavernous sinus, making this an important danger zone. It is advised that injections are placed from lateral to medial, with massage toward the more medial location. Using a cannula may prevent complications. The mid-third dorsal aspect of the nose is considered the safest injection area.

CHEEK

The cheek lies in the infraorbital region, extending laterally from the ear to the nose (above) and mouth (below) in the medial aspect (Figure A.5). African patients have larger cheeks and pronounced

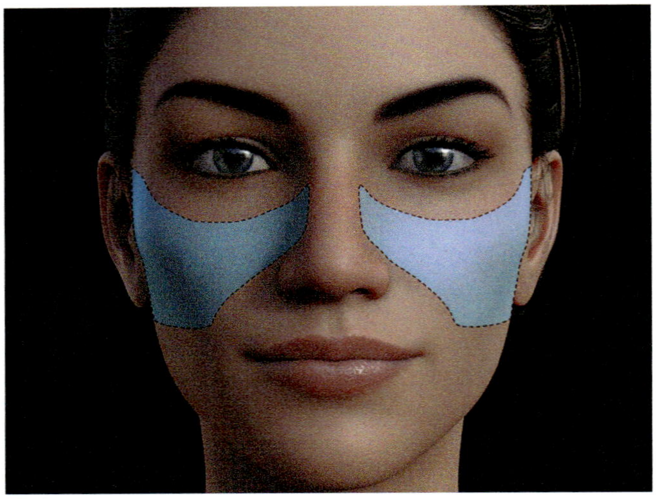

Figure A.5 The cheek area.

zygomatic bones, both frontally and laterally, whilst a prominent central maxilla often prevents a flat-faced appearance.

Asian patients also have pronounced cheekbones, but the flatter nose and small maxillary bones contribute to the typically flatter Asian face. The cheek fat compartment is usually well developed.

With aging, widening of the orbital and nasal cavities and thinning of bone cause soft-tissue sagging, thus enhancing the nasolabial folds, tear troughs and marionettes lines.

The facial nerve originates near the ear lobe, deep to the parotid gland, after which it divides into five branches after emerging from the anterior parotid border. The frontal nerve superficializes above the zygomatic arch, where it accompanies the superficial temporal artery. This represents a danger area.

The facial fat compartments are very well defined and may be divided into superficial and deep groups. Volumizing certain compartments ensures maximal projection, whilst injecting into others may induce sagging (see Cheek chapter). The infraorbital nerve enters the face via the infraorbital foramen which lies 6–8 mm below the infraorbital rim on a perpendicular line at the medial limbus. It is important to avoid intravascular injection by placing injections lateral to the foramen. Avoid embolization into the facial vein, which runs from the mandibular angle to the medial orbital canthus.

LIPS AND PERIORAL REGION

The perioral region comprises the lips and area corresponding to the orbicularis oris muscle (Figures A.6 and A.7).

Whilst the extent of the mouth region does not vary among ethnicities, lip proportions do. African and Mediterranean patients generally have bigger lips, while Asian, North European, and North American patients have thinner lips.

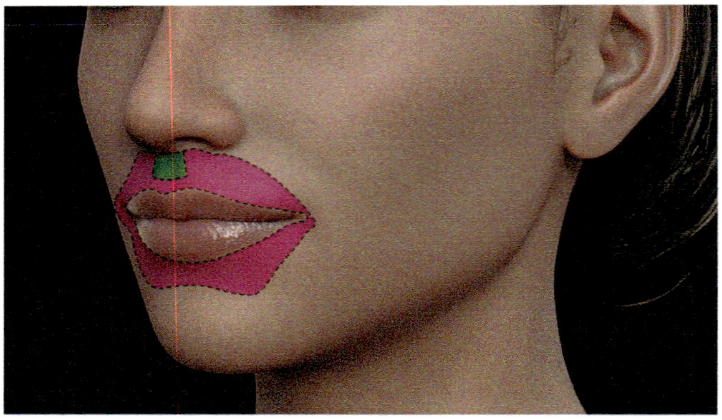

Figure A.6 The perioral area.

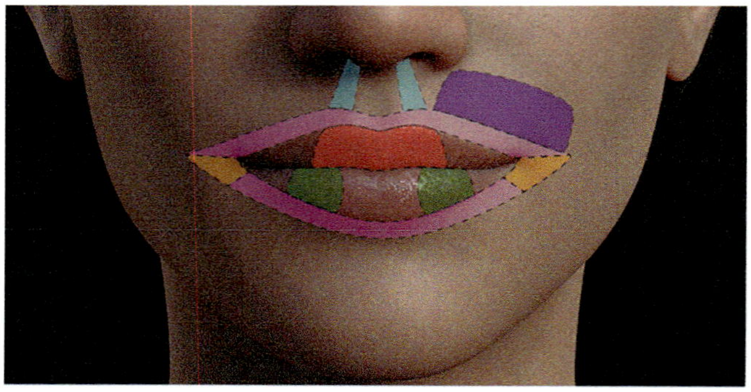

Figure A.7 The lip area.

Elderly patients also present with thinner lips. In the case of total or partial edentulism, there may be moderate to severe alveolar crest atrophy, causing a retraction of the lips and perioral tissue with shortening of the nose-chin length.

Several muscles insert into the modiolus to exert an effect on smiling. Zygomaticus major is stronger in effecting an upwards or zygomatic smile. As the elevators weaken with age, risorius may dominate to cause a more horizontal smile. Eventually, the depressor anguli oris (DAO) may dominate to cause a downwards smile. The zygomaticus minor, levator labii superioris, and levator labii superioris aleque nasi insert into the upper lip.

After passing below the commissure, the facial artery superficializes and divides into superior and inferior labial branches. The superior labial artery penetrates the orbicularis oris to enter the lip, running at the junction of the dry and wet mucosae. The inferior labial artery originates from the facial artery below the commissure, and runs from deep to superficial close to the mucosa. Inferiorly, there is more variation in morphology.

CHIN

The chin lies between the DAO (laterally), inferior margin of the orbicularis oris (superiorly) and mandibular margin inferiorly (Figure A.8). African patients have a wider chin, thicker bone, and more prominent lower maxilla.

Asians often present a retracted maxilla and smaller chin. Apart from soft-tissue sagging, aging does not affect the chin area directly. However, anterior protrusion may result due to loss of occlusion in edentulous patients. Although the chin is a relatively safe area to treat, it is important to note the emergence of the mental nerve just below the two premolars of the mandible. In elderly or edentulous patients, the foramen is usually closer to the alveolar ridge. Injecting the mental nerve may cause permanent dysesthesia, paresthesia, or anesthesia of the lower lip.

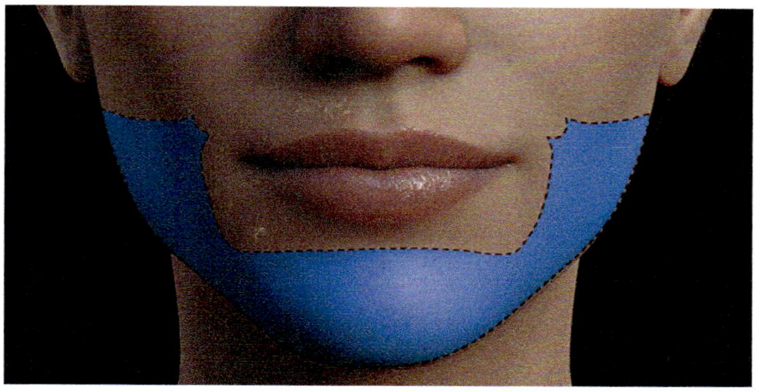

Figure A.8 The chin and jawline area.

JAW

The jaw area extends from the DAO (anteriorly) to the temporomandibular joint posteriorly; inferiorly, it is defined by the bony margin of the jawline (Figure A.9). There are no technically specific aging changes other than soft-tissue sagging. The facial artery crosses the mandible approximately 1 cm anterior to the anterior border of the masseter. The latter is the strongest muscle in the body.

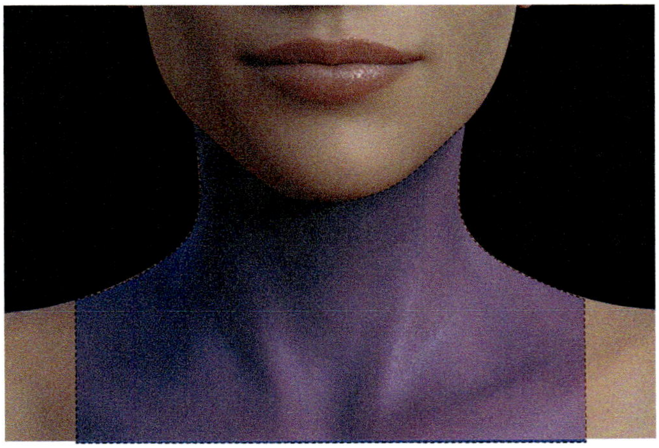

Figure A.9 The neck.

NECK

The neck is defined as the anatomical area originating anteriorly from the inferior surface of the mandible, running to the superior surface of the manubrium sterni. The posterior neck borders are bounded superiorly by the occipital bone of the skull and inferiorly by the intervertebral disc between CVII and T1. The neck is further divided into anterior and posterior triangles. The anterior triangle is bounded by the anterior border of the sternocleidomastoid, the midline of the neck, and inferior border of the mandible. The posterior triangle is defined as the area bounded by the posterior border of the sternocleidomastoid (SCM), anterior border of the trapezius and, inferiorly, the lateral third of the clavicle. The visible anterior triangle is the predominant focus of aesthetic treatments. With aging, the neck develops increased soft tissue laxity, excess skin, fat accumulation and loss of the cervicomental angle.

B FACIAL LAYERS

Eqram Rahman, Yves Saban, Giovanni Botti, Stan Monstrey, Shirong Li, and Ali Pirayesh

The face, with its diverse ability to portray emotions whilst communicating, is one of the most uniquely recognizable areas of the human body. An increasing interest in facial aesthetics, coupled with considerable research, has extended our understanding of the facial layers and the subtle physical variations resulting from underlying bone structure and genetic factors. With progressive aging, the face undergoes asynchronous changes which may present unique surgical challenges. Insightful understanding of facial anatomy as pertaining to the aging process facilitates treatment planning and predictable outcomes [1]. Traditionally the face has been divided into upper, middle and lower horizontal thirds with the upper face extending from the trichion to the glabella, the mid-face from glabella to the subnasale, and lower face extending to the menton.

However, Mendelson and Wong (2013) have posed that a more global understanding is facilitated by distinguishing between functional regions and considering the anatomy in terms of a layered construct bound together by retaining ligaments.

Seven major layers may be differentiated [2] (see Figure B.1):

1. Skin
2. Superficial fat
3. Superficial muscular aponeurotic system (SMAS)
4. Muscle
5. Vasculature
6. Deep fat
7. Bone

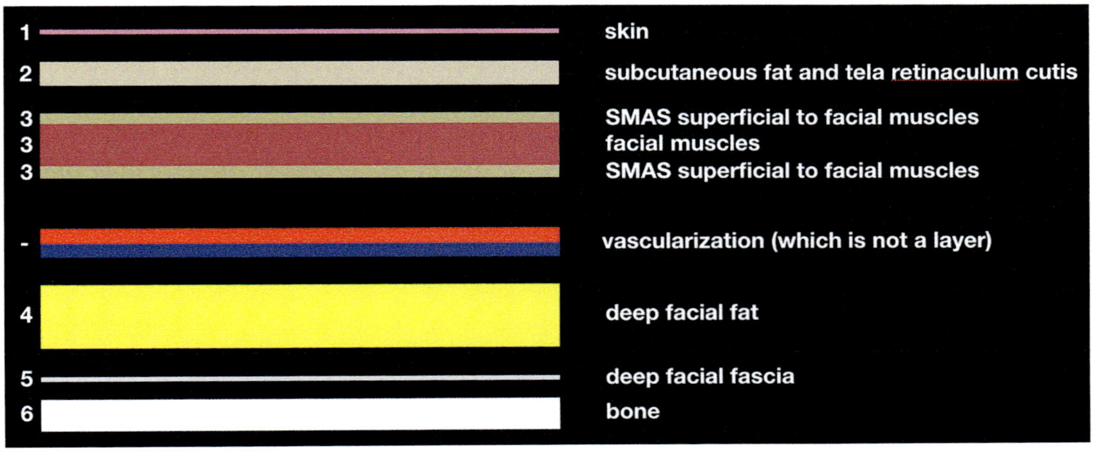

Figure B.1 The schematic illustration of the facial layers.

SKIN

The skin represents the superficial layer of the face and is an important indicator of age. In youth, the skin is smooth, firm, unblemished, and retains a uniform texture [3]. The skin may be histologically divided into epidermis and dermis, with the dermis consisting of collagen, elastic fibers, and ground substance comprising mucopolysaccharides, hyaluronic acid, and chondroitin sulphate [3].

Cutaneous aging often escalates from the fourth decade under the influence of contributory genetic, hormonal, behavioural and environmental factors [3,4]. During soft tissue aging, the two distinct processes of deflation and descent manifest as excess skin [5]. Wrinkles start to appear in the lower eyelids and lateral orbital areas, along with the development of dyschromia, textural changes, pigmentation, dryness, thinning, folds, drooping, and mimetic lines [3]. The midface is particularly susceptible to UV-induced aging, with the subsequent development of rough, wrinkled and leathery skin carrying a higher incidence of telangiectasias, premalignant conditions and malignancies. Other causes of extrinsic aging include smoking, pollution, infrared-A radiation and also visible light [3,4]. Recent advances in the understanding of volume loss as a critical component of facial aging, and the subsequent integration of volume replacement into both surgical and non-surgical treatment algorithms, arguably represents one of the most significant advances in the field of facial rejuvenation [6].

SUPERFICIAL FAT

In youth, the facial fat consists of a diffuse, balanced spread of superficial and deep fat which create the different arcs and convexities of the face. The superficial and deep layers are separated by the superficial muscular aponeurotic system (SMAS). Superficial fat is understood to be separated into unique compartments, which are divided by fascial septae containing vascular structures [2,5]. The major role of the fat layers is as a gliding plane for the facial mimetic muscles [5].

The superficial fat compartments comprise the nasolabial, medial, middle, and lateral temporal-cheek, central, middle, and lateral temporal-cheek (found within the forehead) and superior, inferior, and lateral orbital fat pads. The nasolabial fat, located medial to the cheek fat pads, plays a pronounced role in sagging of the nasolabial fold. The orbicularis retaining ligament (ORL) is situated 2–3 mm below the inferior orbital rim and forms the superior border of both the nasolabial and medial cheek fat compartments. The middle cheek fat compartment, juxtaposed between the medial and lateral temporal-cheek fat compartments, contains a superior fascial border known as the superior cheek septum [2].

The individual fat compartments age at different tempi and vary metabolically, thus contributing to segmental loss of fullness and the stigmata of aging. The periorbital, forehead, malar, temporal, mandibular, mental, glabellar, and perioral sites are prone to volume loss, whilst the nasolabial and inferior jowl compartments may hypertrophy. The infraorbital and malar fat pads often become more prominent, with anterior protrusion of the malar fat causing it to bulge against the nasolabial crease, thus emphasizing the nasal fold [6]. It is important to understand that individual fat pads behave differently after injection with fillers, with inferior displacement of the superficial nasolabial, middle cheek, and jowl compartments after injection. However, injection into the medial and lateral cheek and superficial temporal compartments lead to an increase in local projection without inferior displacement.

SUPERFICIAL MUSCULAR APONEUROTIC SYSTEM (SMAS)

The SMAS, which has been recognized since 1799, is a unique subcutaneous fascia which is continuous with the platysma below and galea above. It acts as an investing fascia for the facial mimetic muscles, thus playing an important role in facial expression [2,5]. The SMAS is firmly adherent to the parotid–masseteric fascia in the lateral aspect, where it is known as the immobile SMAS. The facial retaining ligaments, which originate from either the periosteum (zygomatic and mandibular retaining ligaments) or underlying muscle fascia (masseteric and cervical retaining ligaments) transmit through the SMAS to the overlying skin and serve as barriers between the superficial and deep facial fat compartments [12]. Neurovascular structures, or "facial danger zones," are located between these retaining ligaments [4].

Superiorly, the SMAS passes over the zygomatic arch to meet with the superficial temporal fascia [5]. The SMAS is considerably thicker over the parotid gland, but thins substantially as it courses medially. Superior to the zygomatic arch, the SMAS is known as the superficial temporal fascia where it splits to accommodate the temporal branch of CN VII and the intermediate temporal fat pad [2,7].

Degenerative changes in the viscoelastic properties and three-dimensional structure of the SMAS result in ptosis. Researchers have hypothesized that there is earlier and more progressive aging in the midface due to a decreased amount of SMAS [4]. With increasing age, retaining ligaments are at risk of weakening, thus leading to further ptosis of the masseteric SMAS and resultant jowl formation [2].

Due to the proximity of the SMAS to the temporal branch of CN VII, any dissection in this location should be performed deep to the superficial temporal fascia in order to avoid accidental denervation-related injuries [2].

DEEP FAT

The deep fat comprises the medial and lateral suborbicularis oculi fat (SOOF), and the deep medial cheek fat. Whilst the majority of the SOOF is found inferior to the lateral aspect of the infraorbital rim, it is also found underneath the orbicularis oculi muscle [7]. Other deep fat compartments include the temporal fat pad and a deep addition of this pad known as Bichat's fat pad [3]. The deep, supraperiosteal fat layer is located beneath the SMAS. Although the SMAS is sandwiched between fat layers, there are bilaminar connecting membranes or fusion zones containing neurovascular structures [7]. Compared with the superficial fat layer, the deep fat layer is composed of segmental, large white lobules containing a scant system of thin fibrous septae [3]. With aging, the deep fat layers may disintegrate and descend, resulting in a more prominent appearance of the inferior border of the orbicularis oculi which may accentuate the malar crescent and the nasojugal fold [6]. Post-menopausal changes due to decreased estrogen may cause increased fat deposition in combination with decreased superficial fat [3].

MUSCLE

The facial muscles can be categorized as periocular and perioral and broadly organized into four layers, where CN VII runs between the deepest and third layer. The first, superficial layer consists of the orbicularis oculi, the zygomaticus minor, and the depressor anguli oris. The second layer contains the levator labii superioris alaeque nasi, the zygomaticus major, the risorius, the depressor labii inferioris, and the platysma. The third layer includes orbicularis oris and levator labii superioris. The final, deepest layer consists of the buccinator, the levator anguli oris, and the mentalis [8]. Whilst the major function of facial muscles relates to facial movement, they also play a significant role in maintaining soft-tissue support. The SMAS unites and advances the facial muscles, especially the zygomaticus major and orbicularis oris [2,5].

The mimetic muscles of the cheek are separated into a superficial and deep layer. The superficial layer consists of zygomaticus major and minor, levator labii superioris, risorious, depressor anguli oris, orbicularis oculi, and the orbicularis oris. The deep layer contains the levator anguli oris, buccinator, depressor labii inferioris, and the mentalis [5].

Muscular aging can cause prominent changes such as declining muscle mass and strength. An example of this can be seen in the midface, where the orbicularis oris thins with age while the orbicularis oculi does not. Extensive investigations of facial MRIs at different ages have shown that the midface muscles start to shorten and straighten simultaneously. Researchers have hypothesized that this, in addition to a lifetime of facial contractions, may cause prolapse of the deep midfacial fat compartments [4].

VASCULATURE

Three major arteries originating directly from the external carotid artery or subsequent branches provide arterial supply to the face: the facial, transverse facial, and infraorbital arteries [7,9]. The facial artery, which is the largest, crosses the inferior border of the mandible just anterior to the masseter, where its pulsation may be felt, after which it travels in a coiled fashion towards the pyriform fossa [9]. It runs from deep on the mandible, over the buccinator, beneath risorius and zygomaticus major, under or over zygomaticus minor, crosses the nasolabial fold from medial to lateral at the junction of the proximal third after which it becomes the angular artery which anastomoses with the superficial temporal artery (STA).

The ophthalmic artery is the major artery supplying the orbit. Originating from the internal carotid artery in the middle cranial fossa, this artery traverses the optic foramen and subdivides into numerous branches inside the orbital cavity [7].

The superficial temporal artery represents the final branch of the external carotid artery. This artery arises inside the parotid gland at the point where the maxillary artery branches off the external carotid artery. Bilaterally, this artery supplies a large area of facial skin, including the lateral forehead, the temple, the zygoma, and the ear. One prominent branch that stems from the superficial temporal artery includes the transverse facial artery (also originating from the parotid gland) [7].

The forehead is supplied by the supraorbital and supratrochlear arteries (branches of the ophthalmic artery). The nose has a particularly intricate vascular network of tiny arteries within the alae, tip and columella. Most of this is supplied by the lateral nasal artery (originates from the facial artery) or superior labial artery (also originates from the facial artery). The upper lip is supplied primarily by the superior labial artery, while the lower lip is supplied by three labial arteries. The chin's main vasculature is the mental artery (branch of the inferior alveolar artery) [7].

The majority of veins are located close to the similarly named arteries. After crossing the inferior mandibular border with the facial artery, the facial vein takes a direct path to the medial canthus. The lateral forehead and temporal/parietal regions usually drain via the superficial temporal vein, while the middle forehead and upper eyelid drain via the angular or ophthalmic veins within the cavernous sinus. Venous drainage of the midface is via the infraorbital vein and pterygoid plexus; certain structures, such as the lips and cheeks drain into the facial vein [7].

The location, size and origin of the major arteries may vary between individuals and races [7,9]. With aging, random degenerative changes can occur in individual vessels, including increased diameter, decreased elasticity, and arterial hypertension. These changes can result in elongation and further tortuosity of these arteries [9].

The facial artery crosses the inferior border of the mandible just anterior to the masseter, where its pulsation may be felt, after which it travels in a coiled fashion towards the pyriform fossa [9]. It runs from deep on the mandible, over the buccinator, beneath risorius and zygomaticus major, under or over zygomaticus minor, crosses the nasolabial fold from medial to lateral at the junction of the proximal third after which it becomes the angular artery which anastomoses with the superficial temporal artery (STA).

NERVES

Cranial nerve (CN) VII—the facial nerve—is the main motor innervation of the facial muscles, with damage to CN VII being one of the most dreaded (but rare) complications of surgery. After exiting the stylomastoid foramen, an upper and lower division develops as it passes through the parotid gland before travelling to the facial muscles [3]. This nerve harbors significant clinical implications during facial surgery [5]. Another significant clinical consideration during a mandibular block (CN VII), is potential hemifacial paralysis, otherwise known as Bell's palsy [7].

Other important innervations include CN V (trigeminal nerve), which has three branches as well as additional branches from the cervical plexus.

The greater auricular nerve is found approximately 5 cm inferior to the external auditory meatus, running deep within the superficial cervical fascia. The mental nerve, a branch of the inferior alveolar nerve, exits the mental foramen where it can be seen and palpated when the oral mucosa is stretched. This nerve provides innervation to the lower lip and the mandible. The buccal mucosa and the skin on the cheek is innervated by the buccal branch of the mandibular nerve, while the anterior two-thirds of the tongue is innervated by the lingual nerve (a branch of the mandibular division of the trigeminal nerve) [2].

Face transplants have rapidly blossomed into a feasible management for patients with extreme disfigurements. To help repair damaged facial expression muscles and preserve their function, it is vital also to understand that these muscles do not contain proprioceptive receptors, compared with mastication muscles (which are innervated by the trigeminal nerve and thus contain proprioceptors) [7].

BONES

Youthful features have been said to be optimally present at a point in time when a specific set of skeletal proportions are ideal for their soft-tissue envelope. The skeletal framework forms the basis on which unique facial characteristics are built, rendering underlying bone vital in providing and preserving ideal soft-tissue relationships.

Important facial bony constituents include the frontal, maxillary, zygomatic, palatine, nasal, temporal, lacrimal, ethmoidal and mandibular bones. Bone provides structural support and attachment sites for the muscles of facial expression and mastication, and also protects certain structures such as the eyes.

The facial skeleton undergoes both expansion and selective resorption throughout life, with the pyriform and orbital apertures being particularly susceptible to age-related resorption. Maxillary recession and a 10° decrease in the maxillary angle have been noted after 60 years of age [11]. Midface skeletal involution also occurs from the sixth decade, occurring more frequently in women than men [4]. Skeletal regression of particularly the inferolateral orbital rim and alveolar ridges, contributes to loss of midfacial support and also loss of overall facial height.

Age-related changes within the nasal aperture, paired nasal bones, and ascending processes of maxillae may lead to prominent changes, including nasal lengthening, sagging of the tip, and posterior displacement of the columella and lateral crura [11].

Selective resorption of the upper jaw may lead to a subsequent loss of dentition, with Bartlett et al. [13] demonstrating that decreasing height of the maxilla and mandible correlate strongly with eventual loss of dentition.

Loss of teeth generally affects the mandible more than the maxilla, with women at a higher risk of this loss [4].

Individuals with prominent bony features, including a supraorbital bar, strong cheekbones, and prominent jawlines have been said to age more favorably [11].

CONCLUSION

The face is unique in its profound ability to communicate, express emotion and masticate. As a result of this intricate functionality, it is imperative that medical practitioners have an insightful understanding of applicable anatomy. Each facial layer is morphologically and clinically distinct and may be differentially affected by the aging process. This layered structure provides an intricate canvas, adding to the functional and artistic imagery required during aesthetic treatments.

By first breaking the anatomy down into basic layers, it is easier to visualize the integral structural an functional components before attempting to brainstorm novel aesthetic solutions.

References

1. Kumar N et al. *Plast Reconstr Surg Glob Open.* 2018;6(3):e1687.
2. Prendergast PM. Anatomy of the face and neck. In: *Cosmetic Surgery: Art and Techniques.* Shiffman, MA and Di Giuseppe, A. eds. Springer: Belin, Heidelberg, 2013.
3. Khazanchi R et al. *Indian J Plast Surg.* 2007; 40(2):223–9.
4. Wulc AE et al. The anatomic basis of midfacial aging. In: Hartstein M et al., eds. *Midfacial Rejuvenation.* New York, NY: Springer; 2012: 15–28.
5. Barton FE. *Aesthetic Surg J.* 2009;29(6):449–63.
6. Coleman SR and Grover R. *Aesthetic Surg J.* 2006;26(1S):S4–9.
7. Von Arx T et al. *Swiss Dent J.* 2018;128:382–92.
8. Freilinger G et al. *Plast Reconstr Surg.* 1987; 80(5):686–90.
9. Soikkonen K et al. *Br J Oral Maxillofac Surg.* 1991;29(6):395–8.
10. Mangalgiri A et al. *Indian J Otolaryngol Head Neck Surg.* 2015;67(1):72–4.
11. Mendelson B and Wong CH. *Aesthetic Plastic Surgery.* 2012;36(4):753–60.
12. Rohrich R et al. *Plast Reconstr Surg Glob Open.* 2019;7(6):2270.
13. Bartlett SP et al. *Plast Reconstr Surg.* 1992;90(4): 592–600.

C AGING OF SKIN, SOFT TISSUE, AND BONE

Daria Voropai, Steven Dayan, Luis Fernando Botero, Chiara Botti, Leonard Miller, and Ali Pirayesh

Facial aging is a complex, multifactorial process involving multiple facial layers. Changes in the skin, skull, and soft tissues play contributory roles. Loss of collagen and elastin, combined with epidermal thinning, contributes to the appearance fine rhytides. Distributional changes in the superficial and deep fat pads, in addition to bone remodeling, constitute key morphological factors and result in the characteristic inverted heart shape of the aging face. Understanding these multifactorial aging pathways facilitates effective aesthetic treatments.

The main function of the facial skeleton is to protect the brain and important sensory organs of smell, sight, and taste, and to provide a foundation for the face. The skull is subdivided into two main parts: the cranial vault, which protects the brain and houses the middle and inner ear structures, and the facial bones, which form the support for the soft tissues of the face, the nasal cavity, the eyeballs, and the upper and lower teeth.

The adult skull comprises 22 separate bones, of which only one, the mandible, is mobile and not fused as a single unit. In order to understand the aging process of the skeletal base, it is of great importance to know the relationships between the different bones, transitions, and landmarks.

The face may be divided into thirds (upper face, midface, and lower face) in order to identifying important bony and soft tissue landmarks (Figure C.1).

The upper face consists of mainly the frontal bone, which forms the upper third of the anterior adult skull giving the forehead an aesthetically pleasing curvature. The frontal bone can be divided into three parts (see also Chapter 1, Forehead):

1. Squamous part of the frontal bone
2. Glabella and nasion
3. Supraorbital ridge

The important aesthetic landmark of the upper third is the nasion, defined as the suture between the frontal and nasal bones in the midsagittal plane. Together with the nasion, the glabellar angle (the line connecting the maximal glabellar prominence with the nasofrontal suture, as compared to the horizontal or nasal-sellar line) is used

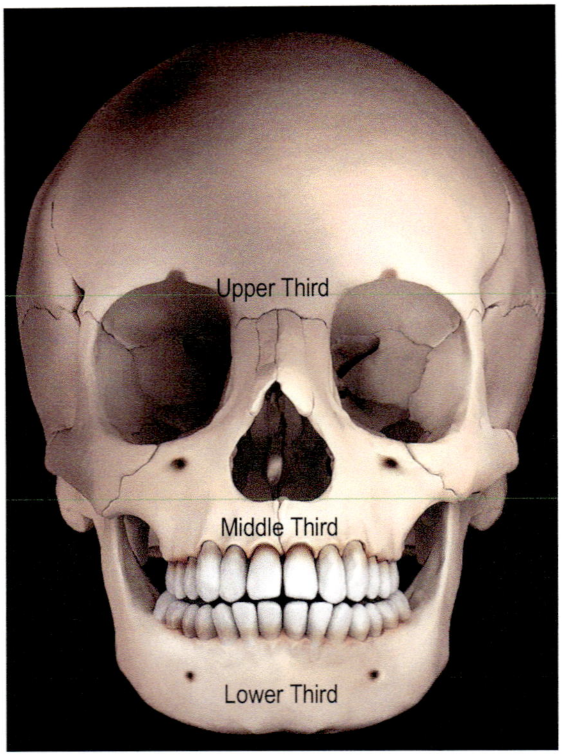

Figure C.1 Facial bone sutures.

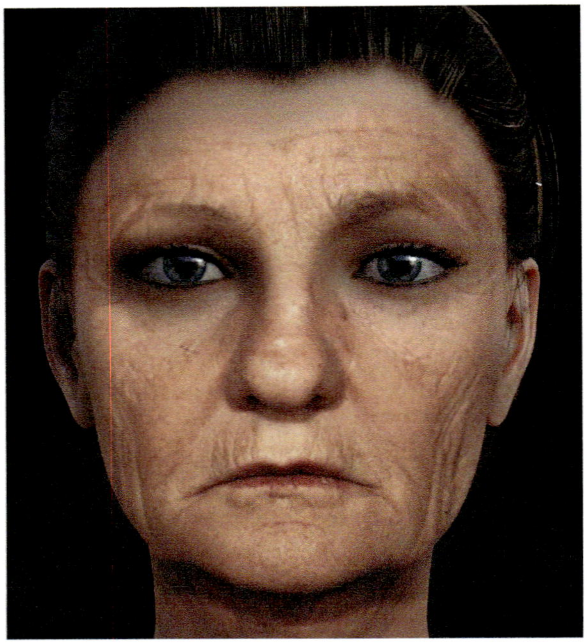

Figure C.2 Skeletonized facial features.

as an anthropometric measurement in facial and cephalometric analysis.

There is no clear understanding as to which aging changes occur in the cranium and the upper face. A well-researched change is the decrease in glabellar angle [2,3]. However, Cotofana et al. [1] studied computed tomographic multiplanar scans of 157 Caucasian individuals between the ages of 20 and 98 years and found significant results, which complemented the results of Yi's [8,9] study looking at aging changes of the frontal eminence and the concavity of the forehead (however, limited to the Korean population). Yi's study concluded that in both genders, aging was associated with increasing length of the concavity (Figure C.2). Cotofana [1] documented a decrease in sagittal diameter in men (−2.24%), an increase in transverse diameter in both women and men (1.97% vs 2.22%), and a decrease in calvarial volume in men and women (5.4% vs 5.1%) (Figure C.2). Furthermore, lateral expansion of the skull [1] could also contribute to the more skeletonized appearance of the face of the older individual, hence the prominent lateral orbital rims, temporal crest, and zygomatic arch.

Soft tissue changes in the aging upper face are also of note. A well-accepted theory is that of volume loss due to lipo- and muscle atrophy [3]. Foissac et al. [11] looked at magnetic resonance imaging scans of 85 female Caucasians (age 18 to >60 years) to analyze the volume and distribution of the central forehead and the temporal fat compartments. They concluded that there is an increase in fat volume in the older group, with an increased basal expansion of the compartments (central fat compartment increasing by 155% and temporal fat compartment by 35.5%). Combinations of these findings result in visual aesthetic implications for the aging upper face, which include enhanced forehead concavity, brow ptosis, temporal hollowing, and a more prominent supraorbital ridge due to a decreased glabellar angle.

The midface is a merging of the following bony structures: nasal, lacrimal, ethmoid, maxillary, zygomatic, and palatine bones [5]. The main function of

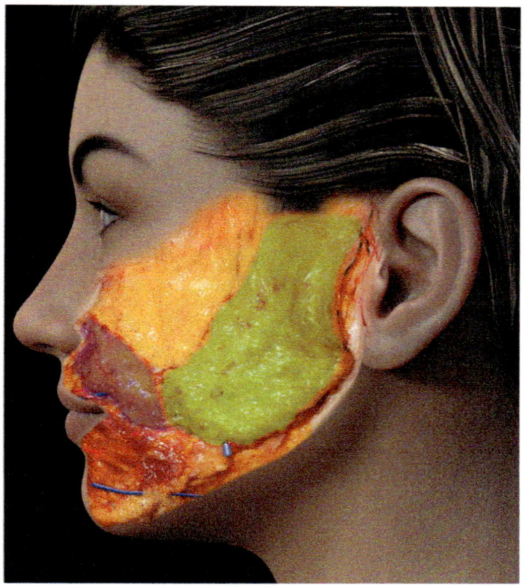

Figure C.3 Midfacial fat.

the midface is to house the eyeballs within the orbit and the teeth within the maxilla, which then transmits masticatory forces to the skull base. The midface also provides a scaffold for the main facial tissues (see Figure C.3).

One of the key points in midface analysis is the bizygomatic distance, or most exterior bilateral point of the zygomatic arch, which is widest part of the face. The midface anthropometric measurement landmarks are the maxillary angle (the angle between the sella-nasion and the line between the superior and inferior maxilla) and the pyriform angle (nasal bone to lateral inferior pyriform aperture, divergent from the sella-nasion line) [3].

Facial skeletal aging is most prominent in the midface, but the rate of bone resorption is not uniform; the maxilla is more prone to bone loss compared to the zygoma [4]. Therefore, it is helpful to analyze the important midface features separately (orbit, maxilla, pyriform aperture, and zygomatic arch).

Maxillary recession is most evident in the anterior aspect [12]. Studies found a decrease of the maxillary angle of 10° between the young (<30 years) and old populations (>60 years). This finding can be causative for the loss of support of the inferior orbital rim [2–4] and loss of projection of the maxilla. The zygomatic arch suffers a posterior and anterior remodeling, which leads to increased temporal hollowing.

Aging changes in the orbit are characterized by an increase in aperture and width. However, there is no uniform resorption; research has proved that the superomedial and infralateral aspects recede more [12,13]. This leads to an expansion of the orbit. A similar process occurs at the pyriform aperture, with lateral widening as the edges of the nasal bone recede with age [4] and an increase in the pyriform angle.

In the lower face, there is only one bone, the mandible, which carries the lower dentition. Important anatomical landmarks are the pogonion, the most anterior point of the chin, and the gonial angle, located at the posterior border at the junction of the lower border of the mandibular ramus.

There are numerous controversial theories regarding aging changes of the mandible. Alvero et al. [10] examined 241 forensic skulls and observed a posterior and superior bone formation in the older population, with anterior and inferior resorption. As a result of this resorption, there is an increase of the mandibular angle, where it becomes more robust compared with the acute angle of youth. Equally, the chin area undergoes changes as a consequence of bone remodeling, where the mandible loses its vertical projection and the chin becomes shorter and more oblique [10]. These processes are accelerated in edentulous individuals and apply to both maxilla and mandible.

Bony changes lead to loss of soft tissue support and therefore changes in facial aesthetics. Decreased mandibular height and length, and an increase in the mandibular angle, contribute to a loss of definition of the jawline and development of jowls.

Loss of maxillary support and projection and the mandible will result in morphological changes, and soft tissue changes also contribute to the saggy appearance in older individuals. Rohrich and Pessa [7] described a compartmentalization of the superficial and deep fat pads divided by septae, fasciae, ligaments, or muscles.

With aging, there is deflation and loss of the normal anatomic subcutaneous facial fat compartments, which give the appearance of increased skin laxity or prominent folds around the nasolabial region, periorbital region, and jowl [7]. One can use the deep and superficial fat pads as a map for facial aging: the deep fat pad of the periorbital area is affected first (the transition between the medial suborbicularis oculi fat and the superior edge of the malar fat pad is lost), which creates a concavity between the thin medial eyelid skin and thicker cheek skin, resulting in a tear trough deformity [14]. Subsequent further deflation of the deep medial cheek fat leads to ptosis of the overlying superficial malar fat pad and further deepening of the tear trough deformity with hollowing of the centromedial cheek. Wysong et al. [15] found that the most dramatic loss of facial fat occurs from the third to the sixth decade, after which depletion stabilizes.

However, there is not only volume loss but also hypertrophy. Donofrio et al. [6] found slight hypertrophy of the submental, jowl, nasolabial, and lateral malar fat pad, which aligns with morphological changes in those areas, characterized by sagging tissues and the appearance of folds (see Figure C.4).

Together with volume loss in fat pads, there is also lack of support and stability of the ligaments because of the repositioning of their points of origin, followed by ligamentous weakening due to continuous stretching. Ligaments function as a hammock for the fat compartments and promote the appearance of sagging when there is a lack of structure [14]. More detailed aesthetic implications and treatment proposals will be elucidated in the chapters to follow.

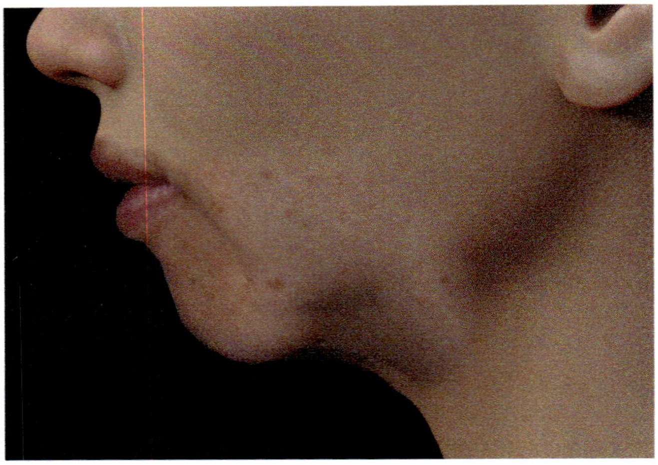

Figure C.4 Sagging submental tissues.

References

1. Cotofana S et al. *Aesthet Surg J.* 2018;38(10):1043–51.
2. Pessa JE. *Plast Reconstr Surg.* 2000;106(2):479–88.
3. Shaw RB Jr and Kahn DM. *Plast Reconstr Surg.* 2007;119(2):675–81.
4. Mendelson BC et al. *Aesthet Plast Surg.* 2007;31(5): 419–23.
5. Schünke M et al. *Kopf, Hals und Neuroanatomie.* 2nd ed. New York: Thieme; 2016.
6. Donofrio LM. *Dermatol Surg.* 2000;26(12):1107–12.
7. Rohrich RJ and Pessa JE. *Plast Reconstr Surg.* 2007;119(7):2219–27.
8. Flowers RS. *Clin Plast Surg.* 1991;18:689–729.
9. Yi HS. *Arch Craniofac Surg.* 2015;16(2):58–62.
10. Toledo Avelar LE et al. *Plast Reconstr Surg Glob Open.* 2017;5(4):e1297.
11. Foissac R et al. *Plast Reconstr Surg.* 2017;139(4):829–37.
12. Wong CH and Mendelson B. *Plast Reconstr Surg.* 2015;136(5S):44S–48S.
13. Farkas JP et al. *Plast Reconstr Surg Glob Open.* 2013;1(1):e8–15.
14. Cotofana S et al. *Facial Plast Surg.* 2016;32(3):253–60.
15. Wysong A et al. *Dermatol Surg.* 2013;39(12):1895–902.

D MYOMODULATION

Mauricio de Maio and Izolda Heydenrych

The definition of modulation is the exertion of a modifying or controlling influence on something.

Clinical observation over the past two decades has shown that injectable fillers may, in addition to addressing volume loss, also profoundly influence muscle dynamics. With aging, structural deficiencies in either bone or fat pads may precipitate abnormal muscle movement. As the indications for facial injectable fillers have evolved from the mere treatment of lines and folds, through three-dimensional facial volumizing, to the current sophisticated paradigm of modifying muscle movement by the use of hyaluronic acid (HA) fillers, it has become possible to consciously complement the mechanism of neurotoxins by the use of HA fillers.

Despite a paucity of literature detailing scientifically measurable muscle strength, case studies offer irrefutable evidence of the potential clinical impact of injectable fillers on muscle function in both the presence and absence of volume deficiency. It is clear that various factors may be instrumental in either facilitating or reducing muscle movement, making this a fascinating field for ongoing study [1,2].

The treatment of facial palsy and asymmetry is complex and mandates insightful, detailed mastery of both anatomy and technique in order to achieve reproducible results [3]. Developing expertise in this field often requires many years of experience, making consistent and reproducible transfer of knowledge a challenging aspect. The first publication on myomodulation highlighted the ability of injectable fillers to influence facial muscle action in a reproducible manner by addressing the muscle imbalance resulting from structural deficiencies with and without substantial volume loss [1]. The evolution of innovative treatment paradigms is offering new treatment methods—and hope—for patients with facial palsy [4].

TERMINOLOGY

The succinct new language of the MD Codes, also encompassing MD ASA and MD DYNA Codes, was conceived in order to refine and standardize description of both facial assessment and technique, and constitutes an invaluable teaching tool [1]. It is important to understand that these points should be applied according to clinical indication and expertise and, as such, constitute a set of accurately defined placement points rather than a rigid prescriptive method.

The MD Codes divide the face into structural units and depict target structures, injection technique, product choice, and danger areas in a detailed and standardized manner through the use of symbols. Placement points and symbols are briefly illustrated in order to facilitate the methodology later in this chapter (Figures D.1, D.2 and Table D.1).

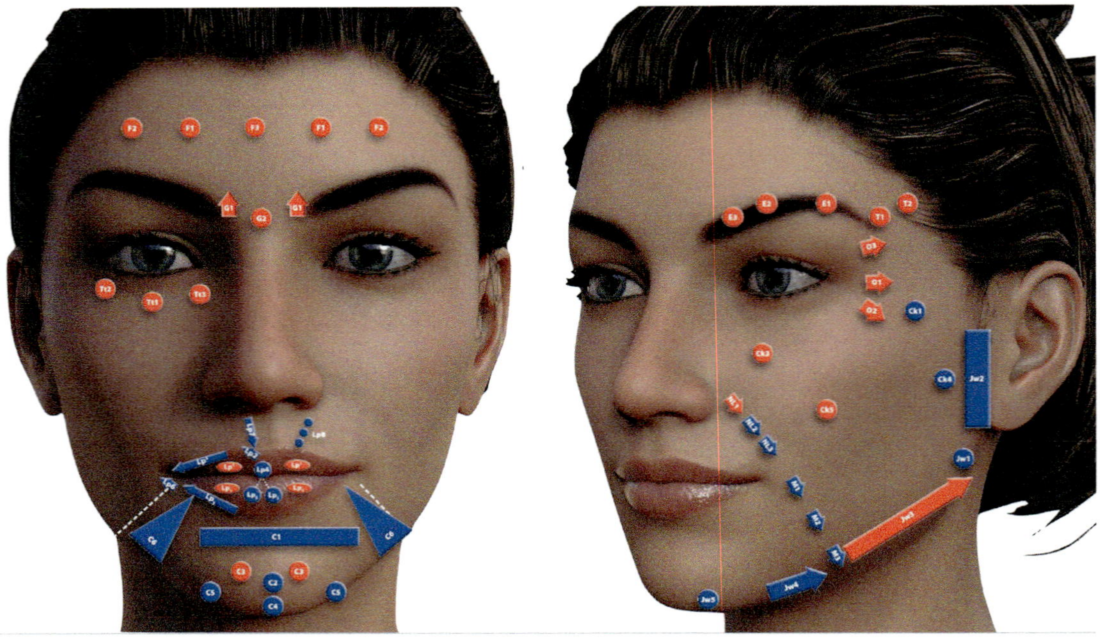

Figure D.1 Illustration of the MD Codes placement and terminology.

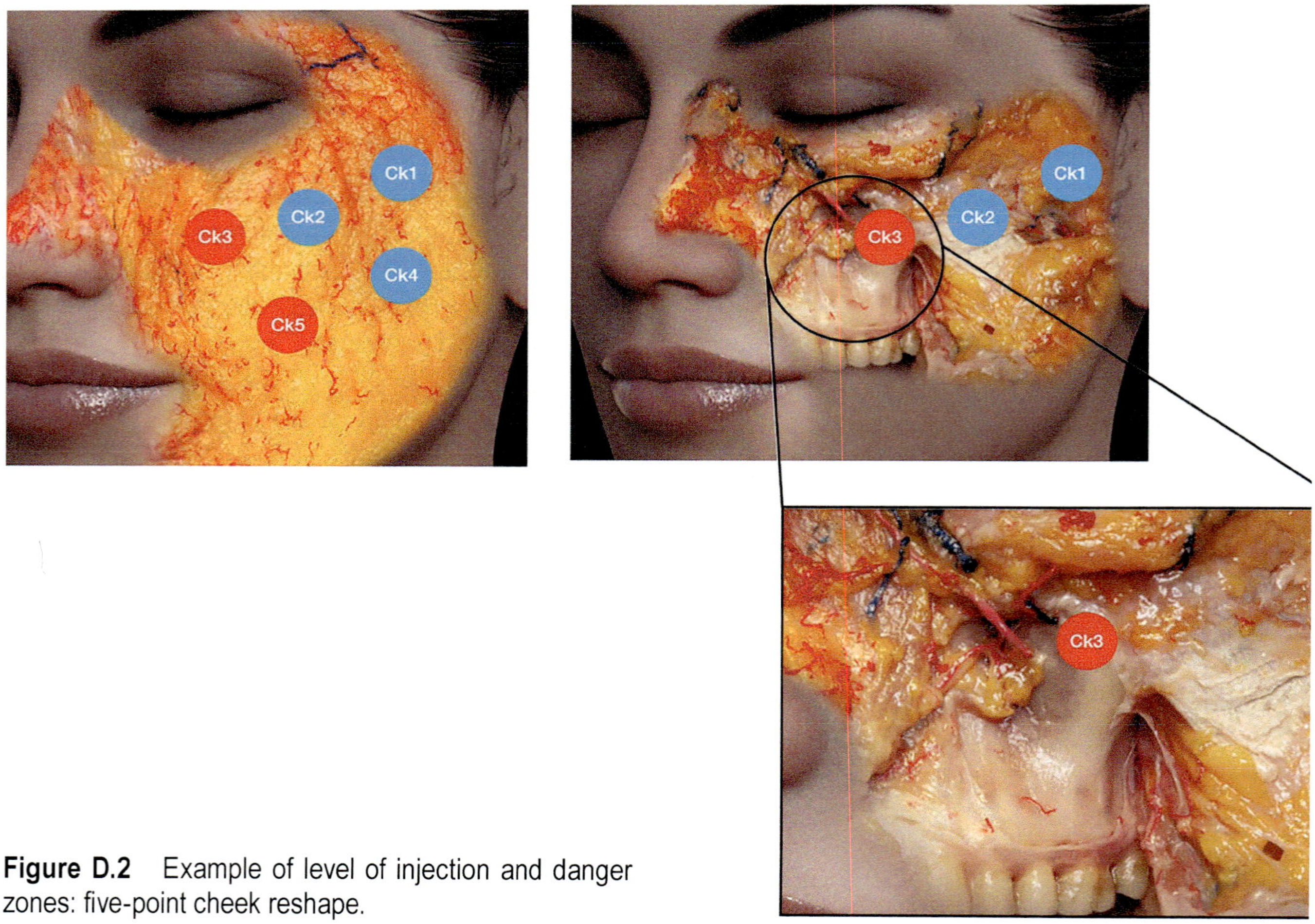

Figure D.2 Example of level of injection and danger zones: five-point cheek reshape.

Table D.1 The Five-Point Cheek Reshape: Injection Areas and Effects

Code	Injection Area	Effect of Injection	Aim
Ck1	Zygomatic arch	Lifts the cheek Gives support to eyebrow and lower eyelid	Bone structure and lateral suborbicularis oculi fat (SOOF)
Ck2	Zygomatic eminence	Provides projection of the cheek and shortening of the palpebral-malar sulcus	Bone structure and lateral SOOF
Ck3	Anteromedial cheek-midcheek	Improves the medial lid-cheek junction and softens the tear trough	Bone structure, deep malar fat pad; medial SOOF
Ck4	Lateral lower cheek/parotid area	Addresses the sunken area at the parotid level and volume loss; lifts the jawline	Subcutaneous
Ck5	Submalar	Addresses the sunken area and improves volume loss in the submalar area	Subcutaneous

The choice of injection device should be based on individual experience and preference (Tables D.2 and D.3) [5].

The targeted structures are specified as:

- Dermal
- Mucosal
- Subcutaneous
- Fat pads
- Supraperiosteal

MD DYNA Codes detail the muscles implicated in facial muscle excursion and suggest specified placement sites for both neuromodulator and/or HA filler. Accurate knowledge of muscle origin and insertion is essential, as is knowledge of the muscular anatomical plane. Insightful knowledge of functional groups and muscle synergism/antagonism is vital in planning product placement; the injector is encouraged to reflect critically on the desired effects of placement above, below, or within muscles and to define a strategy encompassing placement, product choice, and method of delivery before embarking on treatment (Figures D.3 and D.4).

Table D.2 Considerations in the Choice of Injection Device

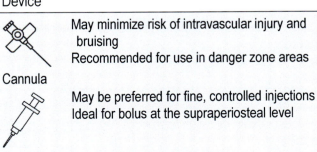

 Cannula	May minimize risk of intravascular injury and bruising Recommended for use in danger zone areas
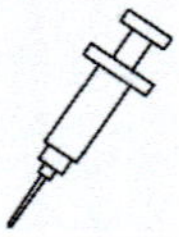 Needle	May be preferred for fine, controlled injections Ideal for bolus at the supraperiosteal level

Table D.3 Details of Injection Delivery

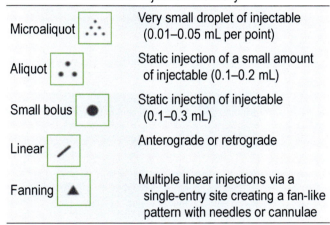

Microaliquot	Very small droplet of injectable (0.01–0.05 mL per point)
Aliquot	Static injection of a small amount of injectable (0.1–0.2 mL)
Small bolus	Static injection of injectable (0.1–0.3 mL)
Linear	Anterograde or retrograde
Fanning	Multiple linear injections via a single-entry site creating a fan-like pattern with needles or cannulae

MECHANISMS

The factors influencing the effect fillers may exert on muscle action (mechanical myomodulation) (see Figure D.5) include:

- Functional muscle groups
- Agonist and antagonist pairs
- Tissue resistance
- Volume loss

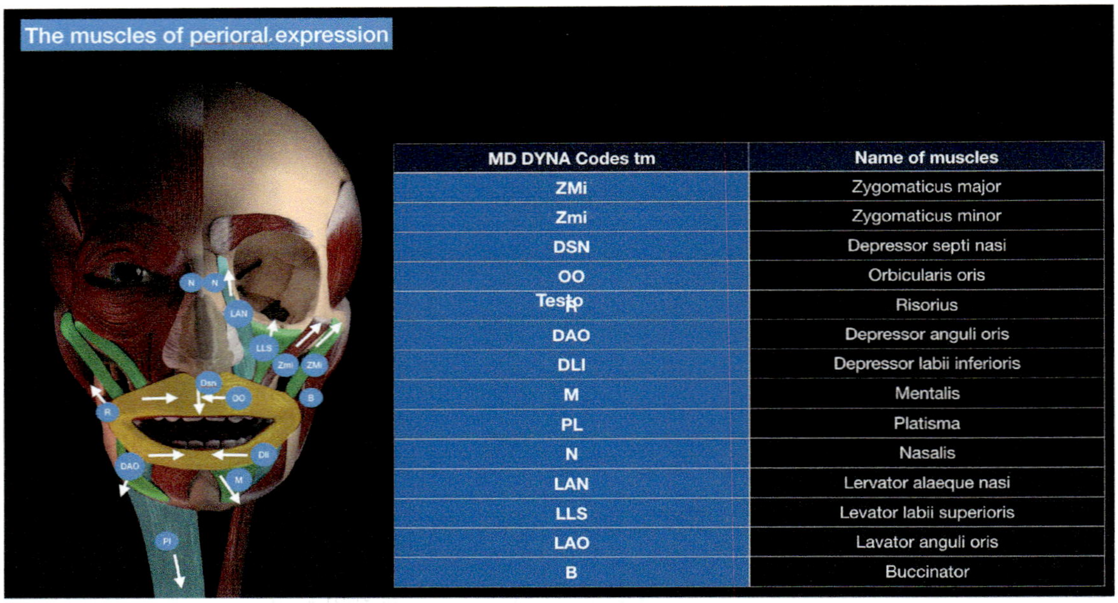

MD DYNA Codes tm	Name of muscles
ZMi	Zygomaticus major
Zmi	Zygomaticus minor
DSN	Depressor septi nasi
OO	Orbicularis oris
R	Risorius
DAO	Depressor anguli oris
DLI	Depressor labii inferioris
M	Mentalis
PL	Platisma
N	Nasalis
LAN	Lervator alaeque nasi
LLS	Levator labii superioris
LAO	Lavator anguli oris
B	Buccinator

Figure D.3 The MD DYNA Codes detailing the specific muscles implicated in facial muscle excursion.

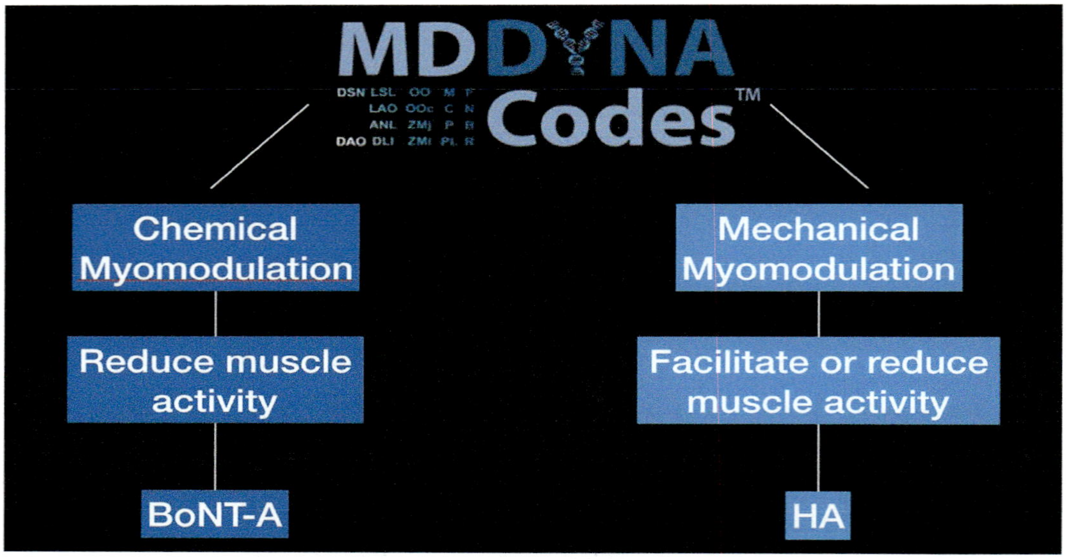

Figure D.4 The MD DYNA Codes differentiating chemical and mechanical myomodulation.

- Superficial muscolar aponeurotic system (SMAS) expansion

Factors potentially inhibiting muscle strength include:

- Adding tissue resistance above the muscle
- Injecting directly into the muscle to create a muscular block

Factors potentially facilitating muscle strength include:

- Injecting beneath a muscle to create a "pulley effect"
- Increasing tensile strength by stretching the muscle
- SMAS expansion

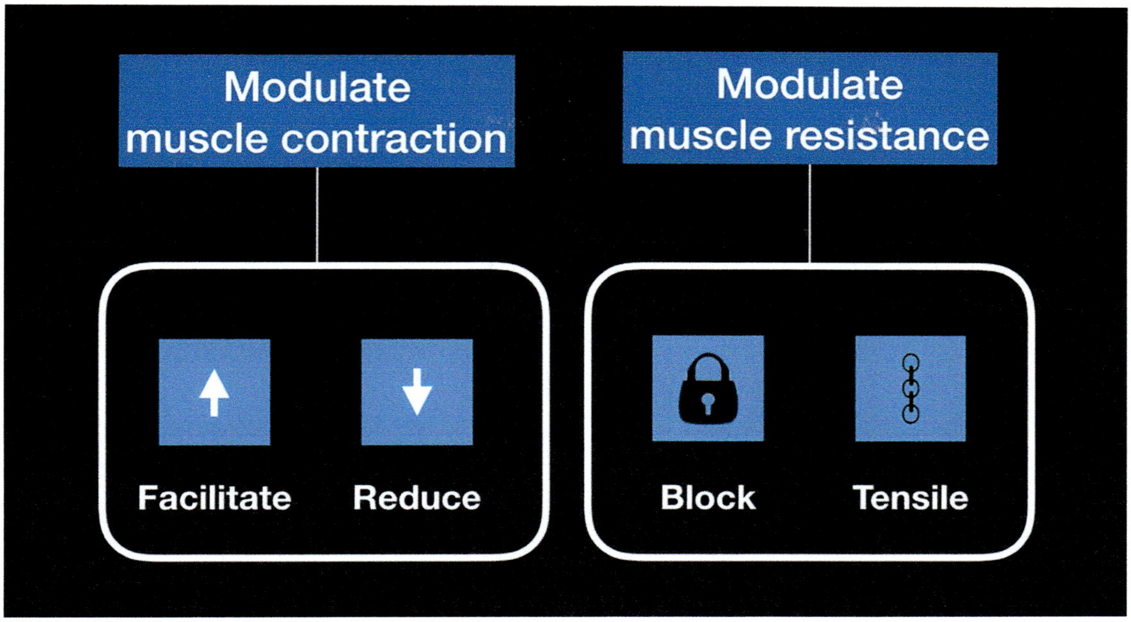

Figure D.5 Mechanisms of myomodulation.

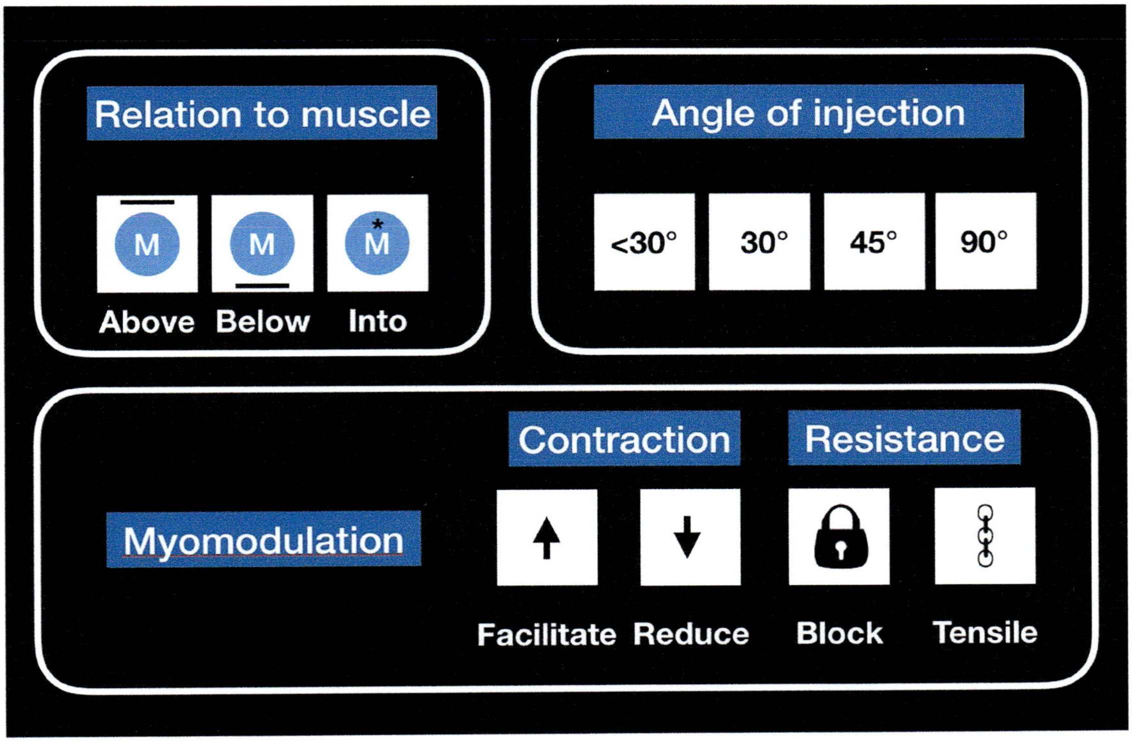

Figure D.6 Language of the MD DYNA Codes specifying placement relative to muscle, angle of injection device relative to skin and proposed mechanism of action: M, muscle.

The MD DYNA Codes specify both the placement for the desired mechanism (above, below, or in the muscle) and required technical details (angle of needle or cannula to the skin) (Figure D.6).

FUNCTIONAL ANATOMY

It is important to know the origins and insertions of the facial muscles (see Tables D.4–D.6) [6].

The skull insertion points [10] are shown in Figure D.7.

It is imperative that the injector have knowledge of anatomical layers and an understanding of the differential effect of injecting above or below a muscle. This is especially important in the midface, where incorrect placement may negatively impact animation and upper-lip length. The layers of the midface comprise:

- Skin
- Subcutaneous fat
- Orbicularis oculi
- SOOF
- Levators of upper lip
- Deep malar fat pad
- Bone

Functional Muscle Groups

Agonist and antagonist groups function synergistically, with levators and depressors working in opposition for normal, balanced facial expression (Figures D.8 and D.9) [11]. Levator strength generally predominates in youth, thus maintaining the position of soft tissue structures and counteracting downward gravitational pull and depressor antagonists. In youth, this balance may be disrupted by underlying structural deficiencies, while loss of bone and/or soft tissue become an increasing problem during

Table D.4 Muscles of the Upper Face [7]

Muscle	Origin	Insertion	Function
Temporalis	Temporal lines on the parietal bone of skull and the superior temporal surface of the sphenoid bone	Coronoid process of the mandible	Functions to elevate and retract the mandible
Elevators			
Frontalis	Galea aponeurotica along the coronal suture	Superciliary skin, where it interdigitates with the brow depressors	Inferior: elevates the brow Superior: causes descent of anterior hairline
Depressors			
Procerus	Periosteum of the nasal bone near the medial palpebral ligament	Glabellar or mid-forehead dermis; merges with frontalis	Depressor of brow with two contraction patterns 1: Lowers lateral end of brow 2: Produces lateral eyelid crow's feet
Depressor supercilii	Nasal portion of the frontal bone	Dermis beneath medial head of brow	Moving and depressing brow
Corrugator supercilii	Medially and deep along nasofrontal suture/supraorbital ridge of frontal bone	Interdigitating with frontal muscle and inserting in the midbrow skin	Approximation and depression of brows; creating vertical glabellar lines
Orbicularis oculi	Medial orbital margin, medial palpebral ligament, anterior lacrimal crest	Preseptal segment inserts into dermis of upper eyelid and brow	Thick orbital part closes eyelids tightly; thin palpebral part closes eyelids lightly

Table D.5 Muscles of the Midface [8]

Muscle	Origin	Insertion	Function
Levator labii superioris alaeque nasi (LLSAN)	Upper frontal process of maxilla, medial infraorbital margin	Skin of lateral nostril and upper lip	Dilates nostril, elevates and inverts upper lip "Elvis muscle"
Levator labii superioris	Broad sheet, medial infraorbital margin; extending from side of nose to zygomatic bone	Skin and muscle of upper lip	Elevates upper lip
Zygomaticus minor	Lateral part of zygomatic bone medial to zygomaticus major	Skin of lateral upper lip; extends to nasolabial sulcus	Pulls the upper lip backward, upward, and outward Aids in deepening and elevating the nasolabial sulcus
Zygomaticus major	Temporal process, anterior zygomatic bone	Temporal process, anterior zygomatic bone	Elevates and draws angle of mouth laterally
Risorius	Pre-parotid fascia	Modiolus	Draws back corner of mouth

Table D.6 Muscles of the Lower Face [9]

Muscle	Origin	Insertion	Function
Depressor labii inferioris	Line of mandible between mentonian symphysis and mental foramen	Orbicularis muscle and skin of lower lip	Depresses lower lip
Depressor anguli oris	Oblique line of the mandible and mandibular tubercle	Modiolus	Depresses corners of mouth
Mentalis	Upper mentonian symphysis and mental fat compartments	Orbicularis oris and skin of lower lip	Elevates and projects lip outward
Platysma	Deep fascia of upper thorax	Lower border of mandible	Depression of mandible

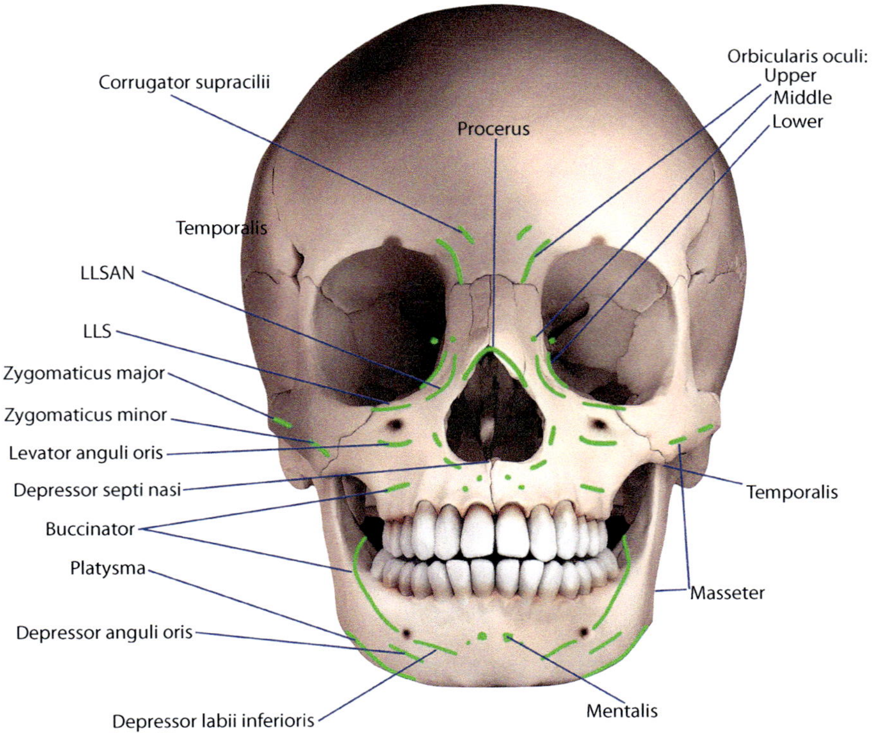

Figure D.7 Points of muscle insertion on the skull.

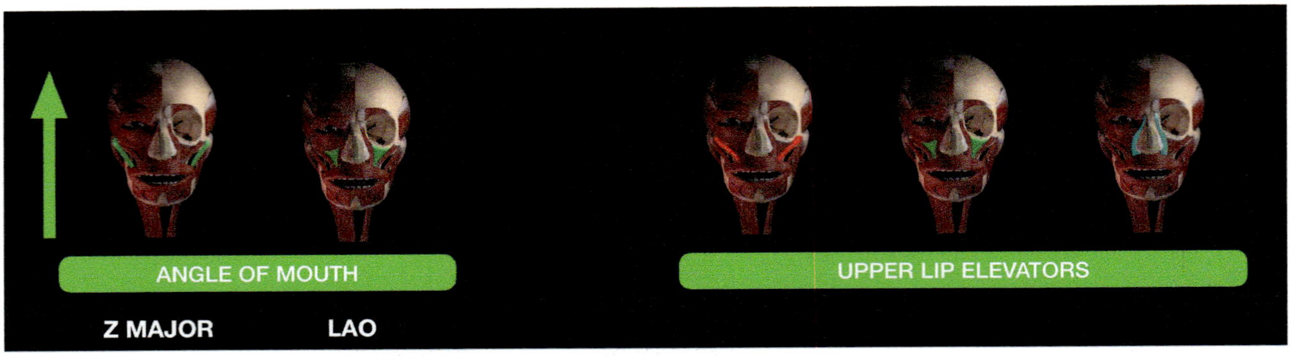

Figure D.8 Midface levators and synergists.

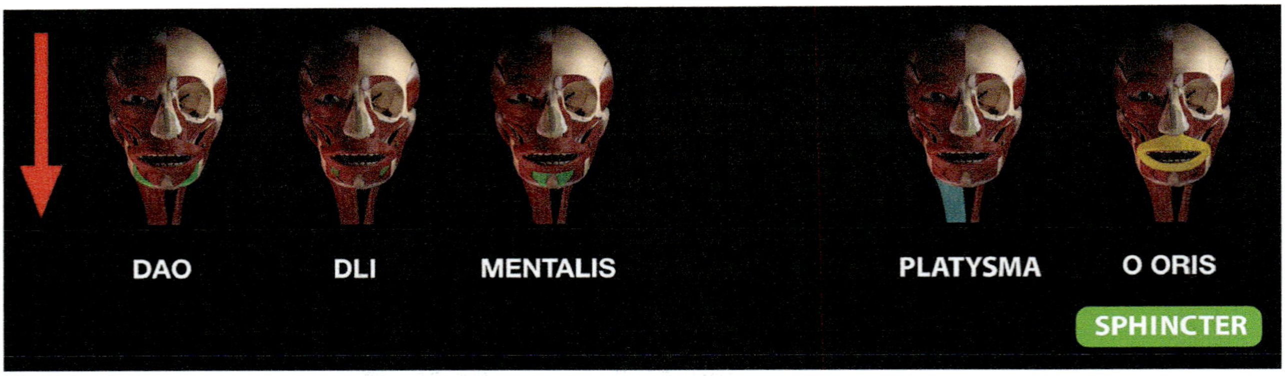

Figure D.9 Lower face depressors.

the aging process. With the loss of levator strength, depressors are more likely to predominate [12].

Factors Influencing the Angle of the Mouth/Smile

In youth, the zygomaticus major plays a critical role in tilting the angle of the mouth when smiling. When zygomaticus major lifting power is reduced due to a lack of underlying structural support, the relative role of the risorius muscle increases, producing a more horizontal smile. On further diminution of zygomaticus major lifting capacity, the depressor anguli oris (DAO) predominates with a resultant "DAO smile" (downturned angles of the mouth; Figure D.10). The lack of tissue resistance leading to a DAO smile may be age-related or secondary to structural deficiency in youth.

The Periorbital Area

As with muscles elsewhere in the face, the periorbital muscles are connected by the SMAS. Lending support to one periorbital area—for example, on the temporal bone beneath the orbicularis oculi—may therefore impact both adjacent and distant areas, thus impacting brow position and horizontal frontalis lines.

In addition, orbicularis oculi and levator palpebrae superioris function as antagonists. Supporting a weakening orbicularis oculi—for example, by placing volume on the temporal bone or lateral zygoma—may effect improved upper eyelid function, improve lateral scleral show, and reduce compensatory frontalis action. Lateral cheek support may also facilitate eye closure, thus serving great practical purpose in facial palsy patients.

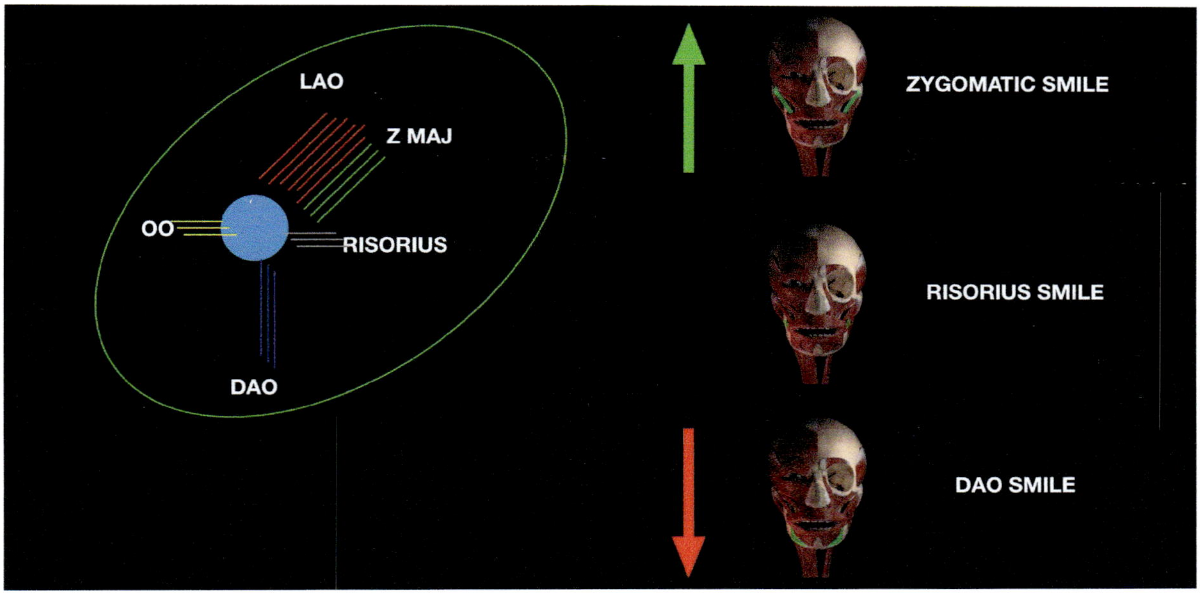

Figure D.10 Smile patterns as mediated by the relative balance of elevators and depressors. Blue circle, modiolus.

Indirect effects of treating the lateral zygoma (Ck1,2) include:

- Shortening the lid–cheek junction
- Improving the intercanthal angle
- Normalizing the position of the brow
- Enlarging eye size
- Improving horizontal forehead lines
- Improving the nasolabial fold
- Improving the jawline

See also Figure D.11.

The Perioral Area

Adding tissue resistance over the mentalis muscle (C1) inhibits upward rotation of the chin, increases vertical height and may also influence lower-lip eversion, as illustrated in a recent study detailing reduction in size of thick Asian lips by adding volume to the chin area [13]. Adding resistance over the DAO inhibits its downward traction, while layering product over the orbicularis oris and DAO are invaluable methods for balancing the perioral region in facial

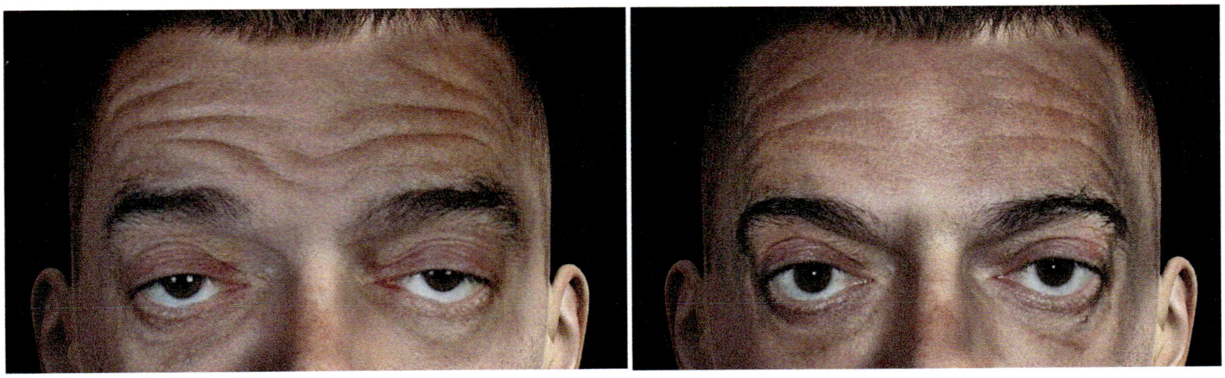

Figure D.11 The indirect effect of filler placement in the deep temporal region (T1), lateral zygoma (Ck1), and lateral cheek (Ck4) on adjacent and distant muscles. Note the improvement in upper eyelid function and the reduction in forehead lines. No botulinum toxin was used. (Left) Before; (right) after.

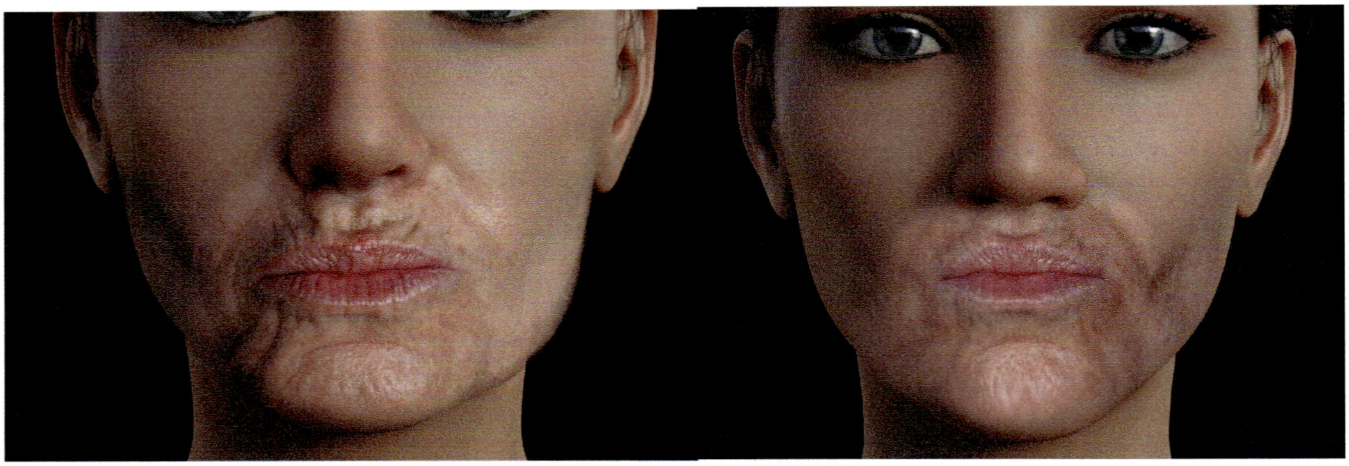

Figure D.12 Improvement of upper lip rhytides after layering HA over the DAO and orbicularis oris. (Left) Before; (right) after.

palsy patients where asymmetry on smiling and phonation may drastically reduce quality of life. Adding resistance over the orbicularis oculi may inhibit upper lip rhytides (Figure D.12).

The upper lip levators function as a synergistic group. Strengthening zygomaticus major and minor function by adding support in the lateral cheek (Ck1,2) may thus indirectly improve a gummy smile by inducing relaxation of the LLSAN.

When treating the upper cutaneous lip (Lp8), also treat Lp[1] where indicated to provide deep support and prevent undue flattening of the vermilion lip.

When balancing a "joker's smile" (overactive zygomaticus major):

- Treat Ck4 to stretch the risorius, thus improving its tensile strength.
- Place Ck1 points posterior to the bony suture, facilitating less strengthening of the zygomaticus major.

HOW I DO IT

For chin wrinkling/expressing disappointment, see Figure D.13.

For gummy smile, see Figures D.14–D.16.

For perioral lines, see Figure D.17.

For the treatment of facial palsy with toxins:

- Document meticulously with photographs and videos both at rest and in animation.
- Assess for underlying residual facial nerve function on the palsy side, e.g., platysma, zygomaticus major.
- Treat the hyperdynamic side of the face with toxins in order to counter the Hering-Breuer reflex; proceed conservatively in the perioral area to minimize functional discomfort.
- Follow up at 2 weeks for possible top-up with toxins.
- Caution that phonation and chewing may initially be affected and warn against inadvertent lip biting and drooling.

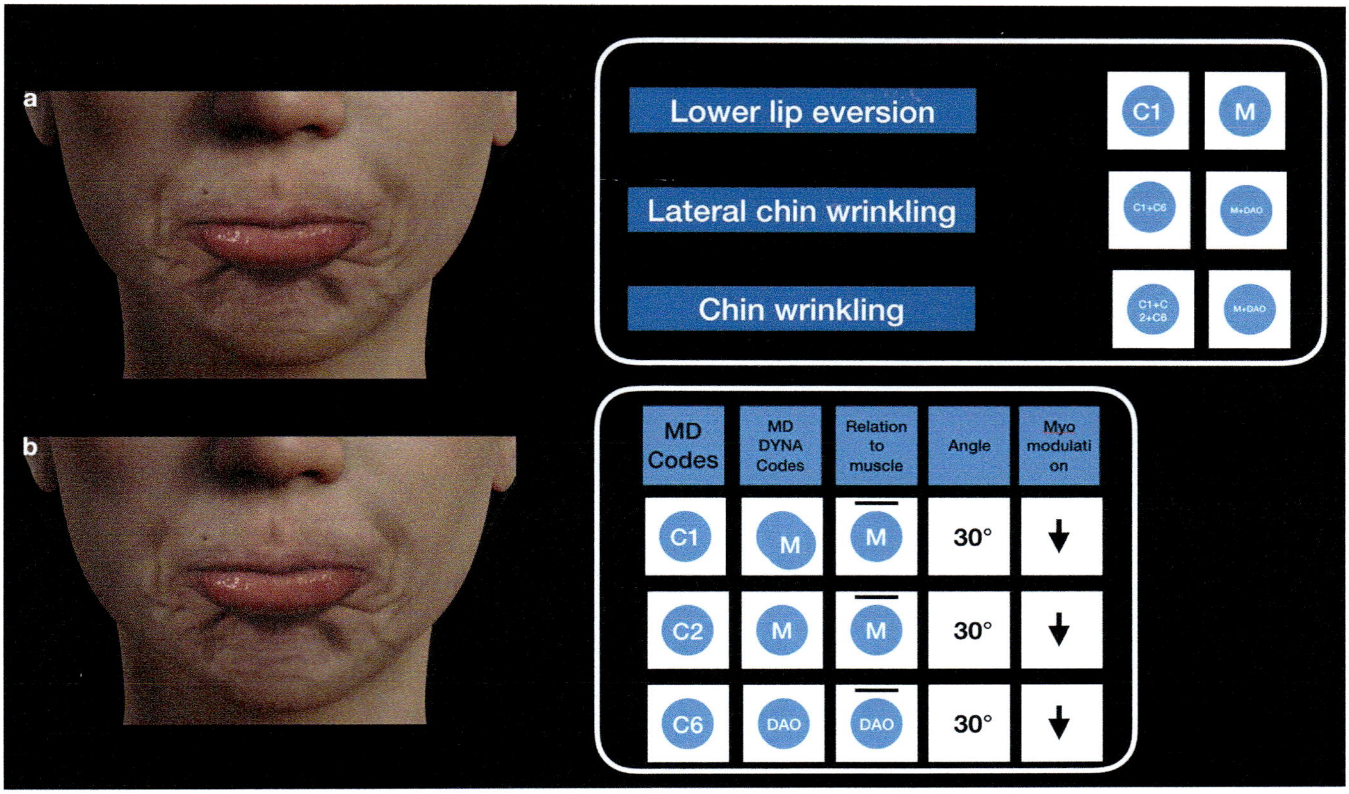

Figure D.13 (a) Codes; (b) technique.

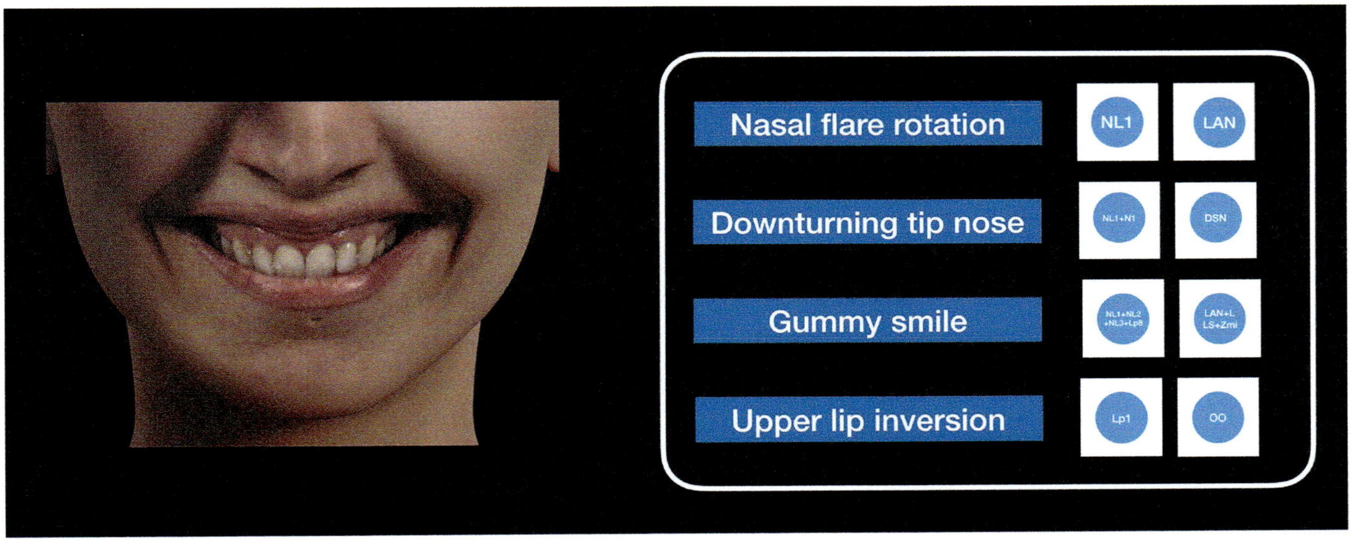

Figure D.14 Codes for gummy smile.

- Encourage chewing on the weaker side in an attempt to recruit muscle strength.
- Myomodulation with fillers may be attempted at 1 month after toxin treatment. See also Figure D.18.

Fillers may be used to rebalance the face in cases of facial palsy, thus contributing significantly to quality of life. Figure D.19 illustrates salient clinical observations over a 6-month period before and after a single

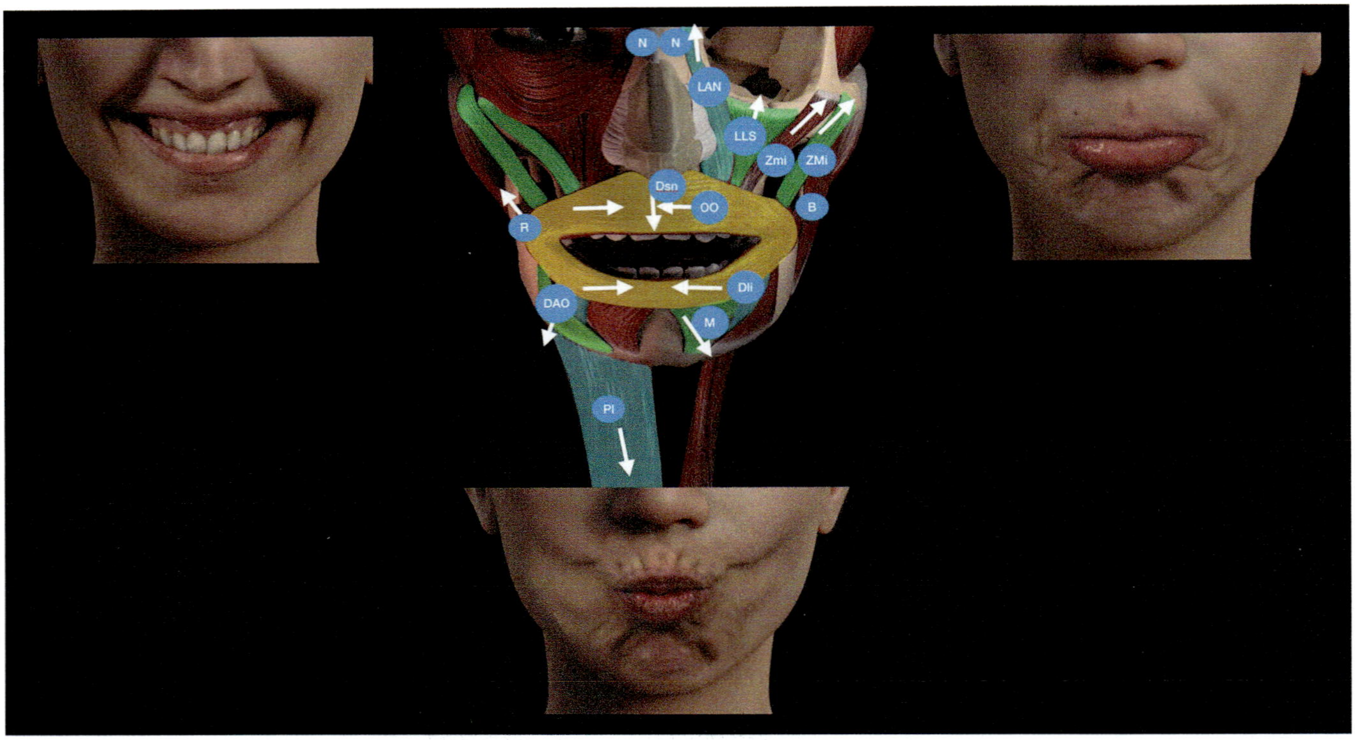

Figure D.15 Muscle vectors to consider when treating a gummy smile.

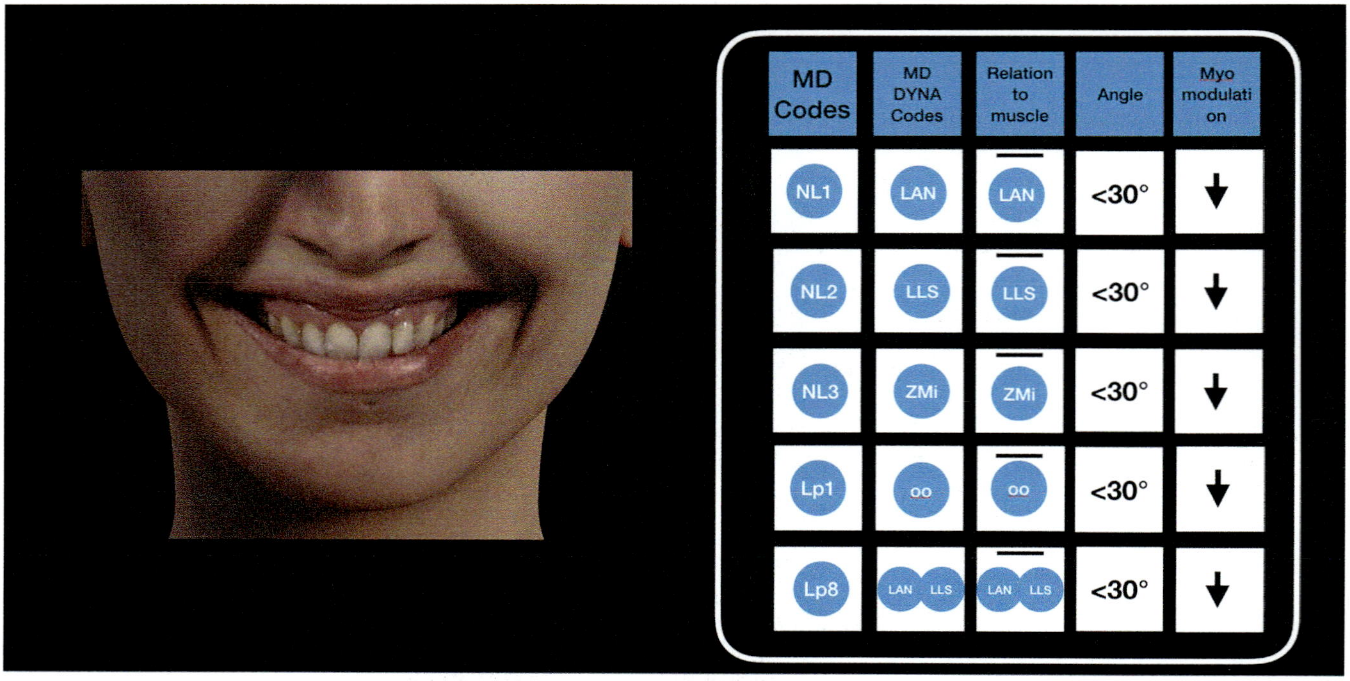

MD Codes	MD DYNA Codes	Relation to muscle	Angle	Myo modulati on
NL1	LAN	LAN	<30°	↓
NL2	LLS	LLS	<30°	↓
NL3	ZMi	ZMi	<30°	↓
Lp1	oo	oo	<30°	↓
Lp8	LAN LLS	LAN LLS	<30°	↓

Figure D.16 Treatment Codes for addressing a gummy smile.

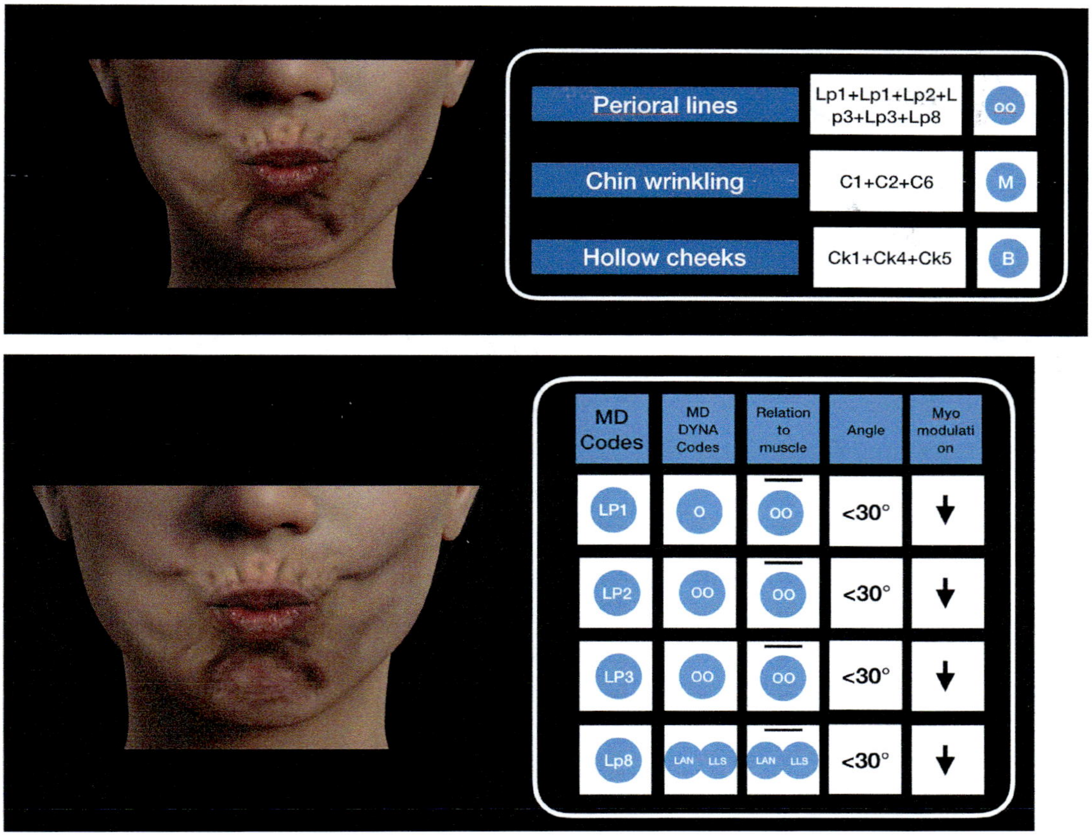

Figure D.17 Codes and technique for perioral lines.

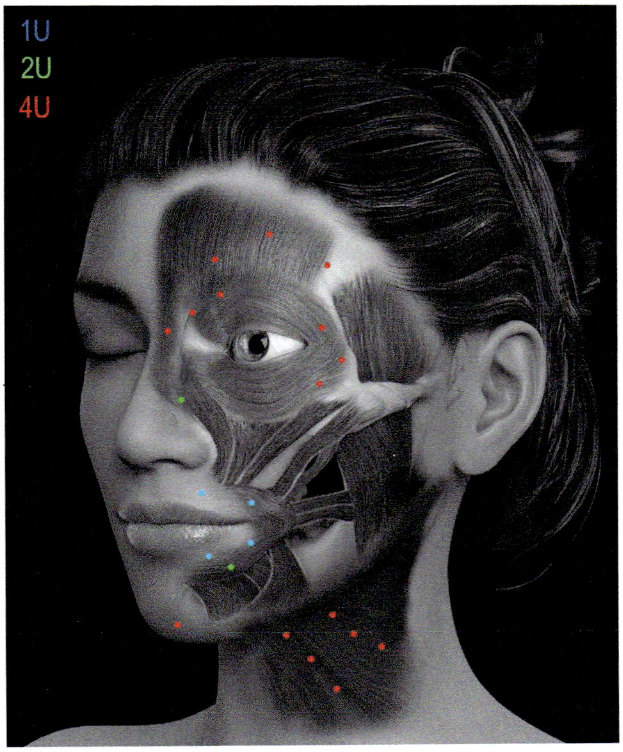

Figure D.18 Potential botulinum toxin treatment areas in facial palsy.

treatment with fillers based on myomodulation principles. Note that no toxins were used.

The main details before treatment are shown in Table D.7.

Treatment was according to the principles of myomodulation (Figure D.20).

The main details after treatment are shown in Table D.8.

COMPLICATIONS

- Injecting filler above the upper-lip levators may lead to an undue lengthening of the upper lip, especially in patients with structural deficiencies and a lengthened upper lip at baseline.

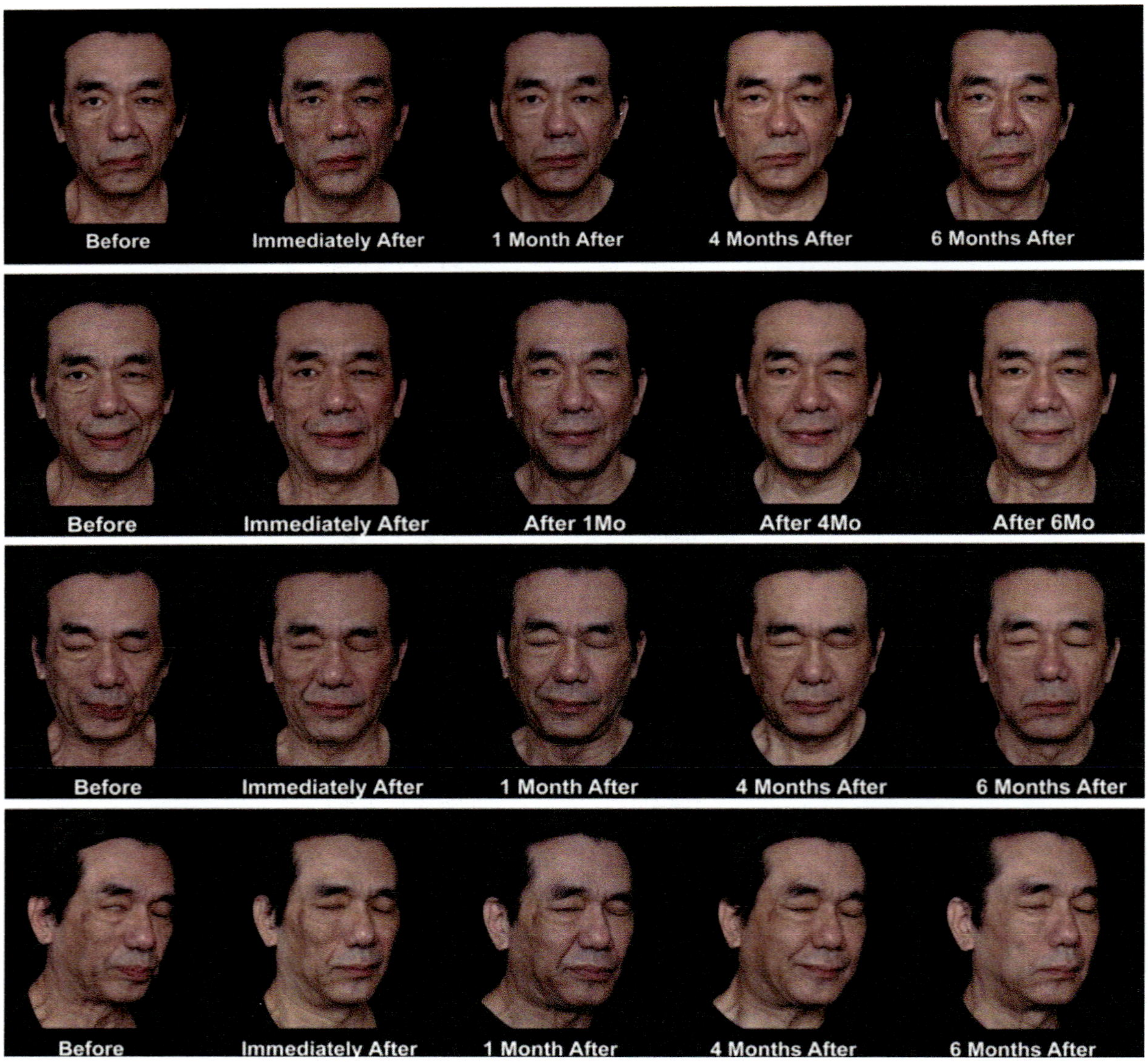

Figure D.19 The evolution of facial symmetry and muscle function upon smiling during the 6 months following treatment with mechanical myomodulation in a patient with facial asymmetry post-surgery for an acoustic neuroma.

Table D.7 Clinical Details of Patient's Left and Right (Palsy) Sides Before Treatment

Left Side	Right Side (Palsy Side)
• Deviation of mouth/oral commissure to L • Prominent nasolabial fold • Narrower eye	• Scleral show as patient tries to close eyes • Excessive activation of orbicularis oris and platysma activity on attempting to close eyes • Some platysma activity on smiling, signaling residual VII activity

- Injecting below the upper-lip levators may increase muscle action, aggravating a gummy smile.
- Injecting over the muscles of phonation (DAO, depressor labii inferioris, mentalis, and upper-lip levators) may initially influence speech; it is prudent to warn patients beforehand.
- Large volumes placed above the upper-lip levators may lengthen the upper lip or induce an unnatural smile.

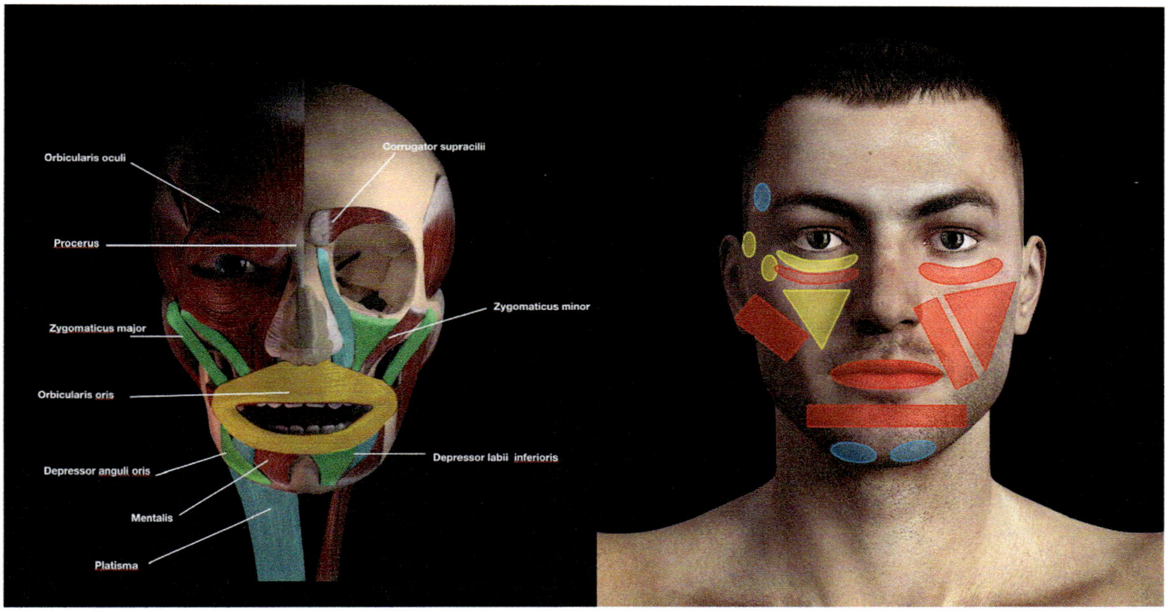

Figure D.20 Treatment areas and target muscles. Injection depth is indicated by red (superficial to muscle), yellow (under muscle), or blue (structural injections).

Table D.8 Clinical Details of Patient's Left and Right (Palsy) Sides After Treatment

Left Side	Right Side
• Reduction in the upper lateral excursion of the zygomaticus major muscle on his left side • Improved facial symmetry • Oral commissures more balanced	Immediately after treatment • Better positioning of the oral commissure, upper and lower lips • Deeper NLF on R due to increased lever effect on Upper lip levators • Less scleral show • Better alignment of the oral commissures One month after treatment • Contraction of zygomatic muscles facilitated • Less recruitment of platysma At 6 months • Closing eye with less recruitment of zygomaticus major

- Treating NL1 and Lp8 will block levator anguli oris (LAO), thus improving a gummy smile, but lengthening the upper lip in patients with a long upper lip.
- Placement below the upper-lip levators will strengthen muscles, thus elevating and everting the upper lip, but may worsen gummy smile.

TOP 10 TIPS

1. In complex asymmetry, consider using HA fillers as an adjunct to treatment with botulinum toxin.
2. Fillers may either facilitate or reduce muscle activity, thus differing from botulinum toxin, which promotes a temporary flaccid paralysis.
3. Always treat the lateral vectors (Ck1, Ck4) first in order to mitigate the gravitational sagging which weakens elevators, thus facilitating depressor action.
4. Work consciously with the concept of synergists and antagonists.
5. The upper-lip elevators function synergistically. Strengthening one muscle (e.g., zygomaticus major) may induce relaxation of others

(e.g., LAO), thus improving a gummy smile by treating the lateral cheek vectors first.

6. Boluses injected with a needle on bone usually facilitate muscle movement via a lever or pulley effect.
7. Fanning with a cannula above muscles in the subcutaneous zone usually reduces muscle movement by stretching fibers and adding tissue resistance. However,
8. Exceptions to this rule include
   - Muscle block with needle on bone in LLSAN, e.g., when treating a gummy smile.
   - Increasing tensile strength of risorius when fanning over buccinator.
9. Be aware of the angle of needle/cannula when applying myomodulation principles.
   In the midface,
   - A $\sim$30° cannula angle to skin will lead to placement in the SOOF (i.e., superficial to upper-lip levators).
   - A $\sim$60° cannula angle will facilitate deposition in the deep malar fat pad (i.e., deep to upper-lip levators).
10. Respect your learning curve; do not attempt treatment of facial palsy patients unless you are able to correct asymmetry in normal patients. This holds true particularly for addressing the smile.

References

1. De Maio M. *Aesthetic Plast Surg.* 2018;42(3):798–814.
2. Swift A & Remington BK. The mathematics of facial beauty. In: Jones DH & Swift A, eds. *Injectable Fillers: Facial Shaping and Contouring*, 2nd ed. Wiley: Oxford; 2019, pp. 29–61.
3. De Maio M. *J Cosmet Laser Ther.* 2003;5:216–7.
4. De Maio M & Bento RF. *Plast Reconstr Surg.* 2007;15(7):917–27.
5. Alam M & Tung R. *J Am Acad Dermatol.* 2018;79(3):423–35.
6. Hutto JR & Vattoth S. *Am J Roentgenol.* 2015;204(1):W19–26.
7. Sykes JM et al. *Plast Reconstr Surg.* 2015;136(5):204–18.
8. Cotofana S et al. *Plast Reconstr Surg.* 2015;136(5 Suppl):219S–34S.
9. Humphrey S et al. *Plast Reconstr Surg.* 2015;136:235–57.
10. Prendergast PM. Anatomy of the face and neck. In: Shiffman MA & Di Giuseppe A, eds. *Cosmetic Surgery: Art and Techniques*. Springer: Berlin; 2013, pp. 29–45.
11. Eskil MT & Benli KS. *Comput Vis Image Underst.* 2014;119:1–14.
12. Coleman SR & Grover R. *Aesthet Surg J.* 2006;26(1S):S4–9.
13. Peng PHL & Peng JH. Adding Volume for Reduction of Thick Lips in the Asian Patient. *Dermatol Surg.* 2018;44(2), pp. 296–298.

E BOTULINUM TOXINS

Massimo Signorini, Alastair Carruthers, Laura Bertolasi, Neil Sadick, Wolfgang G. Philipp-Dormston, and Dario Bertossi

MOLECULAR STRUCTURE AND MODE OF ACTION

Clostridium botulinum is an anaerobic, gram-positive bacterium that secretes an extremely large neurotoxic molecule (900 kDa), which produces food poisoning or botulism. It is now also used in medicine to treat diseases according to Paracelsus's paradigm that the difference between a poison and a drug lies in the dose. Although seven different serotypes of the bacterium (A to G) are known, type A is the one mostly used for the production of clinical formulations. Type B also has clinical applications for those patients who may have developed clinical resistance to type A, but this is seldom the case in aesthetic treatments.

Of the 900 kDa natural molecule, only the central 150 kDa segment (the neurotoxic core) is responsible for its biological activity. The surrounding portions have no pharmacological activity and simply act as a protective shield ensuring unchanged toxin absorption from the host's gastrointestinal tract. These surrounding molecules are named accessory proteins and are both hemagglutinin and non-hemagglutinin in nature. Once the toxin has entered the host by ingestion or injection, the biological role of the accessory proteins is largely terminated and the 150 kDa neurotoxin comes into play. Here again, the structure is complex and each portion of the segment plays a relevant role.

The 150 kDa neurotoxic protein is divided into a 100 kDa heavy and a 50 kDa light chain. The heavy chain has a two-fold action. The first part (binding domain) links to the specific receptors at the level of the axonic presynaptic endings; the second (translocation domain) then carries the light chain through the membrane and into the actual nerve ending. Once there, the light 50 kDa chain accomplishes its task by cleaving a group of proteins, named SNARE, which are responsible for the release of the neurotransmitter acetylcholine. Inhibition of acetylcholine release impairs muscular contraction and flaccid paralysis ensues. The effect of botulinum toxin is only temporary, and within a few months neuromuscular efficacy is spontaneously reestablished.

The details of this process have not been fully elucidated. For the purposes of this chapter, however, it should be made clear that regeneration always and completely occurs.

Interruption of neuromuscular transmission is not the only medical application of the drug. Indeed, receptors for botulinum toxin are widespread in the human body and reach far beyond only neuromuscular junctions. Accordingly, the indications for the treatment have widened tremendously since its introduction 30 years ago. However, it is beyond the scope of this chapter to examine the present status of botulinum toxin in medicine, and from here onward, only aesthetic applications will be considered.

THE MUSCLES OF FACIAL EXPRESSION

With few exceptions, these muscles, often defined as mimetic, are the target of our treatments. Their role is to animate the face, thus allowing communication of feelings and emotions to the outside world. Most mimetic muscles feature a bony origin and a cutaneous insertion. During muscle exertion, the skin is tractioned toward the skeletal origin, causing wrinkles, lines, and furrows to appear on the surface with repeated contraction. Other mimetic elements have both origin and insertion on the skin, but here again, contraction generates surface irregularities. Muscles seldom function independently and more often interplay synergistically and variably with other muscles. This determines the unlimited nuances of facial expressions. Mimetic muscles are divided into two functional groups: elevators and depressors.

How does botulinum toxin step into the field? The answer is simple. In youth, the skin has full elastic properties and recovers promptly after each contraction, and the wrinkles and lines generated by the muscles of facial expression are accurately defined as dynamic. Over time, however, skin elasticity, strength, and resistance decrease, and muscle action eventually produces wrinkles, lines, and furrows that remain at rest. A static component thus becomes increasingly visible, harboring increasing aging.

Botulinum toxin treatment of mimetic muscles, also termed chemodenervation, requires a thorough knowledge of muscle anatomy. While routine aesthetic practice may require treatment of 20 to 30 muscles, treatment of patients with facial palsy may require treatment of additional muscles. The closely adjacent facial muscles lie mostly within the superficial muscolar aponeurotic system (SMAS) of the face and have a distinct three-dimensional structure and orientation. Precise injections of the drug are therefore essential in maximizing efficacy and minimizing complications. The dose is equally important. The injected units should ideally saturate the specific target receptors, leaving no unbound molecules free to move to nearby unwanted muscles. The clinician needs to understand that delivering suboptimal doses will negatively affect duration of result, although not giving rise to complications. Conversely, higher-than-recommended doses may significantly increase the rate of side effects.

Precision in botulinum toxin treatments is key to success. The injector must know the exact localization and depth of the target muscles and the ideal dose for combining efficacy and result. Another extremely important safety-related issue is diffusion rate. Ideally, the formulation with the lowest diffusion potential would guarantee the highest safety margin. In Europe, North America, and many countries, only three different formulations are available. Each of them has a robust literature claiming similar or better performances than its competitors, including the lowest diffusion profile. However, most of the papers are company sponsored and may lack objectivity. Although highly experienced injectors all have personal preferences, it is fair to state that these are often based on subjective impressions only and that to date there is no clear-cut superiority of one formulation over the others in terms of general performance. This is especially true when it comes to the diffusion rate. As long as a licensed product is preferred and correctly administered, efficacy and safety are guaranteed.

RECONSTITUTION

Presently, all licensed formulations are supplied as powders and require reconstitution with saline immediately prior to use. Although physicians are free to dilute according to personal preference, there are well-tested and universally accepted company recommendations. In Europe, licensed formulations are marketed in 50 U vials (Allergan's Vistabel and Merz's Bocouture) and in 125 U vials (Galderma's Azzalure). This raises the vital point that botulinum toxin units are not interchangeable between companies because the biological potency assay tests differ. This is an unfortunate confusion factor for novice injectors. However, there is general agreement that Allergan and Merz dosage units are reasonably comparable (1:1), and that Galderma units are equivalent to Allergan and Merz units in a 2.5:1 ratio. Thus, the Azzalure vial containing 125 U is more or less equivalent to the 50 U vial of Vistabel and Bocouture. Company recommendations from Allergan and Merz suggest diluting the 50 U vial with 1.25 mL of plain saline. This yields 4 U per 0.1 mL of solution. Galderma, on the other hand, has historically recommended a dilution of 0.63 mL per 125 U vial, thereby rendering a solution twice as concentrated as its competitors. It is beyond the scope of this chapter to discuss this rationale. It is fair to state, however, that the double concentration requires considerable extra care for dose precision and may thus obviate an otherwise excellent product. Recent literature has compared the efficacy and safety of Azzalure diluted at 0.63 mL versus 1.25 mL. The results with the 1.25 mL dilution have been as good, if not better, than with the double concentration. This allows the injector to dilute all three formulations with 1.25 mL of saline and to consider the potential of the resulting solution comparable to the others.

A few words should also be spent discussing injection pain. Although generally well tolerated, delivery of the drug may be unpleasant. In part, this is due to the needle, and the thinnest possible gauge size will help to minimize this component. While many injectors use a 30G, the 31–33G sizes may be preferable, although they dull quickly and require frequent changes. However, it is the solution that is mostly responsible for pain during injections. Some authors recommend nerve blocks, but these are possibly more aggressive than necessary. If available, preserved saline (NaCl 0.9% + benzyl alcohol 0.9%) should be used for dilution because the solution is almost pain-free without losing any of its pharmacological properties. Another option is to use plain saline + lidocaine for dilution. This will not impair the effect of the treatment and does reduce pain to some extent; however, preserved saline seems to be the best option.

Although companies recommend keeping the reconstituted solution at 4°C and injecting within 24 hours, both clinical experience and significant literature suggest that the solution remains active for weeks.

MANAGING PATIENT EXPECTATIONS

Careful patient assessment clarifies both the possibilities and limitations of individual treatments. Matching clinical assessment with realistic patient expectations is key to successful practice as careful pretreatment explanation will be generally well accepted, while belated explanations may be construed as excuses. Although botulinum toxin may lead to drastic improvement of facial lines, there may not always be complete eradication. Repeated treatments have been documented to enable longer-lasting results. Patients with very deep or resting frown lines should be realistically informed during initial consultation, and adjunctive treatments, such as careful intradermal injection of hyaluronic acid microdroplets, discussed upfront. Honest and straight-forward physician information helps to establish trust and develop sustainable patient relationships.

TREATMENT OF FROWN LINES (GLABELLAR LINES)

Reduction of frown lines was the first FDA-licensed indication for chemomodulation with botulinum toxin (2002), and the benefit of softening harsh expressions soon became evident. Glabellar target muscles comprise the procerus and paired corrugators. The bony origin of the corrugator is close to the midline, at the level of the medial head of the brow. The fibers course superolaterally and insert to the dermis above the middle third of the brow. Individual variations in the lateral extent and elevation of the fibers are common. An inexperienced injector may safely use the traditional five points. However, best results are reached when the injections are tailored to individual patient features. Dynamic assessment of the frown lines yields precious information as to the bony origin and the direction and the lateral extent of the fibers, and it informs a customized treatment plan. Dynamic assessment also yields important information regarding muscle mass, muscle strength, and optimal dose. It enables the expert injector to predict the anticipated improvement and subsequent necessity of touch-ups with hyaluronic acid. When injecting the **corrugators**, the physician should always keep in mind their three-dimensional structure. The **medial injection** targets the bony origin and should therefore be deep, possibly as **close to the bone** as possible without touching the periosteum. The thumb of the non-injecting hand elevates the soft tissues, helping to keep the solution away from the orbit. The **lateral injections** target the dermal insertions of the fibers and are therefore **superficial**. This reduces the risk of diffusion to the levator palpebrae muscle.

The bony origin of the procerus is at the junction of the nasal bones with the upper lateral cartilages. Fibers are directed superiorly and insert to the dermis of the central forehead, a few centimeters above the glabella.

The classic **procerus** injection point is in the midline at, or just above, the intercanthal level. The correct **depth is halfway between the skin and the bone.**

The classic five-point pattern of injection for frown lines suggests **4 U aliquots per point** (0.1 mL when the 1.25 mL dilution is used), **the total dose being 20 U**. This modality is an excellent guide for beginners. However, individualized patterns and doses will ensue with increasing experience. There are two golden rules for the treatment of frown lines: The first is to inject deeply at the bony origin of the medial corrugator, with the lateral injections being placed superficially. This will significantly reduce the risk of eyelid ptosis. The second is to keep the corrugator injection points close to the brow in order to minimize diffusion to the lower frontalis fibers. This will preserve brow position, preventing brow ptosis.

TREATMENT OF CROW'S FEET LINES (CFLs)

This is the second licensed indication for aesthetic botulinum toxin treatments. The **target** muscle is the **lateral portion of the orbicularis oculi**. Dynamic assessment of the patient is extremely important, as in some patients, CFLs are equally distributed above and below the lateral canthus, whereas in others, they lie mainly above or below. The typical three-point injection pattern is thus tailored to the individual. The orbicularis oculi is extremely superficial, and there is virtually no subcutaneous tissue between its fibers and the skin. Therefore, **intradermal injections** are suggested as the solution will easily reach the muscle. Intramuscular placement increases the chance of bruising and does not improve the result. **The recommended dose is 12 U per side (3 injections, 4 U each)**. The needle should point away from the eye and enter the skin **2 cm lateral to the bony orbit**. In patients with a history of lower eyelid edema, or in those who feature lower eyelid laxity, injections below the lateral canthus should be avoided. When CFLs are very deep, some authors add two additional points lateral to the previous ones. Care should be taken not to chase the CFLs that extend caudally toward the cheek as these are usually generated by the zygomatic muscles, and injections at this level would interfere with the smile.

Combining the treatment of CFLs and frown lines is an excellent strategy, not only for improving wrinkles and softening expressions, but also for brow elevation.

FOREHEAD LINES

The FDA has recently approved the treatment of forehead lines, which now allows on-label injection of the full upper face. The two frontalis muscles are responsible for forehead lines. These are large, flat muscles with no bony origin. Inferiorly, their fibers insert in the deep dermis and subcutaneous tissue of the brows, while the superior origin is from the galea at the approximate level of the hairline. Fibers run upward, generating horizontal lines at right angles with their direction. Functionally, the lower part of frontalis muscles elevate the brows, while the upper part depresses the hairline. The fibers of the paired muscles may remain parallel or may converge as they rise cranially. More often, they divert superolaterally to leave an empty triangle in the central forehead. Fortunately, in contrast with the variable position of the medial margins, the lateral margins are usually at the level of the temporal crest, or temporal fusion line. The forehead may vary significantly in height, with forehead lines localized to either the lower or upper segment, or evenly distributed. The visibility of the frontalis muscles may vary widely between individuals.

Dynamic assessment, which is one of the golden rules to successful botulinum toxin treatment, is possibly even more important at this level. The injector must evaluate several factors, some of which are in reciprocal contrast.

First, precise localization of the muscles must be determined. During contraction, the presence or absence of midline fibers can be easily seen. Injecting where there is no muscle is a waste of product. Dynamic assessment also informs the injector of muscle strength at different levels.

Second, brow position must be carefully evaluated and is possibly the most important factor in forehead treatment. Chemomodulation of frontalis muscles is often a trade-off, as erasing forehead lines and elevating the brows at the same time is simply not possible. In the past, the main, if not only, goal of treatment was maximal reduction of horizontal lines as requested by patients. Leading injectors soon realized that eradication of all lines produced frozen, expressionless faces and also possible brow ptosis. Current expert opinion is that correction of forehead lines should not interfere with brow position. This implies lower dosage and higher injection points placed well above the brows. Patient education is vital in achieving agreement on treatment goals. Many patients still focus on the lines in lieu of brow position. This quandary may be simply resolved by asking the question, "Shall we erase forehead lines as much as possible, or shall we consider brow position as well?" Clearly, patients with a low brow position and deep lines all across the height of the forehead are the most difficult to treat successfully. Another consideration in utilizing low-dose forehead treatment is the dose:duration efficacy. Full doses usually yield results lasting 4–5 months, whereas half doses seldom exceed 3 months. If a patient is treated with full doses for glabella and CFL, with only half doses for the forehead, repeat treatment of the forehead area may be suggested approximately 3 months after the initial session.

Treatment planning is of paramount importance. Dynamic assessment and forehead height will guide toward a single row of four injection points placed at least 2 cm above the brows, or a two-row "M" shaped pattern of six points. The usual 1.25 mL dilution is mostly accepted. As for CFL treatment, it is best to inject subdermally (and not intramuscularly) to minimize bleeding. Typically, aliquots of 0.05 mL are injected (2 U each), giving a total of 8–12 U.

Although facial asymmetries are common, many patients are unaware of them, despite their being clearly visible, especially at brow level. Any pre-injection asymmetries should be thoroughly discussed and well documented photographically in order to avoid any subsequent blaming of treatment. The expert injector may effectively improve brow asymmetry by using individualized doses on each side, although no promises of perfection should be made.

Compensatory action of untreated muscle segments is an important principle in botulinum toxin treatment. This is seldom true of small muscles, as the halo of diffusion tends to involve the whole unit, but in large muscles this possibility may cause side effects. In the forehead, this can occur when only the medial frontalis is injected, leaving the lateral portions untreated. The brain records the central loss of function and recruits laterally for compensation. The consequence is the so-called "Mephisto" or "Spock" look, due to steep elevation of the lateral brow. This unattractive defect is easily corrected by injecting 1–2 U into the point of maximum lateral brow elevation on the affected side.

Finally, physicians should be wary of treating patients with deep forehead lines, strong muscular activation, and high brow position. In many cases, this denotes a compensatory reflex due to underlying eyelid ptosis or dermatochalasis. Such patients require full frontalis action to elevate the brows, thus compensating for the upper visual field obstruction determined by their underlying condition. Chemodenervation of their frontalis muscles would impair this ability and upper visual impairment could be significant. These patients should be corrected surgically and botulinum toxin treatment withheld.

BROW LIFT

Elevating the brow is an important aesthetic goal and may be the main treatment motivation for some patients. In addition to treating the glabella and the CFL, further lateral elevation may be mediated by injecting 2 U aliquots very superficially just below the brow, one at the tail, and another 1 cm medially. Care must be taken not to inject higher to preserve full action of the lower frontalis. The goal is to reduce the sphincteric action of the upper lateral fibers of the orbicularis oculi, which lower the lateral portion of the brow.

LOWER EYELID INJECTIONS

Injecting the lateral portion of the lower orbicularis oculi has two different applications, the first being to widen the eye aperture and the second to correct muscular hypertrophy if present. Patient assessment is important in avoiding complications. A snap-back test should be performed to verify lower eyelid tone. The technique for the aforementioned indications implies a single 1–2 U intradermal injection lateral to the mid-pupillary line, 4–5 mm below the lid margin.

BUNNY LINES

Bunny lines are generated by the nasal part of the transverse nasalis muscle. Although they may be visible at rest, dynamic assessment is essential to appreciate their precise extent. Treatment is quite straightforward and a single 2–3 U aliquot in the middle of the bunny-line area usually solves of the problem. Avoid injecting laterally to prevent involvement of the levator labii superioris alaeque nasi, as this would lead to alteration of the smile and lengthening of the upper lip.

ELEVATION OF THE NASAL TIP

The target muscle here is the depressor septi nasi. The bony origin is from the maxilla at the level of the canine tooth, and the skin insertions are along the columella up to the nasal tip. Patients with a low nasal tip will not benefit from this treatment if the defect is caused by a long inferior projection of the nasal septum. Local examination will quickly clarify this. A single 2–3 U subdermal injection at the base of the columella will gently elevate the nasal tip when the indication is correct. Further improvement may be achieved by injecting hyaluronic acid in a deeper plane to open the nasolabial angle to some extent, and in selected cases, this combination is quite successful.

CORRECTION OF THE GUMMY SMILE

Overaction of the upper-lip elevators leads to excessive exposure of the gums when smiling. Treatment with botulinum toxin can be very effective in mild to moderate cases, but when gum exposure is more than 50%, the treatment should be surgical. Patient assessment must take this into account and also consider upper lip length and lip asymmetries. Chemomodulation of upper-lip elevators will lengthen the upper lip and this may become a problematic issue. Patients with a short upper lip are therefore the ideal candidates. Preexisting lip asymmetries should be carefully evaluated, discussed, and photographically documented.

The treatment is usually performed in two sessions. Initially, **the levator labii superioris alaeque nasi muscles are injected with 2–3 U each, just lateral to the nasal ala and about 1 cm above the white lip**. Penetration is one half of the standard 12 mm needle. Some authors also inject the depressor septi nasi as described previously at the same session. The patient is reassessed after 2 weeks. If required, the levator labii superioris muscles are treated at this stage, each with a 2 U aliquot injected 1 cm lateral to the previous points.

Lengthening of the upper lip and lip asymmetries are not uncommon following gummy-smile treatment. The innovative concept of myomodulation, based on the reduction of muscular overaction with the use of hyaluronic acid, is reported to be effective, longer lasting, and possibly with fewer side effects to correct the gummy smile.

PERIORAL WRINKLES ("BARCODE" LINES)

Perioral wrinkles should be treated with four points (two per side) of 1 U each to the superficial dermis.

Perioral Wrinkles (Bar Code)

Use of botulinum toxin in this area requires experience to select the patients, determine the dose and the injection points. This treatment is not suggested in the older patient with a thin muscle mass.

The target muscle is the orbicularis oris, the perioral spincteric muscle of labial occlusion. Its function is therefore essential. Over time it generates perioral wrinkles, one of the most unwanted signs of aging. Chemomodulation of this muscle at high enough doses can certainly reduce the bar code dramatically, but this most likely entails unacceptable side effects at the level of lip function. The key message is that botulinum toxin can help to correct the bar code, but cannot do the job on its own. Indeed, this is the perfect area for the association with Hyaluronic Acid, usually performed in two sessions.

Botulinum toxin at very low dose is used first. The targets are only the most superficial fibers of the muscle, thus leaving the main body undisturbed to preserve function. Two injection points for each side of the upper lip are determined dynamically, keeping the medial one at least 4 mm away from the peak of the Cupid's bow, and the lateral one at least 5 mm away from the oral commissure. Both points lie 1 mm above the vermillion border. The dose range is 0.5–1 units per point, and must be delivered intradermally with the bevel of the needle facing up and the syringe held almost flat to the skin surface.

Patients should be informed that in the first 10–15 days lip function may sometimes be mildly hampered. Aliquots of 0.5 units will keep the treatment on a safer side. Some injectors also prefer a double concentration to prevent diffusion to the deeper fibers.

At the second session (10–15 days later), a soft and moldable hyaluronic acid is used to deposit a very thin layer of product just below the dermis of the white lip, in order to mildly lift and stretch the skin. Small volumes only should be used, usually no more than 0.25 mL per side, to reach the effect without significantly changing lip shape and size. The results of this association are usually very good.

Complications

Impairment of lip function (prevention: avoid treating older patients and/or very thin muscles; treatment: none).

Depressor Anguli Oris (DAO)

The bony origin of this triangular muscle is at the anterior portion of the margin of the mandibular body, the skin insertion at the oral commissure. It generates expressions of sadeness, disapproval and reproach.

Hypertony of the DAO at rest downturns the commisures and confers a sad look. Also, when the soft tissues of the midface begin to sag with age, the DAO may contribute to some extent to the marionette line.

Botulinum toxin may be used to lift and align the commisures with the horizontal axis of the lips.

Unfortunately, the origin of the DAO lies just below the origin of the depressor labii inferioris (DLI). The fibers of DAO and DLI part as they direct upwards to their skin insertions, the former supero-laterally to the commissure, the latter supero-medially to the lower lip. However they have significant overlapping in their lower half, the DAO lying just above the DLI. This very close proximity can be responsible for the diffusion of botulinum toxin to DLI when DAO is injected, with significant consequences on the smile. This complication is not rare and has been experienced by top injectors also. Some of them actually do not inject the DAO any more.

Due to the particular anatomy, correct points of injection and doses are critical for the outcome. Unfortunately, there is no fool-proof injection site. In the lower half of the muscle the underlying DLI can be affected by the injection, in the upper half the dangerous neighbor is the orbicularis oris. Our prefered landmark for a single subdermal 3 units injection is 12 mm above the mandibular margin, 1 cm lateral to the commissure.

Finally, it should be kept in mind that botulinum toxin alone is not a recommended treatment for Marionette lines. These are a multifactorial condition in which DAO plays a role, but even more so soft tissue sagging and volume loss. Hyaluronic acid is the cornerstone to correct marionette lines, but botulinum toxin in synergy may give a valuable contribution in selected cases.

Complications

DLI impairment (prevention: careful landmarks, careful depth of injection; treatment: none).

Hypertonicity of the Chin

The bony origin of the mentalis muscle is from the prominence of the alveolar process between the medial incisor and the canine, its fibers are directed perpendicularly to the surface of the chin. In normal conditions, it elevates the soft tissues of the chin and projects the lower lip upwards and forward. Overaction of the muscle produces irregularities of the skin surface, a condition colourfully described in the literature as "golf ball chin", "popply chin" and "peau d'orange". It also flattens the soft tissues against the bone compromising chin projection.

Treatment is performed with a single 6–8 units injection in the midline, 1 cm above the lower chin margin, into the deep subcutaneous tissue. In large chins, the same dose can be divided into two paired injections, each 5 mm from midline. If injected more laterally, the solution could reach the DLI and interfere significantly with the smile. Minor touch-ups are sometimes necessary to improve the result, usually with superficial microdroplets for residual surface irregularities.

Treatment of the mentalis muscle often improves the lower third of the face very significantly.

Complications

DLI impairment (prevention: midline injection only, or paired paramedian injections not further than 5 mm from midline; treatment: none).

Treatment of the Platysma

This is an extremely wide, long and thin muscle with a complex anatomy and function. It runs from the upper chest vertically to the lower face with parallel fibers. Bony origins and skin insertions are localized at both extremities: at the chest level the 2nd, 3rd and 4th rib and the skin of the deltopectoral region; in the lower face, the mandibular bone and the skin of the cheek, chin and oral commissure. Functionally it is an elevator of the soft tissues of the upper chest and lower neck, and a depressor of the soft tissues of the lower face. Hypertony of the platysma becomes an issue with aging as it produces vertical bands, the most prominent at the level of the medial margin. Patient selection is critical for the outcome. Ideally, the muscular component of the bands should be well palpated and skin laxity should be absent or mild. Patients with increased degrees of laxity will not respond to treatment and should undertake a surgical neck lift.

Platysma bands are marked dinamically, and injection sites placed every 2 cm all along the extent of the band. Aliquots of 2 units are injected into each point in a very superficial plane. Indeed, the muscle is extremely thin and if the needle reaches across, the solution may affect deeper structures of the neck. Serious complications may arise, such as dysphagia and dysphonia. Keeping the syringe almost flat to the skin surface and inserting the needle at a very acute angle is a good technique to avoid deep injections.

Another application of platysma injections is to assist in soft tissue elevation of the lower and midface. Indeed, the fibers reaching the lower face with the SMAS are active depressors of the soft tissues. Injecting in two parallel rows, above and below the mandibular margin, in a multiple w pattern, will reduce this component and may assist lower and midface elevation. A 4-point row is placed 1 cm above the mandibular margin, another 4-point row 1 cm below it. The 2 units aliquots are delivered subdermally. Please note that the most medial point of the upper row will affect the DAO as well, so extra care should be taken to avoid affecting the DLI with a deep injection.

Complications

No result (prevention: correct patient selection; treatment: surgery).

Dysphagia, dysphonia (prevention: proper plane of injection; treatment: none).

Masseter Hypertrophy

The masseter is not a muscle of expression, it is a purely functional muscle involved in mastication. Treating the masseter with botulinum toxin therefore has nothing to do with wrinkles, lines or furrows. The goal is to reduce the muscle mass through a relative atrophy in patients who complain of regional hypertrophy. This is a basic concept that must be immediately understood by clinicians, because results will only be seen several weeks after the treatment, versus the few days necessary to reach the outcome on mimic muscles.

Not surprisingly, this application was pioneered in the far east where masseter hypertrophy is a common but also unwanted racial feature. There should be no concern about masticatory function after the treatment, as the temporalis and pterygoid muscles will compensate for the reduction of masseteric function. This treatment can also be applied to cases of bruxism, although this indication is beyond the purpose of this chapter.

The masseter is a strong quadrangular muscle divided in two parts, superficial and deep. The superficial part is the largest, its fibers arise from a thick tendinous aponeurosis along the anterior 2/3 of the antero-inferior margin of the zygomatic arch. The fibers are directed postero-inferiorly to the region of the mandibular angle and to the external surface of the lower half of the mandibular ramus. The deep part is smaller, its fibers arise from the medial aspect of the lateral third of the zygomatic arch, and are directed vertically down to the supero-lateral surface of the mandibular ramus and to the coronoid process.

It is quite simple to outline the limits of the muscle. The superior, posterior and inferior margins are precisely localized along the zygomatic arch, the mandibular ramus, and the inferior mandibular margin at the angle. The anterior margin is also easily identified by palpation as the patient bites tightly. Considering that the upper third of the area is tendinous, the injections should be evenly distributed in the lower two thirds of the outlined masseter.

According to the extent of the area three to five sites are established, mainly closer to the angle and the lower margin of the mandibular body. The needle must be able to reach all the way down to the external surface of the mandible, therefore a 25 mm length is preferable to make sure that both the superficial and deep parts of the muscle are injected. It is also advisable to keep the anterior points several mm lateral from the anterior margin of the muscle, to avoid interference with the risorius. Doses are quite variable according to masseter bulk. In the caucasian patient, a total of 20–25 units per side are usually adequate at the initial session (evenly distributed at each injection site). However, in cases of very significant masseter hypertrophy 50 units per side or more may be required.

At two weeks after treatment, palpation of the masseters when the patient bites strongly can give the injector a clue about the degree of chemomodulation achieved. However the esthetic goal, i.e. reduction of soft tissue protrusion at the mandibular angle, can not be appreciated before 8 weeks.

Only at this time the injector should decide whether or not to increase the botulinum toxin dose, and if sio usually by 50%. Once again, evaluation of the touch-up should be at no less than 2 months. With customized follow-ups, the goal is to reach a regimen of 2 sessions per year to keep the desired correction stable.

Complications

Asymmetry of the smile (prevention: keep injections away from the anterior margin of the masseter; treatment: none).

Hernia-like bulging of the deep muscular component when clenching the teeth (prevention: inject both deep and superficial muscular component; treatment: inject the deep muscular protrusion).

Bibliography

Braz AV & Sakuma TH. Patterns of contraction of the frontalis muscle: A pilot study. *Surg Cosmet Dermatol.* 2010;2:191–4.

Brin MF et al. Safety and tolerability of On a botulinum toxin A in the treatment of facial lines: A meta-analysis of individual patient data from global clinical registration studies in 1678 participants. *J Am Acad Dermatol.* 2009;61:961.e1–970.

Carruthers A, Carruthers J & Cohen J. A prospective, double-blind randomized, parallel-group, dose-ranging study of botulinum toxin type A in female subjects with horizontal forehead rhytides. *Dermatol Surg.* 2003;29:461–7.

Carruthers JDA & Carruthers JA. Treatment of gabellar frown lines with C. botulinum-A exotoxin. *J Dermatol Surg and Oncol.* 1992;18:17–21.

Cohen JL, Dayan SH, Cox SE, Yalamanchili R & Tardie G. On a botulinum toxin A dose-ranging study for hyperdynamic perioral lines. *Dermatol Surg.* 2012;38:1497–505.

Dayan SH. Complications of botulinum toxin A use in facial rejuvenation. *Facial Plast Surg Clin N Am.* 2003;11(4):483.

De Maio M & Rzany B. *Botulinum toxin in aesthetic medicine.* Springer-Verlag, Bersli.

Flynn TC. Periocular botulinum toxin. *Clinics in Dermatol.* 2003;21:498–504.

Goodman GJ. The masseters and their treatment with botulinum toxin (Botox). In: Carruthers A, Carruthers J, eds. *Botulinum Toxin (Botox).* 3rd ed., Saunders, Philadelphia, PA.

Klein AW. Complications, adverse reactions and insights with the use of botulinum toxin. *Dermatol Surg.* 2003;29:549–56.

Polo M. Botulinum toxin type A (Botox) for the neuromuscular correction of excessive gingival display on smiling (gummy smile). *Am J Orthod Dentofacial Orthop.* 2008;133:195–203.

Sundaram H, Signorini M & Liew S. Global Aesthetics Consensus: Botulinum Toxin Type A—Evidence-Based Review, Emerging Concepts, and Consensus Recommendations for Aesthetic Use, Including Updates on Complications. *Plast Reconstr Surg.* 2016;137:518–29.

F ABSORBABLE SOFT TISSUE FILLERS: CORE CHARACTERISTICS

Ali Pirayesh, Colin M. Morrison, Berend van der Lei, and Ash Mosahebi

INTRODUCTION

The increasing popularity of minimally invasive cosmetic procedures in recent years has caused a surge in the use of soft-tissue fillers. Minimally invasive cosmetic procedures have increased 300% from 2000; among the most utilized minimally invasive cosmetic procedures, soft-tissue fillers rank second, behind neuromodulators [1].

Hyaluronic acid (HA) products are currently the most utilized soft-tissue fillers. Adequate working knowledge of individual products, injection techniques, and anatomic principles is vital to improve outcomes and to prevent and minimize complications.

There is a plethora of literature detailing the use and safety of soft-tissue fillers. Each company is keen to highlight unique and proprietary characteristics which set their product apart from the competitors. The sheer choice and volume of different soft tissue fillers flooding the market may be overwhelming for novice and even seasoned injectors.

The aim of this chapter is to allow an unbiased description of common HA and non-HA absorbable soft-tissue fillers as a rough guide for decision making. This chapter is not intended to be exhaustive as this would be beyond the scope of this book in which we endeavour to cover "the essentials for injections". Basic rheology, HA manufacturing processes and short review of injections and layering principles by region are discussed with a focus on patient safety.

Prevention of complications and management of paramount importance when utilizing soft tissue fillers are covered in a different chapter.

HYALURONIC ACID FILLERS

HA is a naturally-occurring component of the extracellular matrix. It is a glycosaminoglycan (GAG) polymer consisting of repeat disaccharide units of glucuronic acid and N-acetylglucosamine. Approximately 50% of the body's total HA is in the skin [2]. HA acts as a scaffold for the extracellular matrix, providing rigidity, hydration and turgor whilst allowing cellular movement and regeneration [3]. It is also important in protecting the skin from free radical damage, particularly against UVA and UVB. HA is rapidly metabolised in the tissues, with one third of total body HA being turned over daily [4,5].

HA from animal sources generally has longer polymer chains than in those from bacterial sources (usually from the *Streptococcus equi* species); they are forbidden in Europe as soft tissue fillers. Bacterial fermentation is generally preferred as a source for HA because it is less likely to be antigenic, being free from foreign proteins and easier to purify [6,7].

HA SOFT TISSUE FILLERS

HA soft tissue fillers consist of long chains of hyaluronic acid. Most dermal filler products will consist of HA crosslinked with a chemical such as 1,4-butanedioldiglycidyl ether (BDDE) for Restylane®, Belotero®, Teosyal®, Hyabell®, Stylage® and Juvéderm® and suspended in a physiological or phosphate-buffered solution [8].

The process of crosslinking (Figure F.1) adds a molecule to link the polymer chains to each other, thus modifying their physical properties to make them longer-lasting and less likely to be degraded. The most commonly used crosslinker is 1,4-butanediol diglycidyl ether (BDDE); BDDE has a significantly lower toxicity than other crosslinking agents (e.g., divinyl sulfone or formaldehyde) and is biodegradable [9–11].

The product is then processed "sized" into smaller, crosslinked domains to allow for injection through a needle into the skin as a homogeneous gel or a suspension of particles in gel carriers.

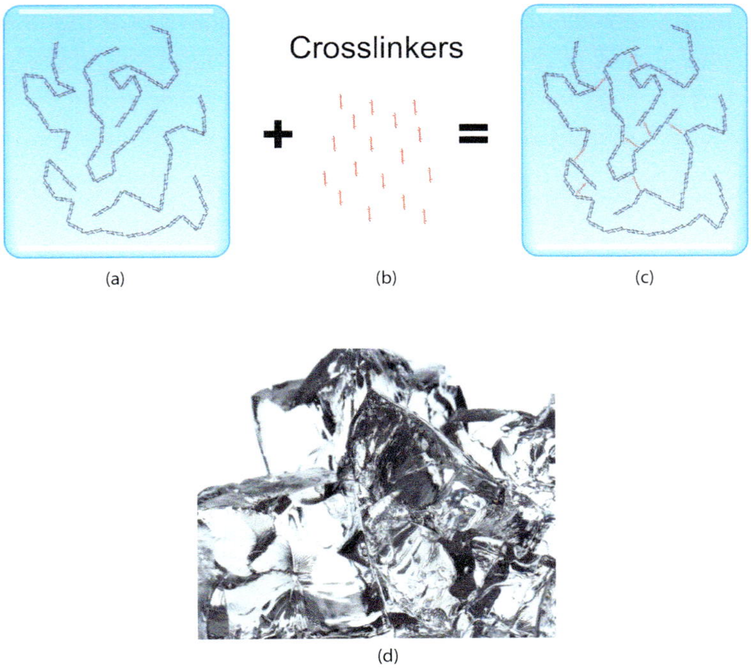

Figure F.1 Crosslinking HA polymer chains transform the HA solution (a) into a gel (c). Crosslinker molecules (b) bind individual HA polymer chains to create a network (c), which manifests macroscopically as a gel mass (d). (Adapted with permission from Tezel A & Fredrickson GH. *J Cosmet Laser Ther.* 2008;10(1):35–42.)

Variability in methods used to manufacture HA fillers have given rise to differences in properties such as degree of cross-linkage, particle size and concentration. These properties are vital in determining the clinical performance of the filler [12].

The HA filler manufacturing process usually consists of the following steps:

- Dilution of HA powder in basic medium
- Mixing of BDDE (ratio is important for quality)
- Cross-linking reaction (heating)
- Dilution of gel in basic medium (addition of lidocaine)
- Purification
- Mixture of purified cross-linked (and sometimes uncross-linked HA)
- Degassing, then filling the syringes
- Gel sterilization
- Blistering and packaging

HA fillers can be classified according to their particulate forms: either monophasic or biphasic gels. Monophasic gels consist of a single 'phase' of HA. They can be either monodensified - HA is mixed and cross-linked in a single step (e.g., Juvéderm and Teosyal) - or polydensified - HA goes through two stages of cross-linking (e.g., Belotero). Biphasic gels such as Restylane and Perlane consist of two 'phases' of HA - cross-linked HA of a specific size which is then suspended in non-cross-linked HA acting as a carrier [13,14].

Controversy remains over the relative clinical effectiveness of monophasic vs biphasic hyaluronic acid fillers; it is likely that no single method is superior to another, rather that the different physical properties of dermal fillers are more suitable for different clinical indications.

DERMAL FILLER RHEOLOGY

"Rheology" is the study of the physical characteristics that influence the way materials behave when subject to deforming forces. Once injected, fillers are subject to shearing, vertical compression and stretch from muscle movements, compression, and gravity [15].

It is our role as practitioners to understand the way fillers will behave when injected into a particular area or layer of the skin and to choose the most appropriate dermal filler to achieve the desired aesthetic result. Fillers used to treat different parts of the face have very different desirable qualities. For example, when treating the deep supra-periosteal layers of the chin or jawline, it is important that the filler gives good volume and projection without spreading through the tissues. Conversely, when injecting into superficial dermal layers, it is important that fillers can easily spread through the tight connective tissue in order to sit smoothly in the upper layers of the skin.

A number of factors affect the physical characteristics of HA dermal fillers. These include:

- **Elastic modulus (G')**: The ability to recover the original shape after shear deformation. Elasticity is the ability of a material to return to its original shape after being deformed [16].
- **Viscous modulus (G'')**: The inability to recover the original shape after shear deformation. Viscosity is a measure of the resistance of a fluid, which is being deformed by either shear or tensile stress [16].
- **Complex modulus (G^*)**: The total ability of material to withstand deformation. It is defined as the sum of the elastic modulus (G') and viscous modulus (G'') [16].
- **Tan δ**: The ratio between the viscous modulus and the elastic modulus corresponds to the loss tangent (loss factor) tan δ, and thus describes the ratio between the elastic and the viscous share of a polymer fluid. If the loss tangent δ is greater than 1, the material is predominantly viscous, and if it is smaller than 1, the material is predominantly elastic.
- **Cohesivity**: The cohesivity of a filler is the strength of the cross-linking adhesion forces that hold the individual HA units together. Cohesivity

is determined by the concentration of HA and the degree of cross-linking. High cohesivity helps the filler maintain vertical projection [15].

A gel must be cohesive in order to avoid any migration. Visco-elastic properties and crosslinking determine how cohesive the gel is. A gel with low cohesivity is suitable for delicate and superficial treatments. A gel with high cohesivity has more volume and lifting capacity for structural contouring. The extrusion force of the gel is also important and differs amongst various fillers.

- **Lift Capacity**: The lift capacity of a filler is its ability to oppose deformation and flattening and affects its suitability for different applications, whether for more superficial correction of fine lines or deeper use for wrinkles and folds, volumizing, and contouring. G′ has usually been previously used to predict and describe the lift capacity of a filler [15,17–19], but lift capacity has also now been treated as a function of both elastic modulus (G′) and gel cohesivity and will differ among products using proprietary manufacturing processes [19].
- **Resistance to Deformation**: This phenomenon - the ability to mould a filler in order to achieve a desired effect - is important for the clinician. The resistance to deformation of a filler is a function of the physical properties of its chemical composition, including cohesivity [17].
- **Tissue Integration**: Tissue integration - the way the filler integrates with or distributes into surrounding tissue - is an essential parameter for clinical and marketing purposes and also by which to assess products under development [18]. When injected, HA fillers tend to spread within the reticular dermis and to distribute between the dermal fibers, but different HA dermal fillers behave differently if different crosslinking technologies have been used to create specific viscoelastic properties. Several studies have investigated the behavior of different crosslinked dermal fillers, whether injected intradermally or in the subcutaneous layer [15,18,19]. Histology is usually employed to give a qualitative measure of tissue integration.

Rheology is not sufficient by itself to completely understand filler performance but it is useful for an evaluation of different fillers of similar composition [18]; animal models have been developed to allow such comparative evaluations among fillers. The results indicated that biological interaction has an important role to play in the filler's clinical performance [18].

HA fillers can be dissolved with hyaluronidases, increasing their "safety" when compared to non-HA fillers. HA levels are determined by the balance between enzymes that create it (synthase HAS1, HAS2 and HAS3) and those that break it down (hyaluronidases HYAL1, HYAL2 and HYAL3) [20]. Hyaluronidases are enzymes licensed for enhancing penetration of subcutaneous or intramuscular injections, local anaesthetics and infusions and reduce swelling [21]. However, they are also widely used "off-label" in aesthetic medicine to dissolve hyaluronic acid fillers. The enzymes can be classified by their mechanism of action: mammalian (endo-Beta-N-acetylhexosaminidase), leech/hookworm (endo-Beta-D-glucuronidase) and microbial (hyaluronate lyase) [22]. The most commonly-used preparation in the UK is Hyalase, derived from sheep; however, microbial and human hyaluronidases appear to have advantages in terms of safety and reduced immunogenicity [21].

CHALLENGES IN FILLER CHOICE IN FACIAL AESTHETICS

Harmony in facial rejuvenation and replenishment requires an understanding of the complex anatomy and dynamic structure of the face and its evolution during the facial ageing. Fillers implanted in the face area subjected to forces such as lateral shear and compression/stretching from intrinsic tissues and extrinsic sources. The challenge in the development of novel fillers will consist of optimizing their tailoring for the ideal mechanical properties for each specific indication and facial region; see further Figure F.2.

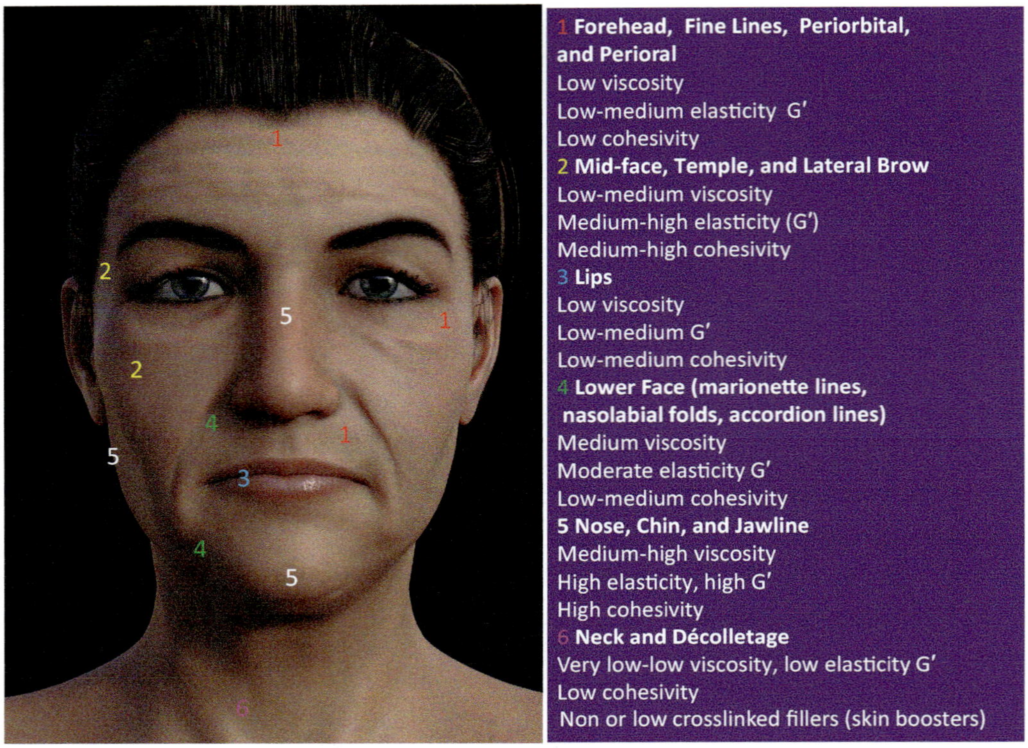

Figure F.2 Basic soft tissue filler rheology.

Area: Forehead, Fine Lines, Periorbital, and Perioral

Aim: To restore volume in intradermal and subdermal planes.

Filler properties: Allows easy moulding and spread of product for smooth effect, non-bulking.

Rheology: Low viscosity; Low-medium elasticity, G′; Low cohesivity with low-to-medium G*. For the tear trough it is important that there is minimal "water attraction."

Area: Mid-face, Temple, and Lateral Brow

Aim: To restore volume, projection, and contour in deep dermal, subdermal, or supra-periosteal injection.

Filler properties: Withstands shear deformation from weight and tension of the overlying soft tissue such as dynamic contraction forces of the lip and cheek elevators; Withstands compression; Minimal displacement; Maintains shape.

Rheology: Low-medium viscosity; Medium-high elasticity (G′); Medium-high cohesivity. Important for minimal separation and displacement cause by repetitive contraction of the overlying musculature.

Area: Lips

Aim: To enhance and provide volume: two distinct types of filler properties may be required to achieve either projection or smoothing or both, since the challenge in this area is to avoid edges and bumps.

Filler properties: Easy moulding and spread of product for smooth effect, non-bulking.

Rheology: Low viscosity, Low-to-medium elasticity G′ with Low-to-medium cohesivity; to contribute to lift capacity or projection.

Area: Lower Face (Marionette Lines, Nasolabial Folds, and Accordion Lines)

Aim: To restore volume in deep dermal or subdermal planes.

Filler properties: Easily mouldable; Minimal projection; Non-palpable.

Rheology: Medium viscosity; Moderate elasticity G′; Low-medium cohesivity.

Area: Nose, Chin, and Jawline

Aim: To restore or enhance projection and/or profile definition; to withstand compression of skin and tight muscle tension over the prominent bony structures.

Filler properties: Minimal lateral spread; Maintaining a sharp vertical projection over time; Maximal vertical projection.

Rheology: Medium-high viscosity (to minimize migration); High elasticity high G′; High cohesivity.

Area: Neck and Décolletage

Aim: To rejuvenate and tighten in intradermal and immediate subdermal planes.

Filler properties: Very easy moulding and spread of product for smooth effect; non-bulking.

Rheology: Very Low-Low viscosity; Low elasticity G′; Low cohesivity; Non or low crosslinked materials (skin boosters).

TECHNOLOGY OF COMMON ABSORBABLE FILLERS

This list, derived from articles indexed in PubMed and from company publications, is by no means exhaustive.

Cohesive Polydensified Matrix (CPM) (Merz-Anteis, Belotero Range)

CPM is based on a dynamic crosslinking process, with two additional steps in the crosslinking process. Introducing an additional amount of HA produces a monophasic polydensified gel that combines a high level of crosslinked HA; and continuation of the crosslinking process leads to a lighter level of crosslinked HA, in a cohesive matrix [23].

Interpenetrating Network Like (IPN-Like) (Vivacy, Stylage Range)

Two or more monophasic HA gels are separately crosslinked and then mixed together, forming an interpenetrating network. An antioxidant—mannitol—is added to protect the HA chains from oxidative stress [23].

Non-Animal Stabilized Hyaluronic Acid Technology (NASHA) (Galderma, Restylane Vital and Vital light, Restylane Lyft/Lyps/SubQ)

A small amount of BDDE is added between polysaccharide chains in specific conditions to allow the formation of a complex matrix of HA gel. A sizing process generates the HA gel particles that are then suspended in a fluid phase. The resulting product range is based on the particle sizes adapted to specific clinical indications of the final product [23].

Optimal Balance Technology (OBT)/ XpressHAn Technology (Galderma, Restylane Refyne/Defyne/ Volyme)

The same concentration of hyaluronic acid is maintained in the entire range, but with different degrees of crosslinking and different sizing for the gel calibration that allows it to be injected through a fine needle [24].

Resilient Hyaluronic Acid (RHA) (Teoxane, Teosyal RHA Range)

RHA range is characterized by a gel with long HA chains stabilized with a low amount of BDDE while minimizing the degradation of the HA during the process. The products in this range differ in the degree of crosslinking as well as their HA concentration [23]. The products allow "strength" for higher G′ and "stretch" for lower G′.

Vycross Technology (Allergan, Juvéderm Vollux, Voluma, Volift/Vollure, Volbella, Volite)

This technology uses a proprietary combination of lower (between 0.5 and 1 MDa) and higher (>1 MDa) molecular weight HA to improve the crosslinking efficiency between HA chains. The increased proportion of lower molecular weight HA allows a higher concentration during the crosslinking and a higher efficiency of the reaction [1].

Monophasic Particle Technology (MPT) (Adoderm, Varioderm® Range, Hyabell® Range)

This technology approach permits to customize the degree of cross-linking (going up to 80% of efficient connections between the molecules of HA chains) and concentrations. Main characteristics of these gels are the difference in concentrations, its balance on rheological values while granting a soft and homogenous extrusion force [25,26].

ProfHilo NAHYCO™ technology (IBSA)

This is a slowly degraded HA without chemical modification, available as intradermal injectable formulations with intended enhanced injectability, longer duration, and high biocompatibility. The hybrid cooperative complexes are supposed to deliver a higher HA amount than the unmodified HA products. The formation of the hybrid cooperative complexes is characterized by a drop in dynamic viscosity that, in clinical practice, allows the clinician to inject very high concentrations of HA. These formulations can be defined "physical gels", in which interactions between long and short HA chains were made, without changing the disaccharides unit structure and without introducing other "chemical compounds". A key feature of the hybrid cooperative complexes is claimed to be prolonged stability to enzymatic attack, despite the absence of chemical cross linking.

Neuvia Organic (Intense, Intense IV, Intense Lips, Intense Rose)

IPN stands for Interpenetrating Polymer Network, a technology to combine two different polymers - HA (from *Bacillus subtilis*) and PEG as the cross linker - in one network to obtain a 3D hydrogel matrix.

Neauvia Organic Stimulate is intended to offer not only filling effect but also biostimulation. It consists of HA with 1% of calcium hydroxyapatite (8–12 microns).

NON-HA FILLERS

There are other popular absorbable fillers available that are not made from HA and are popularised not only as dermal fillers and volumizers but also as biostimulating agents which intend to stimulate collagen in vivo. A possible disadvantage of these fillers is the fact that they cannot be dissolved with hyaluronidase. These include:

Poly-L-Lactic Acid (PLLA)

PLLA is an absorbable polymer which stimulates fibroblast production and generation of collagen; results usually last for around two years [27]. For optimal results, multiple treatment sessions are often required. The main concern with PLLA is a delayed development of palpable nodules. However, a study by Woerle et al. on 300 patients followed-up over five years reported that with adequate dilution, longer hydration time, addition of lidocaine and proper handling of the vials, the incidence of nodule formation is below 1% [28]. Similar recommendations were made by Alessio et al. [29]. The most widely known filler that contains PLLA is Sculptra (Dermik Laboratories), which was approved by the FDA in 2004 for the correction of facial lipoatrophy in patients with HIV [30].

Calcium Hydroxylapatite (CaHA)

Radiesse (MERZ) is the only CaHA filler approved by the FDA; it was approved first in 2006 for the correction of facial lipoatrophy in patients with HIV, and for moderate wrinkles and skin folds [3]. Radiesse is composed of 30% calcium hydroxylapatite microspheres suspended in a 70% gel carrier. It is a synthetic compound, similar in structure to bones and teeth. Radiesse is non-immunogenic, hence does not require patch testing, and is fully degraded and excreted by the body. The corrective results last for approximately 12 months [27].

When used in hyperdiluted form (i.e., 1.5 mL of product plus $\geq$1.5 mL of diluent), Radiesse has a minimal or absent immediate volumizing effect due to carboxymethylcellulose gel dispersion, generating only long-term tissue remodeling by the CaHA microspheres and allowing its injection more superficially for dermal rejuvenation and the treatment of larger areas such as neck, décolletage, buttocks, thighs, arms, abdomen, knees, and elbows.

Polycaprolactone (PCL)

Ellansé (Sinclairpharma) is CE marketed as a biodegradable collagen stimulator, composed of microspheres of a bioresorbable polymer, polycaprolactone (PCL), in an aqueous carboxymethyl cellulose (CMC) gel carrier. PCL biodegradation occur via hydrolysis of the ester linkages that are totally eliminated from the body. Four versions are available: Ellansé-S (short, S version), Ellansé-M (medium, M version), Ellansé-L (long, L version), and Ellansé-E (extra-long, E version), with expected in vivo longevity of 1, 2, 3 and 4 years, respectively.

SUMMARY

Hyaluronic acid is a natural constituent of human skin present in abundance. HA is transformed into soft tissue filler for aesthetic treatments by stabilisation with cross-linking proteins, usually 1,4-BDDE. This makes HA more resistant to degradation and therefore enables it to last several months in the skin.

HA fillers are characterized through a combination of rheology, animal, or clinical performance evaluations to help the clinician better understand the relative performance attributes of different fillers when used in a biological environment.

Emerging technologies used for manufacturing HA dermal fillers with different rheological properties are continuing to come onto an expanding aesthetic market.

Non-HA fillers are intended to have certain advantages such as a longer duration of effectiveness and generation of collagen in the skin but cannot be dissolved with hyaluronidase.

Both novice and seasoned injectors must remain on top of their game to keep up with these technologies, allowing them to choose the filler with the most optimal properties for the patient's indication, providing safe and effective treatments.

References

1. Rohrich RJ et al. *Plast Reconstr Surg Glob Open*. 2019 Jun 14;7(6):e2172. doi: 10.1097/GOX.0000000000002172. eCollection 2019 Jun. Practical Approach and Safety of Hyaluronic Acid Fillers.
2. Reed RK et al. *Acta Physiol Scand*. 1988 Nov;134(3):405–11.
3. Triggs-Raine B & Natowicz MR. *World J Biol Chem*. 2015 Aug;6(3):110–20.
4. Laurent TC et al. *Ann Med*. 1996 Jun;28(3):241–53.
5. Schiller S & Dorfman A. *J Biol Chem*. 1957 Aug;227(2):625–32.
6. Tezel A & Fredrickson GH. *J Cosmet Laser Ther*. 2008;10(1):35–42.
7. Gold MH. *J Cosmet Dermatol*. 2009;8:301–7.
8. Yeom J et al. *Bioconjug Chem*. 2010 Feb;21(2):240–7.
9. De Boulle K et al. *Dermatol Surg*. 2013 Dec;39(12):1758–66.
10. Foureman P et al. *Environ Mol Mutagen*. 1994;23:51–63.
11. Ciba-Geigy Corp. A cutaneous carcinogenicity study with mice on the diglycidyl ether of 1,4-butanediol. 1987.
12. Edsman K et al. *Dermatologic Surgery*. 2012 Jul;38(7pt2):1170–9.
13. Prasetyo AD et al. *Clin Cosmet Investig Dermatol*. 2016;9:257–80.
14. Mansouri Y & Goldenberg G. Update on Hyaluronic Acid Fillers for Facial Rejuvenation. Center for Devices and Radiological Health. Available from: http://www.mdedge.com/cutis/article/101904/aesthetic-dermatology/update-hyaluronic-acid-fillers-facial-rejuvenation
15. Pierre S et al. *Dermatol Surg*. 2015 Apr;41(Suppl 1):S120–6.
16. Kablik J et al. *Dermatologic Surgery*. 2009 Feb;35(Suppl 1):302–12.
17. Stocks D et al. *J Drugs Dermatol*. 2011;10:974–80.
18. Hee CK et al. *Dermatol Surg*. 2015 Dec;41(Suppl 1):S373–81.
19. Dugaret AS et al. *Skin Res Technol*. 2018;27(12):1378–87.
20. FDA. Dermal Fillers Approved by the Center for Devices and Radiological Health, (2011) <https://www.fda.gov/medicaldevices/productsandmedicalprocedures/cosmeticdevices/wrinklefillers/ucm227749.htm>
21. Cavallini M et al. *Aesthet Surg J*. 2013 Nov;33(8):1167–74.
22. Meyer K & Rapport MM. *Adv Enzymol Relat Subj Biochem*. 1952;13:199–236.

23. Micheels P et al. *Drugs Dermatol.* 2016 May 1; 15(5):600–6.
24. Segura S et al. *J Drugs Dermatol.* 2012 Jan;11(1 Suppl):s5–8.
25. Bingöl A & Dogan A. *MÄC.* 2012;6:6–12.
26. Dogan A & Andonovic L. Rheological properties of dermal fillers, Presented at *19th International Master Course on Aging Science IMCAS World Congress*, January 26–29, 2017; Paris, France.
27. Ballin AC et al. *Am J Clin Dermatol.* 2015 Aug; 16(4):271–83.
28. Woerle B et al. *J Drugs Dermatol.* 2004 Jul; 3(4):385–9.
29. Alessio R et al. *J Drugs Dermatol.* 2014 Sep;13(9):1057–66.
30. Kates LC & Fitzgerald R. *Aesthet Surg J.* 2008;28(4):397–403.

G COMPLICATIONS OF ABSORBABLE FILLERS

Maurizio Cavallini, Gloria Trocchi, Izolda Heydenrych, Koenraad De Boulle, Benoit Hendrickx, and Ali Pirayesh

Injectable fillers currently constitute the second most commonly performed aesthetic procedure after botulinum toxin [1]. The tremendous market expansion, coupled with new treatment paradigms and inadequate control of both products and injectors, has heralded a concerning increase in serious adverse events [2,3]. Complication recognition and management have become the most significant unmet needs for filler treatments [4,5].

A multitude of soft tissue fillers are currently available for facial aesthetic indications, ranging from autologous fat, polymethylmethacrylate, calcium hydroxylapatite, poly-L-Lactic acid, polycaprolactone, and hyaluronic acid (HA) [6]. Because HA fillers have the powerful advantage of being completely removable by the use of hyaluronidase, depending on approval in specific countries, they are referred to as reversible [7] and are currently the most widely used dermal fillers. For this reason, this chapter is aimed primarily at complications arising from the use of HA fillers.

The optimal approach to filler complications lies in having practical strategies for their prevention, as well as the insightful knowledge required for timely diagnosis and treatment.

PREVENTION

All injectors should work with an operative strategy aimed at reducing the risk of complications. Careful pre-consideration should be given to the possible confounding factors specific to each procedure. Although by no means comprehensive, the following 10-point plan may be used as a simple pre-injection checklist.

1. History and selection: It is advisable to invest time in a pretreatment consultation, with elucidation of skin conditions, systemic disease, medications, and previous procedures. The treatment plan should ideally be structured over time with due consideration given to pending medical procedures, dental visits, and immunizations. These steps aim to limit inflammatory reactions or hypersensitivities due to a heightened immune system.

Skin barrier disruption due to inflammatory or infective conditions may persist for 3–4 weeks after apparent clearing of skin conditions, thus allowing the penetration of infective agents. Acne, rosacea, and dermatitis should be adequately treated, with an additional 3–4 weeks allowed for repair of optimal barrier function before filler treatments are performed. Increased numbers of resistant *P. acnes* at the edges of topically treated acne areas are thought to play a role in the formation of biofilms via the toll-like receptors (TLR-2), and the "safe distance" for filler placement relative to an area of acne is unknown.

Ascertain the use of current antibiotics and indications thereof as patients with remote infections involving the urinary tract, sinuses, intestinal tract, and oral cavity are best deferred for treatment. Hematogenous spread of normally non-virulent bacteria may lead to binding to the toll-like receptors (TLRs) with possible triggering of an immune response and formation of late-onset nodules many months later. Prophylactic antivirals are advised to prevent virus reactivation if there is a history of herpes simplex infection in the intended area of injection.

Dental procedures, visits to the oral hygienist, and tooth bleaching/whitening are best avoided during the 2–4-week period before and after filler treatment to reduce the risk of hematogenous bacterial seeding and potential development of biofilm.

Filler treatments are contraindicated in active autoimmune diseases such as systemic lupus erythematosus, rheumatoid arthritis, mixed connective tissue disease, and Hashimoto's thyroiditis, but may be performed in burnt out conditions such as end-stage morphoea.

It is preferable to avoid injecting patients with multiple, severe allergies and a history of anaphylaxis. Drug allergies might also preclude optimal management of complications, should they arise. Knowledge of previous surgical and nonsurgical cosmetic procedures is vital as these could cause anatomical repositioning of structures and fixation and scarring of underlying vasculature, thus facilitating intravascular placement. Knowledge of the types and location of previously injected products may help to prevent compatibility issues with minimally degradable fillers.

Patients should be given a pre-filler checklist as an exclusion questionnaire in order to emphasize the importance of having no infective or inflammatory conditions (cutaneous or systemic) at the time of treatment. The checklist should ideally include a list of common anticoagulating compounds (medications and foodstuffs) for avoidance in the week before treatment (aspirin, nonsteroidal anti-inflammatories, salmon oil, vitamin E, gingko biloba, alcohol, dark chocolate, grapefruit, etc.).

Post-Treatment Checklist

- The patient should be furnished with written post-treatment instructions and contact numbers. Common-sense advice such as washing the face with uncontaminated water, using a new lipstick, and applying uncontaminated facial products should be given.
- The injector/clinic should be available via phone for 48 hours post-procedure.
- It is good practice to have a staff member call the patient the next day.

2. Assessment: Consider the intricacies of ethnicity, gender, and generational needs in order to construct an applicable treatment plan.

3. Informed consent: Signed informed consent is crucial in creating awareness of the potential risk of filler-induced complications.

Written pre- and post-treatment instructions help to establish realistic expectations and minimize legal repercussions.

It is wise to obtain informed consent for both the procedure as well as the management of inadvertent complications, should they arise, in order to expedite efficient management. This includes the discussion of possible, albeit rare, ophthalmic complications

4. Reversibility is a powerful advantage when using HA products. Practical knowledge pertaining to locally available hyaluronidases and their effect on locally available HA fillers is of paramount importance as the required dosages may differ. Certain products require more massage than others in order to dissolve adequately.

5. Product characteristics such as HA concentration and proprietary crosslinking should be understood in the context of ideal depth, placement, and duration.

The hygroscopic nature of HA is an important determinant of product-related swelling and needs to be differentiated from procedural swelling. The HA concentration and extent of crosslinking determine the product's characteristics (viscosity, elasticity, resistance to degradation, G′ [elastic modulus], G″ [viscous modulus], and Tan Delta) and ultimately its clinical efficacy and ideal depth of placement.

6. Product layering over late or minimally degradable fillers is discouraged, although layering of HA filler over other HA fillers is generally deemed acceptable. Late or minimally biodegradable fillers may be provoked into reactivity when a second filler such as HA is layered over them, potentially inducing long-lasting complications such as foreign body granulomas. Although HAs remain the most compatible fillers, it is wise to be cautious when considering cross-brand layering.

Accurate knowledge of the types and locations of previously injected products may help to prevent compatibility issues with minimally degradable fillers, and filler types should be meticulously documented after each treatment.

7. Photographic documentation (pre- and post-procedure) is vital for patient monitoring, medio-legal purposes, and as a tool for self-education.

8. Procedural planning and aseptic technique are pivotal in avoiding complications, and it is essential to prevent breaching of the clean workspace. Consider the following:

- Have everything at hand to reduce breaks in the aseptic field and the concomitant risk of injection-related infections.
- A preconceived plan and clear procedural flow help to minimize complications.

Makeup should be removed, and the skin cleansed carefully with, for example, 2% chlorhexidine gluconate in 70% alcohol. Avoid ocular exposure to the disinfectant as chlorhexidine is toxic to the cornea. Beware of soaked or dripping gauze when used near the eyes or perforated tympanic membranes (due to ototoxicity).

- Stringent aseptic technique is mandatory: cleanse, degrease, and disinfect. There are no universally recommended topical antiseptics, but chlorhexidine, chloroxylenol, iodophors, alcohol, iodine, and hypochlorous acid may be appropriate.
- Rinsing the mouth with an antiseptic mouthwash containing chlorhexidine (0.2%) or povidoneiodine adequately disinfects the oral cavity for up to 8 hours and has been suggested as a preventative practice for perioral treatments or patients with a lip-licking habit.
- The treating physician should remove all jewelry, wash their hands with antiseptic cleanser, and use gloves for all cases of injection therapy. The procedure is not deemed sterile as the syringe itself is not completely sterile. Thus sterility is lost once the syringe is handled, making aseptic technique of paramount importance.

- Surgical principles of sterile technique, i.e., not touching any component of the needle or cannula that penetrates the skin, may further reduce infective complications. Constant vigilance against possible contamination is of the utmost importance.
- Cleansing over a sufficiently broad area is imperative as there is a higher infective risk upon inadvertent touching of cannulae on the adjacent skin.
- Frequent needle (and cannula) changes are advised for multiple entry points.
- The use of disposable sterile dressing trays with containers for prep solution, gauze, and disposable sterile drapes enhances a safe, clean work area in an office environment.

9. **Insightful knowledge of injection anatomy** is of paramount importance in avoiding danger areas and serves as the foundation for avoiding disastrous complications. Although the exact position of vessels is highly variable, the plane in which they run is far more predictable. Therefore, knowledge of "safety by depth" is a vital safety tool, as is constant awareness of the early signs of vascular compromise [1].

Seckel has divided the face into various danger zones, knowledge of which is important when treating specific regions [9].

Danger Zone 1

This zone is located by turning the patient's head to the opposite side, palpating the sternocleidomastoid muscle, and drawing a straight line from the caudal edge of the external auditory canal to a point 6.5 cm below on the midpoint of the muscle belly. The area is encircled with an approximate radius of 3 cm.

The zone includes the region in which the **great auricular nerve** emerges from beneath the **sternocleidomastoid muscle**, making it susceptible to injury when dissecting over the muscle. The great auricular nerve originates from the cervical plexus branching off spinal nerves C2 and C3 and provides sensation to the skin on the mastoid area, parotid area, and the outer ear surface. Permanent injury to this nerve results in numbness of or painful dysesthesia (in case of neuroma) of lower two-thirds of the ear and adjacent neck and cheek skin.

Danger Zone 2

This zone is anatomically located by drawing a line from 0.5 cm below the tragus to 2 cm above the lateral eyebrow. Another line is drawn along the zygoma to the lateral orbital rim. The last line is then dropped from the point above the eyebrow through the lateral end of the brow to the zygoma. These lines form a triangle in which the temporal branch of the facial nerve lies on the undersurface of the temporoparietal fascia-superficial muscolar aponeurotic system (SMAS) layer and is more likely to be injured with deep-plane dissections.

This zone includes the region in which the **temporal branch** of the **facial nerve** runs under the **temporoparietal fascia-SMAS** layer. The branch emerges from beneath the parotid gland at the level of the zygoma and innervates the frontalis muscle in the forehead. Temporal branch injury may lead to paralysis of the frontalis muscle. The involved side of the forehead becomes paralyzed with ptosis of the brow and asymmetry of the brows.

Danger Zone 3

This zone includes the **marginal mandibular branch** of the **facial nerve** at its most vulnerable point and also the **facial artery** and **vein**. This zone is located by identifying a point 2 cm posterior to the angle of the mouth and drawing a 2 cm radius circle based on it. At this zone, the platysma-SMAS layer thins, thereby exposing the nerve and nearby facial vessels that are susceptible to injury.

Damage to this nerve leads to significant aesthetic and functional repercussions. At rest, the tone in the normally innervated zygomaticus major muscle will be unopposed by the now denervated DAO muscle, resulting in elevation of that corner of the mouth and the lower lip pulled up over the teeth. During grimacing or frowning, the now denervated DAO muscle cannot depress the corner of the mouth and lower lip, meaning the lower teeth will not show on the affected side.

Danger Zone 4

This zone includes the **zygomatic** and **buccal branches** of the **facial nerve**, which are superficial to the masseter muscle and Bichat's fat pad but deep to the platysma-SMAS and parotid fascia layers. These branches are no longer protected by the parotid gland and therefore are more vulnerable. The danger zone is located in a triangular region bound by the body of the mandible inferiorly, the parotid gland posteriorly, and the zygomaticus major muscle anteriorly. Using surface anatomy, this can be delineated by having a point at the oral commissure, at the highest point of the malar eminence, and the posterior border of the angle of the mandible.

Injury to these nerves can result in paralysis of the zygomaticus major, zygomaticus minor, and levator labii superioris muscles. This results in sagging of the upper lip during rest and a more apparent disfigurement during smiling when the contralateral unopposed zygomaticus major and minor muscles pull the mouth toward the innervated side.

If nerve damage occurs, the muscle paralysis is often not long-term, given the multiple interconnections between branches of the buccal and zygomatic nerves.

Danger Zone 5

This zone lies at the superior orbital rim above the mid-pupil where the **supraorbital (CN V)** and the more **medial supratrochlear (CN V) neurovascular bundles** are found. The supraorbital nerve lies deep to the corrugator supercilii muscle (CSM), and the supratrochlear nerve passes through the CSM. Nerve injury may cause numbness of scalp, forehead, upper eyelid, and nasal dorsum. This danger zone can be identified with a 1.5 cm circle with the supraorbital foramen at its center, which is easily palated at the supraorbital rim at mid-pupil level.

Danger Zone 6

This zone lies in the infraorbital region where the **infraorbital (V2) neurovascular bundle** exits the infraorbital foramen. Nerve injury may cause numbness of the lateral upper nose, cheek, upper lip, and lower eyelid. **Zygomatic branches of the facial nerve** also run in this zone to innervate the levator labii superioris muscle. This danger zone can be identified by drawing a 1.5 cm circle that centers around the infraorbital foramen located 0.8–1 cm below the infraorbital rim at mid-limbus level.

Danger Zone 7

This zone contains the **mental nerve** which carries sensory innervation to the ipsilateral chin and lower lip and is a branch of the **mandibular branch** of the **trigeminal nerve**. The mental nerve exits the mental foramen, which is located at the midpoint of the body of the mandible, in line with the second lower premolar. The mental foramen lies on a sagittal line drawn through the mid-limbus of the pupil, the supraorbital, and the infraorbital foramen.

Implications of nerve damage can be significant, with patients often not noticing when food is dribbling from that side of their mouth. Inadvertent lip biting may ensue while chewing.

10. Technical knowledge of placement and injection depth is cardinal to the success of dermal fillers.

Strategies for optimizing technique include

- Knowledge of injection anatomy.
- Awareness of danger areas.
- Aspiration before injecting where applicable.
- Slow injection speed with the least amount of pressure possible.
- Moving tip with delivery of product where applicable.
- Incrementally injecting small 0.1–0.2 mL aliquots of product.
- Use of small syringe to deliver precise aliquots.
- Use of small needle to slow down injection speed.
- Use of blunt cannulae where indicated.
- Careful consideration of the patient's medical history.
- Stopping injection if resistance is encountered or the patient experiences pain/discomfort.
- It is vital to routinely check perfusion in the treated areas as well as areas with watershed perfusion (glabella, nasal tip, upper lip), ensuring that makeup is not obscuring skin tone.
- Initial signs of vascular compromise may be subtle and fleeting.

CLASSIFICATION OF COMPLICATIONS

Filler complications are traditionally divided into four categories: allergic, intravascular, infective, and late onset nodules/inflammation. They may also be classified by onset, although multiple publications and timeframes currently lead to a lack of consensus. A 2014 consensus led by Signorini proposed a more generalized scheme of early and late-onset events (see Table G.1) [5].

Table G.1 Classification of Soft Tissue Filler Complications by Onset of Adverse Event

Early reactions
Vascular infarction/soft tissue necrosis
Inflammatory reactions (acute/chronic)
Infection
Allergic reactions/hypersensitivity
Injection-related events
Pain
Ecchymosis
Erythema
Bruising
Bleeding
Inappropriate positioning
Distant spread
Late reactions
Inflammatory reactions (acute/chronic)
Infection
Granuloma (typically chronic)
Differential diagnosis
Nodules
Dyspigmentation
Displacement of hyaluronic acid filler material

The South American consensus panel defined three main intervals:

- Immediate onset (up to 24 hours)
- Early onset (24 hours to 30 days)
- Late-onset (after 30 days)

The panel also proposed the term persistent intermittent or cyclic delayed swelling (PIDS). This is defined as edema/swelling occurring in the filler area or vicinity and is often associated with events such as vaccinations, infection, or local trauma [12].

See further Table G.2.

Table G.2 Consensus Recommendations for the Classification of Adverse Events Related to HA with Regard to Onset: Possible Diagnoses

Immediate onset (<24 hours)	Early onset (24–30 days)	Late onset (>30 days)
Vascular damage: embolization, arterial occlusion, etc. Allergic reaction Hematoma Overcorrection Ecchymosis Paresthesia	Vascular damage: ischemia, necrosis, telangiectasia Color changes: persistent, erythema, ecchymosis, Tyndall effect, post-inflammatory hyperpigmentation Systemic changes: infection, inflammation, paresthesia Scars: hypertrophic, atrophic Irregularities: overcorrection, infiltration (cellulite), nodules	Vascular damage: telangiectasia Color changes: post-inflammatory hyperpigmentation, persistent erythema Scars: atrophic, keloid Irregularities: Pile, nodules, late edema

THE CLINICAL SPECTRUM OF MANIFESTATIONS

Certain complications are universal to HA filler treatment in all facial areas (skin discoloration [Figure G.1], hematomas, swelling, edema, allergic manifestations, infections, vascular compromise, etc.), whereas others are more specific to individual facial zones and will be discussed in the individual chapters.

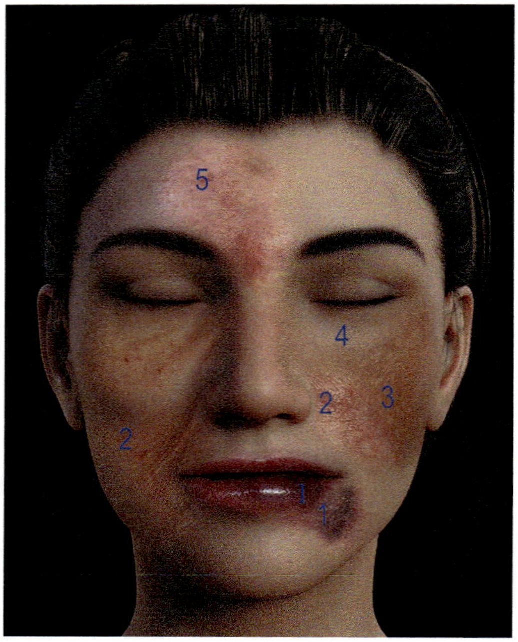

Figure G.1 Causes of skin discoloration include: (1) hematoma/echymoses, (2) neovascularization, (3) hyperpigmentation, the (4) Tyndall effect and (5) ischaemia.

It is important to evaluate patients holistically, exclude underlying systemic conditions (autoimmune disease, sarcoidosis, thyroid disease, etc.) and to approach complications systematically.

In addition to the presence of previous fillers, the differential diagnosis of periorbital edema (Figure G.2) includes

- Inflammatory/allergic conditions
- Renal disease
- Cardiac failure
- Thyroid disease
- Helminthic infections
- Autoimmune disease
  - LE
  - Dermatomyositis
- Previous fillers

For treatment of edema, see Figure G.3.

Hypersensitivity Reactions

Hypersensitivity reactions occur when the filler elicits an immune response. The response may be a type I hypersensitivity reaction, which typically has an early onset (within minutes to hours of injection), or a type IV reaction, which has a delayed onset (1–3 days up to several weeks after injection). The primary diagnostic symptoms of hypersensitivity reactions may

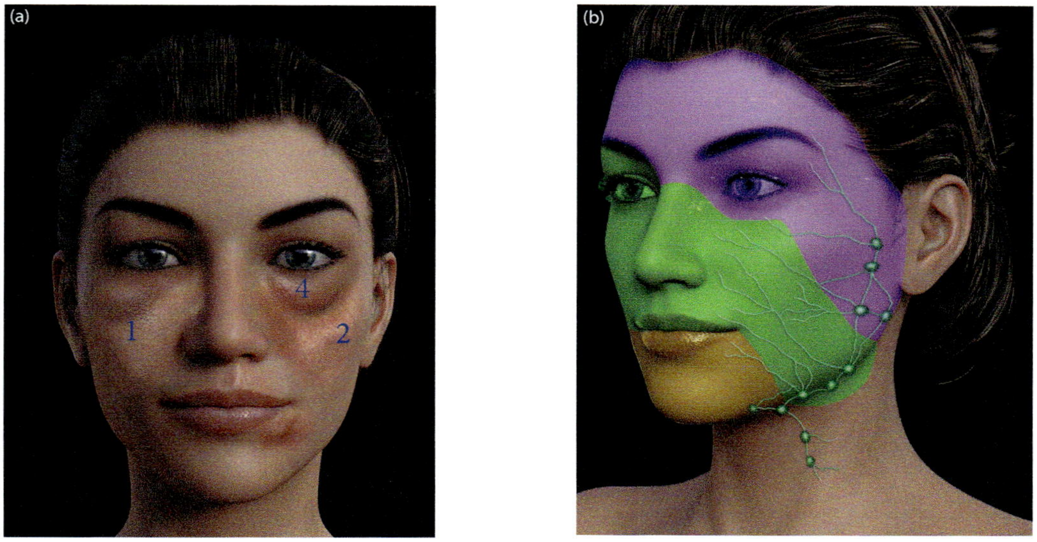

Figure G.2 (a) Other than procedural swelling, causes of post-filler edema include: (1) malar edema, (2) late inflammatory response syndrome (LIRS), (3) late onset nodule, (4) PIDS and (b) schematic representation of facial lymphatic drainage.

include edema (localized or generalized), erythema, pruritus, pain or tenderness (pressure-related), rash, and induration. Delayed reactions may also present with various types of skin lesions, including painful erythematous nodules, abscesses, or cyclic urticarial swelling. In rare cases, acute hypersensitivity reactions may be severe, with cases of anaphylactic shock cited in the literature [10]. See also Table G.3.

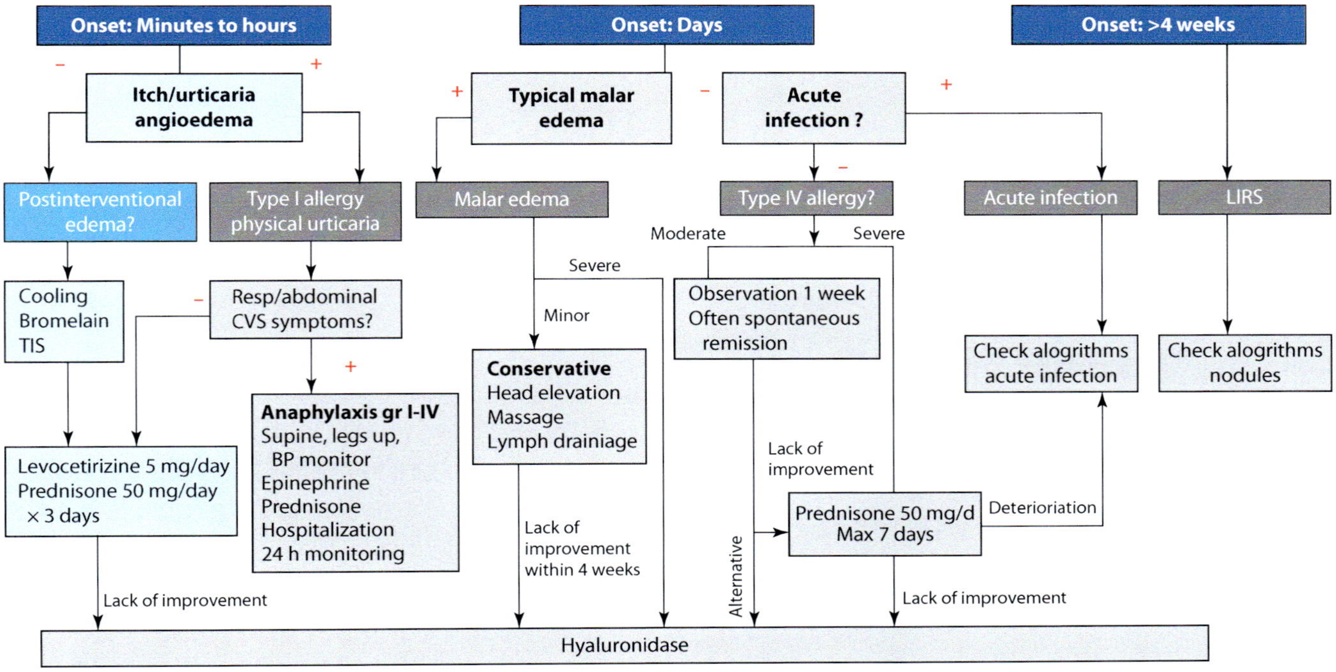

Figure G.3 Treatment of edema algorithms. (Adapted with permission from Snozzi P & Van Loghem JAJ. *Plast Reconstr Surg – Glob Open*. 2018;6(12):1–11.)

Table G.3 Algorithm for Early and Delayed Hypersensitivity Reactions

Hypersensitivity reactions	
Early	**Delayed**
Check vital signs	Cold compresses
Resuscitation measures:	H1-receptor antagonists
Adrenalin	H2-receptor antagonists
Intravenous access	Leukotriene synthesis inhibitors
Fluids	Oral corticosteroids
	Propranolol
	Ibuprofen

Infections

Infections, both acute onset manifestations and delayed onset biofilms, are a risk for filler treatment in all facial areas, thus necessitating stringent aseptic technique. It is vital to remember that infections in adjacent areas (e.g., sinusitis, dental abscess) or even distant infections (e.g., gastrointestinal, urinary tract infections) may import microorganisms into the filler mass. When infections do occur, due diligence is required in diagnosing the causative agent. It is important to have a rationale for the source of infection, to adhere to local macrobiotic guidelines, and to exercise responsible antibiotic stewardship (Table G.4 and Figure G.4).

Table G.4 Antibiotic Choice by Area

Skin	Sinus	Dental	GI
Doxycycline	Doxycycline	Amoxicillin	Metronidazole
Clindamycin	Cephalexin	Clindamycin	Clindamycin
Clarithromycin	Amoxicillin + Clavulanic acid	Cephalosporin	Ciprofloxacin
Azithromycin		Amoxicillin + Clavulanic acid	
Low-grade infections			
Doxycycline			

Vascular Events

The initial symptoms of intravascular placement are often (but not always) pain and skin color change. It is important to realize that initial color change may be fleeting and remote from the injection point, manifesting in areas of watershed perfusion. This necessitates constant awareness of watershed perfusion areas such as the glabella, nasal tip, and upper lip. Initial pain may be masked by the addition of local anesthetics to filler formulations. Although usually immediate, onset has been reported to be delayed up to 24 hours. Red/bluish coloration is generally indicative of venous occlusion. Livedoid discoloration ("fish-net stocking pattern") should always raise the suspicion of vascular compromise.

Later secondary diagnostic symptoms include blisters, pustules, tissue necrosis, and end-stage scarring.

It is important to exclude vascular occlusion in all cases of pustulation occurring in the week after filler treatment, even if there is a history of herpes simplex, especially when occurring on a livedoid background (Figures G.5 and G.6).

TREATMENT

- Stop injecting immediately if there is any suspicion of inappropriate pain, skin blanching, or mottled discoloration.
- Apply warm compresses.
- Injection of hyaluronidase: High-dose pulsed hyaluronidase/HDPH (500–1000 IU) in repeated hourly doses for 3 hours forms the basis of the emergent therapy. The use of a large bore cannula is advisable for subdermal instillation of the hyaluronidase in order to avoid bruising, which would confound the visual feedback of improving skin color.
- Massage the affected area in the direction of smaller arterioles to increase the exposure of product to hyaluronidase.

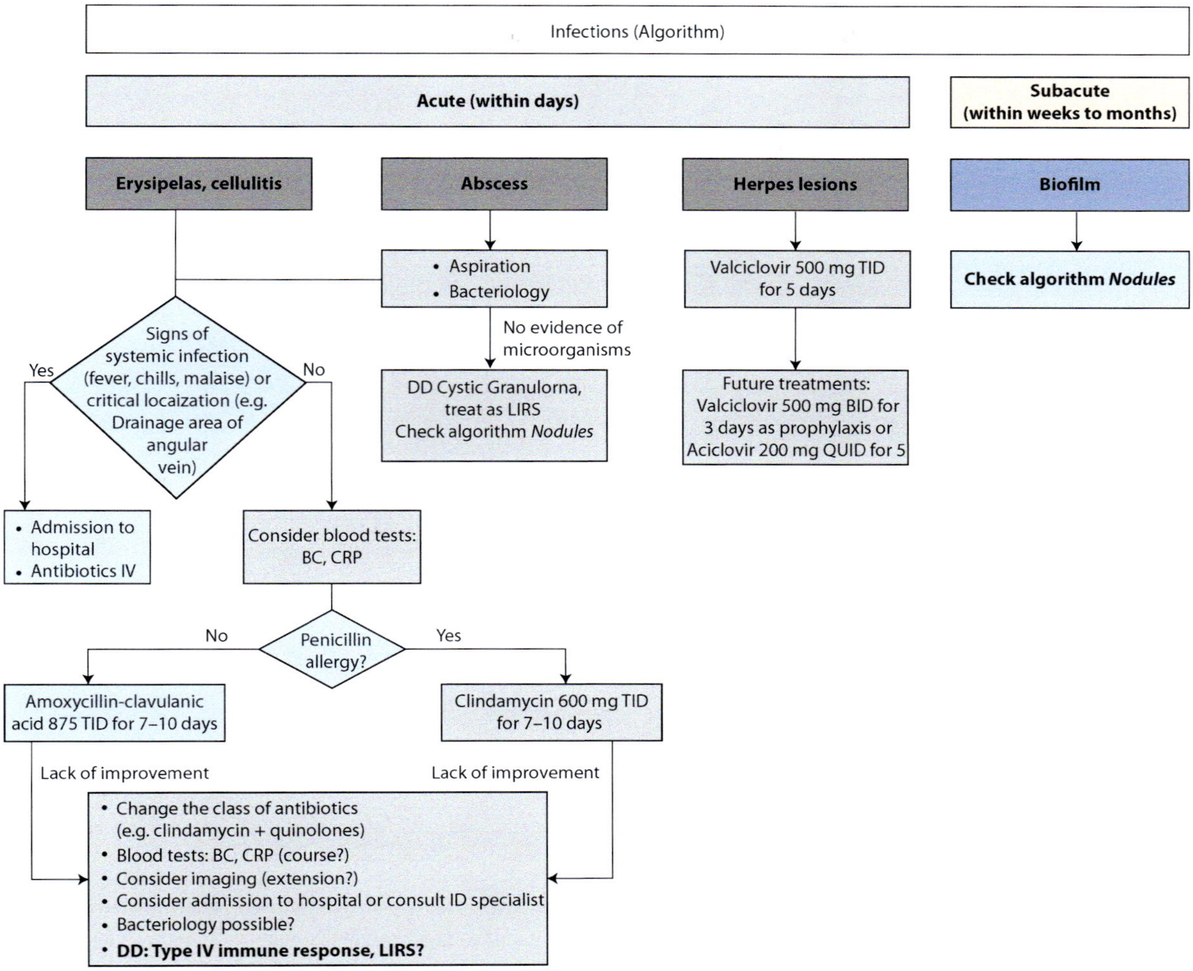

Figure G.4 Infections algorithm. (Adapted with permission from Snozzi P & Van Loghem JAJ. *Plast Reconstr Surg – Glob Open*. 2018;6(12):1–11.)

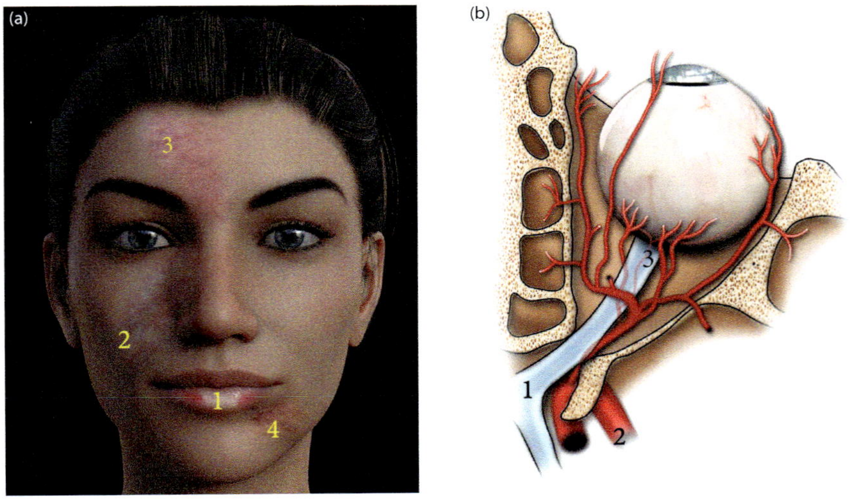

Figure G.5 (a) Clinical examples of vascular occlusion: (1) Early blanching, (2+3) livedoid discoloration; (4) pustulation. (b) Vascular arterial supply of the orbit: (1) Ophthalmic nerve, (2) internal carotid artery, (3) central retinal artery.

Vascular compromise (Differential diagnosis)		
Diagnosis	**Peripheral ischemia with impending necrosis**	**Retinal ischemia**
Clinical presentation and time of occurrence	1. **Blanching phase** • Immediate onset, duration <1 min, sometimes painful 2. **Livedo reticularis phase (marbling)** • After a few minutes (seldom within a few hours), due to lack of oxygen resulting in venous dilation, virtually pathognomonic 3. **Blue-gray phase** • Tans of minutes to hours, due to sustained lack of oxygen. May appear more rapidly in the vermillion. 4. **Blister phase** • After 1-2 days, as a first sign of skin necrosis 5. **Demarcation and ulceration phase** • After days to weeks, healing by secondary intention	• During Injection or immediately after injection: loss of vision, sometimes concurrent eye pain • Over the course sometimes ophthalmoparesis
Differential diagnosis	• Vasoconstriction due to epinephrine containing local anesth. (blanching phase) • Hematoma (blue-grey phase) • Herpes simplex/herpes zoster lesions (blister phase)	• None
Therapy	• High dose hyaluronidase within a few minutes to hours • Warm compresses • Aspirin • Further therapeutic options (low evidence level): Low-molecular-weight heparin (LMWH), pentoxyfillin, hyperbaric oxygen therapy (HBOT)	• Retrobulbar injection of hyaluronidase within 30 minutes • If retrobulbar injection cannot be performed by the injector: immediate referral to e (well-briefed) ophthalmologist • Afterwards hospitalization: possibly PGE1 therapy, consider other medical therapies (HBOT, LMWH, pentoxyfillin) • MRI of the brain to rule out any cerebral ischemia
Prophylaxis	• Use blunt cannulas (25G) in high-risk areas • Small boluses (max. 0.05 mL/bolus) in high-risk areas • Slow injection • Aspiration (needle) • Consider manual compression of the angular artery during injection • Risk factors: previous surgery, scars (including acne scars!), small-gauge needles/cannulas	

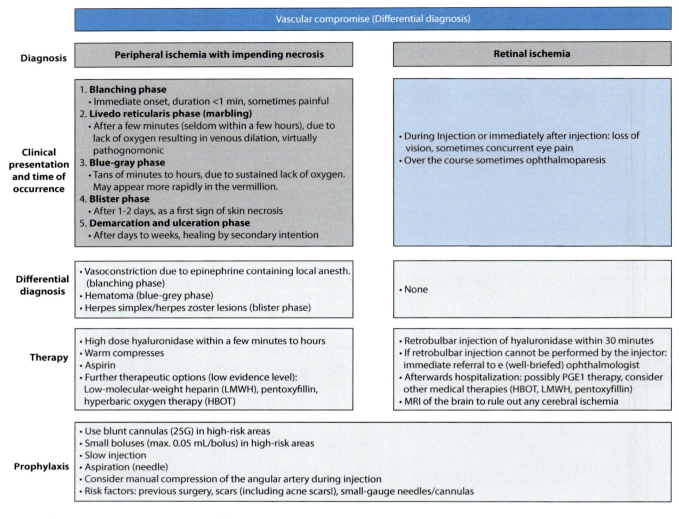

Figure G.6 Vascular compromise differential diagnosis. (Adapted with permission from Snozzi P & Van Loghem JAJ. *Plast Reconstr Surg – Glob Open*. 2018;6(12):1–11.)

- Give patient two tablets (650 mg) of aspirin to chew and swallow.
- Ultrasound, MRI, Doppler, arteriography, or phlebography may help in assessing filler placement and vascular damage, as well as aid in treatment planning.

HYALURONIDASE

Hyaluronidase (Hase) may be used to reverse the effect of HA fillers (and also in some instances aid in reversing unwanted occlusion by non-HA fillers by partially degrading the dermal matrix).

Hyaluronidases are naturally occurring enzymes (endoglycosidases) that can depolymerize HA, leading to its degradation by hydrolyzing the disaccharides at hexosaminidic β-1 through β-4 linkages. This enzyme is often used off-label in aesthetic dermatology for treating undesirable effects of HA and indications include misplaced injections, overcorrection, the Tyndall effect, granulomas, inflammatory reactions, and vascular occlusion.

Hyaluronidase has

- Immediate effect
- A two-minute half-life

- Duration of action of 24–48 hours
- Efficacy lasting longer than it is short half-life due to continuing action despite partial degradation

Hyaluronidase initiates degradation of the crosslinks in the HA dermal filler, causing it to behave like endogenous HA, which has a half-life of 24–48 hours.

Because of individual rheological and crosslinking properties, different HA fillers demonstrate an individual sensitivity to degradation by Hase. Importantly, individual Hase products also vary in activity depending on their source and concentration. Insightful understanding of the variations in locally available Hase products, as well as their differential effect on the multiple HA fillers available, will maximize treatment efficiency should the need for reversal arise. This variation in response was clearly demonstrated in the recent publication by Casabona [11], who stated that there may be a threefold difference in the amount of Hase required for degradation of a given volume of HA. Certain HA products denature more slowly than others, necessitating effective massage in order to break the HA bolus and expose it more efficiently to the Hase.

Dosages for All Indications Except Vascular Occlusion

The amount injected should be titrated to clinical effect, but actual dosages vary. A consensus opinion in the literature states that five to 10 units of hyaluronidase are required to break down 0.1 mL of 20 mg/mL HA, although there may be quite a range [4].

Treatment results may be assessed from 48 hours and repeated at intervals of 48 hours or longer, with the degree of further treatment depending on indication, risk: benefit ratio, treatment side effects, and patient or practitioner expectation.

Vascular compromise: High-dose pulsed hyal-uronidase/HDPH (500–1000 IU) in repeated hourly doses for 3 hours forms the backbone of the emer-gent therapy (Table G.5). It is advisable to use a large bore cannula for subdermal placement of the hyaluronidase to avoid bruising, which would confound the visual feedback of improving skin color.

Table G.5 DeLorenzi's High-Dose Pulse Hyaluronidase (HDPH) Dosage and Protocol for Intravascular Events

High-dose pulse hyaluronidase		
Dosage	Standard dosage	500 IU per area
	Lip, nose, and forehead	Act as multipliers
	Two areas	1,000 IU per hour
	Three areas	1,500 IU per area

Protocol

- Inject at least every 60–90 minutes until skin color has normalized and capillary refill time has normalized.
- Massage to increase embolus contact with the hyaluronidase by propelling the HA distally into thinner walled arterioles
- Aim to complete treatment within 72 hours of onset for complete resolution.
- Keep patient in clinic for observation and treatment until the capillary refill has improved (usually three sessions over 3 hours).

Do not apply nitroglycerin paste until the offending HA has been dissolved (day 2 or 3 of treatment) as dilation of adjacent, non-obstructed vascular pathways may lead to the propagation of the embolus toward the orbit by opening so-called "choke-anastomoses" acting as containment of further damage after a noxious event to tissue.

Source: Adapted with permission from DeLorenzi C. *Aesth Plast Surg*. 2013 May 1; 33(4):561–75.

Although the timeframe for initiation of treatment for vascular compromise (excluding intraocular complications) is given to be as within 72 hours, there is potential benefit to initiating and/or persevering with treatment beyond this time limit should there have been treatment delay or suboptimal response.

For intraocular complications, see further Chapter 5.

It is important to realize that, although rare, allergic and anaphylactic reactions to hyaluronidase are possible. Human recombinant hyaluronidase carries the lowest risk of allergenicity but is not available in all countries.

Practical Points

- The use of high-frequency ultrasound may be useful in elucidating the presence, identity, and location of underlying filler for treatment with Hase.
- Massaging the treated area during and after injecting with Hase may help to optimize effect and to aid mechanical breakdown.
- When feasible, avoid treating with Hase when
    - Botulinum toxin treatments have been performed within the previous 48 hours.
    - There is an area of infected skin unless there is vascular occlusion, and the risks outweigh the benefits.

Intradermal Testing

An intradermal test may be performed except when the indication is for vascular compromise, and a delay could result in further harm to the patient. Intradermal testing entails injecting 20 U of hyaluronidase in the forearm and observing the results after 30 minutes (a positive reaction at lower doses might not be recognized). Positive reactions are identified by a local wheal and itching, minor inflammation, and erythema.

A history of allergic reactions to wasp or bee stings may represent an increased risk of allergic reaction to Hase and constitute a relative contraindication, as the venom of stinging insects might contain hyaluronidase, and this mechanism might be the source of sensitization in affected individuals. Unless there is a past medical history of allergic reaction or anaphylaxis to hyaluronidase or insect bites, previous history of allergy seems unrelated to the safe administration of hyaluronidase and the risk:benefit ratio of treatment with Hase should always be considered.

Doses higher than 300 U may induce inflammation and eosinophil recruitment, thereby increasing the risk of type-1 hypersensitivity reactions such as urticaria and angioedema.

Observe at-risk patients for at least 2 hours after Hase treatment.

It is of vital importance that emergency resuscitation drugs are available and that expiry dates are current. It is highly advisable that dependable reminder systems (e.g., computer prompts) are in place for replacement of emergency drugs.

The use of high-frequency ultrasound may be useful in elucidating the presence, identity, and location of underlying fillers as well as in guiding aspiration and biopsies.

In this regard, we wish to encourage injectors to experiment with the effect of locally available Hase on the HA fillers regularly used in their markets.

LATE-ONSET ADVERSE EVENTS

Late-onset events may be either inflammatory or noninflammatory, presenting variously as edema, induration, nodules, cystic abscesses, or cyclic urticarial swelling. The degree of inflammatory change, manifesting as mild, moderate, severe, or frank fluctuation and infection, will dictate the preferred method of treatment (see Figures G.7 and G.8) [8].

ULTRASOUND DIAGNOSIS

Doppler ultrasound (duplex Doppler) is becoming an important tool in improving the safety of filler injections by

- Identifying the filler location and type in the event of a complication
- Locating important vascular structures before injection
- Identifying previous/unknown fillers in intendant treatment areas
- Guiding aspiration and biopsies

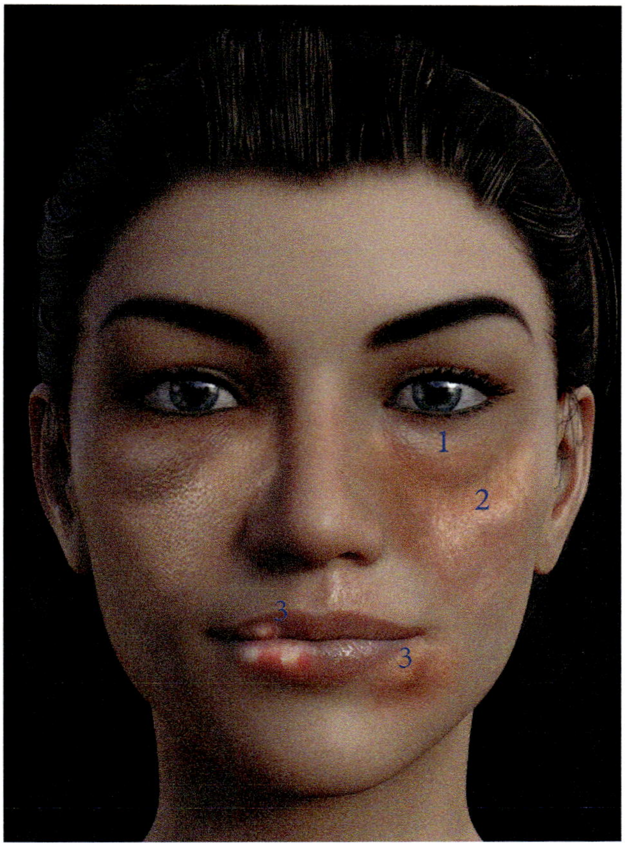

Figure G.7 Examples of late onset adverse events: (1) edema, including PIDS (2) induration and (3) nodules..

The use of duplex Doppler devices allows gross visualization of blood flow as red and blue colors, thus enabling identification of larger vessels and blood flow in conjunction with underlying dermal structures. Duplex is proposed by some injectors to be utilized for identification of vascular structures in the proposed treatment areas, with the aim of minimizing intravascular placement of fillers. However, it must be noted that no imaging modality can substitute for clinical experience and anatomical knowledge in terms of safety and efficacy.

In cases of diagnostic uncertainty, the following special investigations may be of value:

- CRP, an acute inflammation protein, usually associated with bacterial infections, immunohematological alterations, rheumatologic diseases.
- Full blood count and differential white blood cell count.
- Erythrocyte sedimentation rate (ESR).
- Acute-phase reactants, e.g., CRP, ESR, Procalcitonin. These appear to be the most sensitive markers for the presence of autoimmune/inflammatory syndrome induced by adjuvants (ASIA) related to dermal filler use.

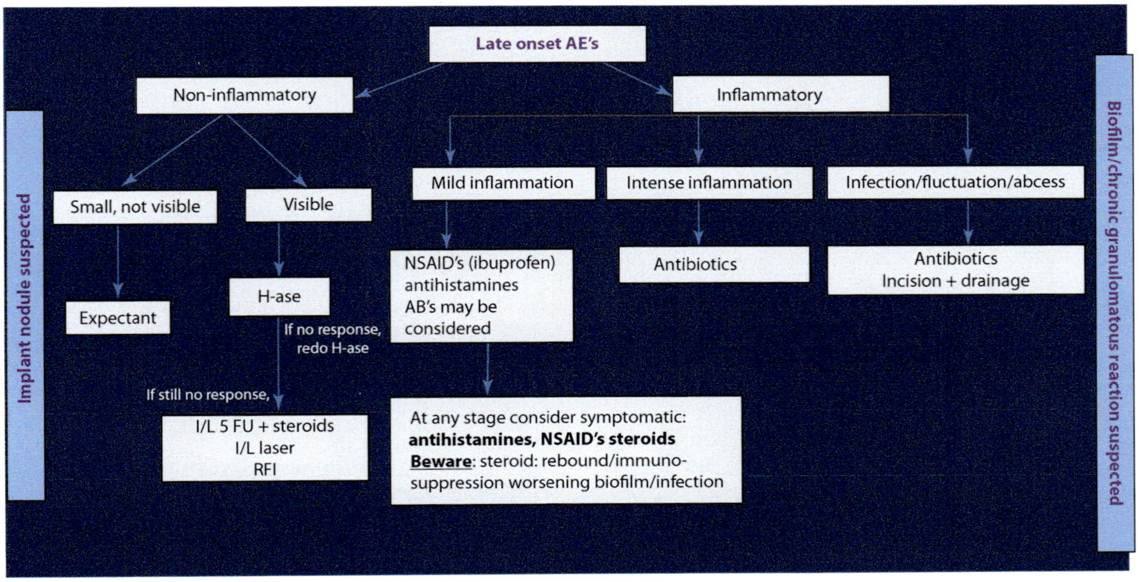

Figure G.8 Differential diagnosis of late-onset adverse events. (Adapted with permission from Batniji RK et al. *Plast Reconstr Surg*. 2020 (in press).)

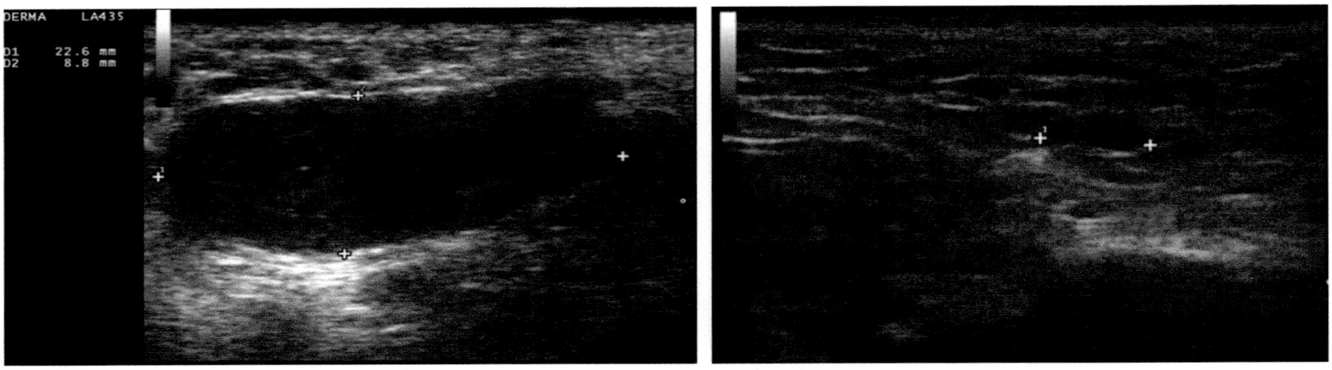

Figure G.9 HFUS shows subcutaneous thickening and swelling with the possible presence of residual deposited filler (from anechoic to hypoechoic).

- For suspected autoimmune disease,
  - ANA (antinuclear antibodies).
  - *ENA*: Antibodies to extractable nuclear antigens such as anti-SSA-Ro, anti-SSB-La (SLE, Sjogren Syndrome), anti-Jo1 (Polymyositis, Dermatomyositis), anti-Scl 70 (Progressive Systemic Sclerosis).
  - RF (rheumatoid factor).
  - ANCAs (anti-neutrophil cytoplasmic antibodies) detected in several autoimmune disorders, particularly with systemic vasculitis.
- Biopsy may identify both underlying foreign body granulomas and filler types.
- Angiotensin converting enzyme (s-ACE) and chest x-ray for suspected sarcoidosis.
- High frequency ultrasound (HFUS) (Figure G.9).
- MRI (Figure G.10).
- Biopsy with differential immunostaining.

CONCLUSION

The field of aesthetic fillers is currently enduring an onslaught on safety. All injectors should work with an operative strategy aimed at reducing the risk of dermal filler complications through conscious awareness and careful pre-consideration of the possible confounding factors specific to each procedure. Algorithms for diagnosis and treatment are constantly evolving, and injectors should ensure that they are up to date with current best practice. It is vitally important that all injectors are aware of the increasing incidence of ophthalmic complications and are aligned with an ophthalmologic specialist adept at treating vascular occlusion as a complication of injectable fillers.

Recently, a combined technique of infrared (IR) facial heating and MRA (3D-TOF MOTSA) was proposed. Images may be acquired on a 1.5 or 3 Tesla (T) full-body MR system, using a dedicated head coil. Additionally, a flexible wrap-around surface coil may be mounted on top of the head coil in order to increase the signal reception from the facial vessels. Before the 3D TOF MRA examination, which is known to be flow dependent, the patient is positioned with closed eyes in front of an IR light source (300 W with an UV filter) for 10 minutes. This should induce vasodilatation and enhance vascular flow. At the same time, the patient is asked to stimulate their facial muscles by slowly moving the lips and forehead and switching between several facial expressions during the exposure time in order to further enhance the arteries (by vascular dilatation and increased flow speed due to muscle activation). An oblique coronal 3D-TOF MOTSA MRA sequence is acquired in an oblique coronal plane. During the acquisition, the patient is asked to remain completely still. A multislab technique is used to reduce the saturation effect of the inflowing blood signal. MIP images are made in

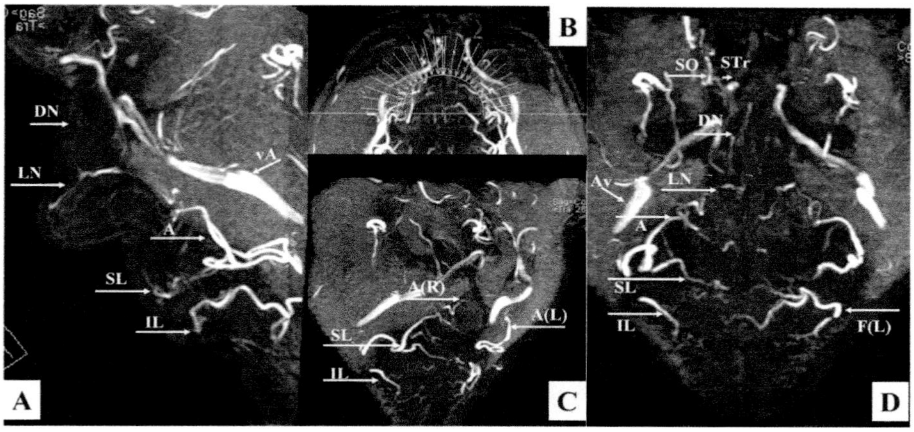

Figure G.10 MRA findings (MIP of 3D-TOF) in a 58 year old male. Superior (SL) and inferior labial (IL), angular (A); lateral nasal (LN); dorsal nasal (DN); supratrochlear (STr); supraorbital (SO) and facial artery (F); angular vein (Av); (R) Right and (L) Left.

a sagittal plane. The MRA allows visualisation of the important facial arteries (facial [F]; angular [A]; superior [SL] and inferior labial [IL]; lateral nasal [LN]; dorsal nasal [DN]; supratrochlear [STr]; supraorbital [SO]; and superficial temporal [ST] artery) (Figure G.10).

Peri-orbital artefacts may hinder the visualization of the periorbital vessels and in patients with dental wires (after having braces), the perioral vessels may be hard to see 1.5T MRA also are more susceptible to motion artefacts due to the longer examination time. Although the reaction of the skin (red colour) to the IR exposure will be visible, no adverse reactions due to the "IR enhancement" are noted, nor mentioned. The only (sometimes confusing) venous structure—running more posteriorly and laterally outside of the field of interest—is the large angular vein.

References

1. Cavallini M & Molinari P. *Managing Errors and Complications in Aesthetic Medicine.* Oltrarno: Officina Editoriale; 2016. 176 p.
2. Heydenrych I et al. *Clin Cosmet Investig Dermatol.* 2018;11:603.
3. De Boulle K & Heydenrych I. *Clin Cosmet Investig Dermatol.* 2015 Apr 15;8:205–14.
4. Hirsch RJ et al. *J Cosmet Laser Ther.* 2007; 9:182–5.
5. Signorini M et al. *Plast Reconstr Surg.* 2016; 137(6):961e–71e.
6. Kapoor, KM, Kapoor, P, Heydenrych, I, & Bertossi, D. Vision Loss Associated with Hyaluronic Acid Fillers: A Systematic Review of Literature. *Aesth Plast Surg.* 2019 Dec 10; 1–16.
7. DeLorenzi C. *Aesth Plast Surg.* 2013 May 1; 33(4):561–75.
8. Batniji RK et al. *Plast Reconstr Surg.* 2020 (in press).
9. Seckel B. *Facial Danger Zones: Avoiding Nerve Injury in Facial Plastic Surgery.* Thieme; 2010. 1–49 p.
10. Snozzi P & Van Loghem JAJ. *Plast Reconstr Surg – Glob Open.* 2018;6(12):1–11.
11. Casabona G et al. *Dermatologic Surg.* 2018;44(11):42–50.
12. Casabona G et al. *Surg Cosmet Dermatol.* 2017;204.

Further Reading

Alijotas-Reig J et al. *Clin Rev Allergy Immunol.* 2013;45(1):97–108.

Taylor GI et al. *Plast Reconstr Surg.* 2017;140(4): 721–33.

1 FOREHEAD

Izolda Heydenrych, Fabio Ingallina, Thierry Besins, Shannon Humphrey, Steven R. Cohen, and Ines Verner

INTRODUCTION

The forehead is an anatomic area with distinct contours and creases: contours indicate underlying bone and fat pads whilst creases predict underlying vasculature. An in-depth understanding of the location of neurovascular structures is vital when performing forehead injections. The most balanced enhancement and rejuvenation in the forehead is achieved by combining relaxing toxin injections and reshaping or volumizing filler treatment.

BOUNDARIES

The boundaries of the forehead are the frontal hairline (superiorly), the eyebrows and nasal root (inferiorly), and laterally, the temporalis crest at the temporalis muscle insertion (Figure 1.1). In patients with hairline recession, the superior extent of the forehead is at the superior border of the paired frontalis muscles. The transition between the forehead and the temporal region is at the temporal crest where the fascial planes fuse to form the conjoined tendon (Figure 1.2).

AGING

The hallmarks of a youthful forehead include a subtle convexity, smoothly outlined contours, lack of furrows, and even skin tone and texture. In the female patient, the ideal forehead should have a gentle convex curve 12°–14° off vertical. Ideal forehead height and brow shape count among the seven features of true facial beauty, but forehead shape and contour are extremely variable and compounded by ethnicity and gender. Although forehead height cannot be altered by injectables, the contour may be optimized by use of fillers, and both brow shape and position are supremely treatable with toxins and fillers.

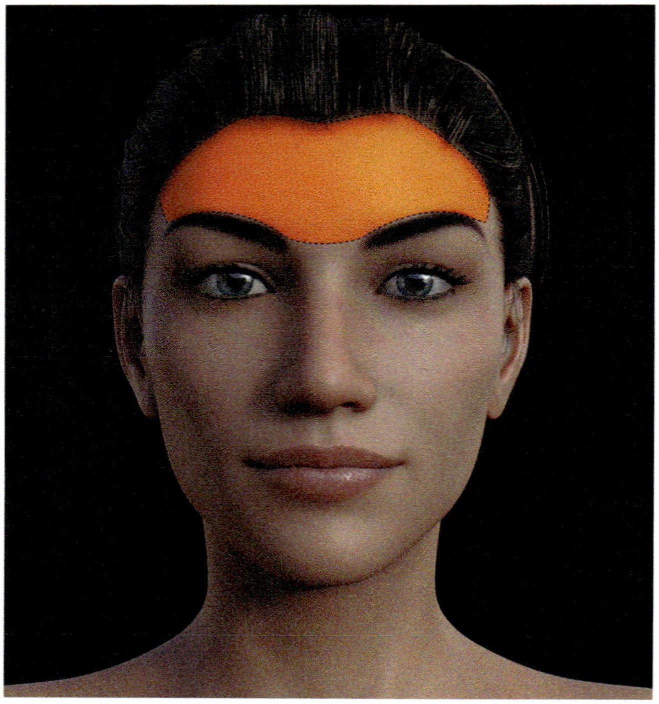

Figure 1.1 The boundaries of the forehead are the frontal hairline (superiorly), the eyebrows and nasal root (inferiorly), and the temporal crest (laterally).

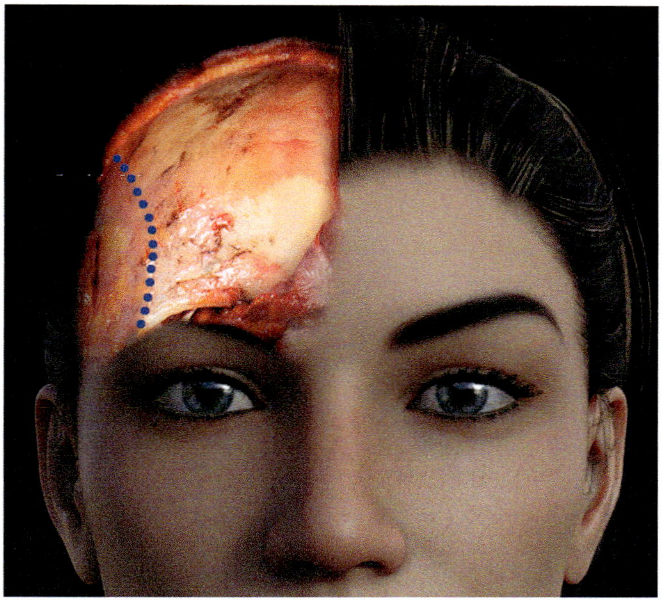

Figure 1.2 The temporal crest marks the lateral forehead boundary; a deep branch of the supraorbital nerve runs 1 cm medial to this line.

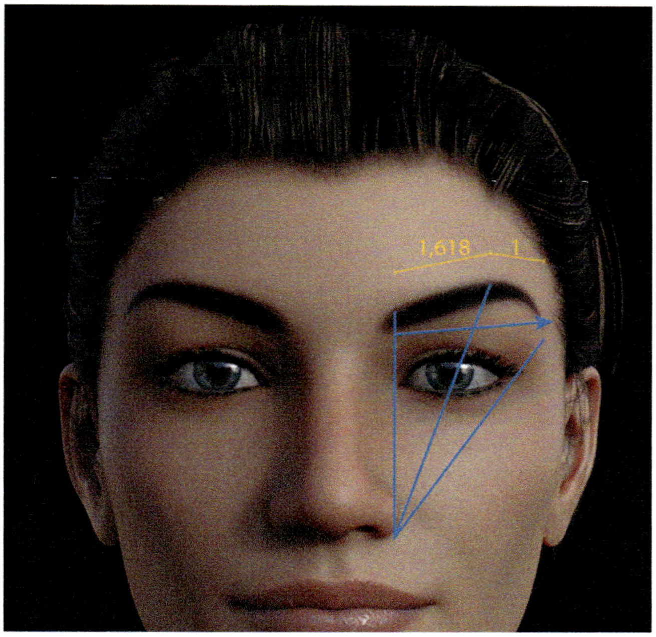

Figure 1.3 The proportions of the ideal female brow.

Figure 1.3 shows the ideal female brow, which should be situated above the orbital rim and has the following characteristics:

1. The head of the brow should be in a vertical line with medial canthus.
2. The brow should raise at a 10°–20° angle.
3. The brow should peak above the lateral limbus.
4. The distance from medial canthus to the peak should be in the "phi" or "golden ratio" (1:1.618) to distance from peak to tail.
5. The tail of the brow should be higher than the medial head.

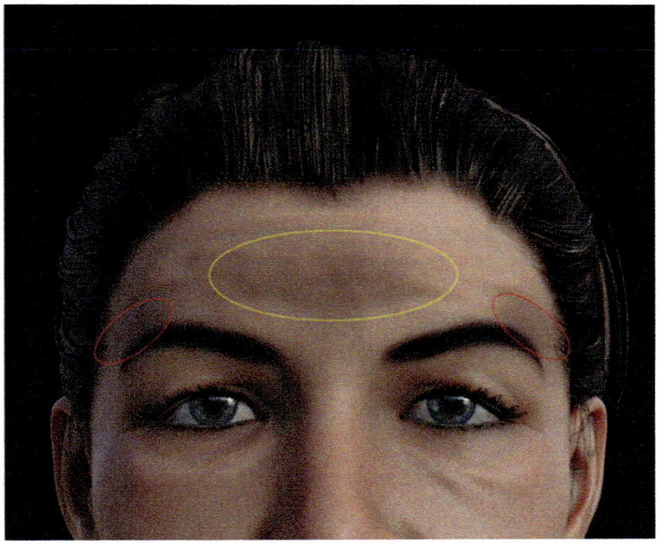

Figure 1.4 The aging forehead: Note central and suprabrow volume loss and horizontal forehead lines.

In addition to intrinsic and actinic aging, there are changes in bone and soft tissue, with site-specific aging of facial fat pads leading to skeletonizing and accentuation of the brow muscles. Overall, widening of the orbital aperture, a more acute glabellar angle, and loss of bony support contribute to the formation of wrinkles (Figure 1.4).

The face conveys valuable information regarding health and age while the forehead and brows render

ASSESSMENT

The upper face should be assessed for volume loss, eyebrow position, the presence of static lines (rest) and dynamic lines (animation) and baseline asymmetry.

CAUTION

- Glabellar toxin will not eradicate resting lines.
- Excessive frontalis muscle inactivation with toxin may accentuate brow ptosis and upper-lid heaviness.

clues as to underlying emotions. Repetitive muscle movements induce static lines which contribute to the stigmata of aging (Figure 1.5).

The aesthetically desirable female eyebrow should be situated above the supraorbital margin. The medial aspect (head) should be slightly lower than the lateral aspect (tail) and the peak at a line vertical to the lateral limbus of the iris. Even distribution of volume along the entire length should obscure sharp bony edges. The male eyebrow is lower and flatter and lies at the supraorbital margin.

CAUTION

- There are multiple danger areas in the forehead and conscious avoidance of vessels is mandatory.

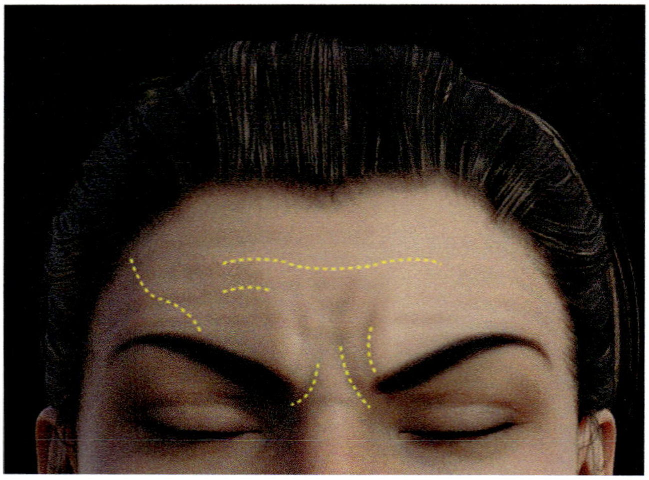

Figure 1.5 Patient with static glabellar and forehead lines. These factors should be discussed before toxin treatment, as should brow position and any baseline asymmetry.

The aging forehead has the following characteristics:

1. Static lines: Glabellar and transverse forehead lines (TFLs)
2. Remodeling of the periorbital bone in the superomedial and inferolateral directions, resulting in an altered and vertically lengthened orbital aperture
3. Increased susceptibility to excess upper eyelid skin and contour deformities
4. Bone loss leading to a more acute glabellar angle
5. Hollowing of the mid-forehead and suprabrow areas, with possible brow ptosis, cautioning against the use of neuromodulators in the lower forehead
6. Compensatory elevation of the lateral forehead (Figure 1.6)

CAUTION FOR BOTULINUM TOXIN TYPE A (BONT-A) TREATMENT

- Narrow forehead, compensatory raising of the lateral brows, age >60 years (Figure 1.6).
- These patients are best not treated with frontalis toxin as treatment will unmask underlying brow ptosis.

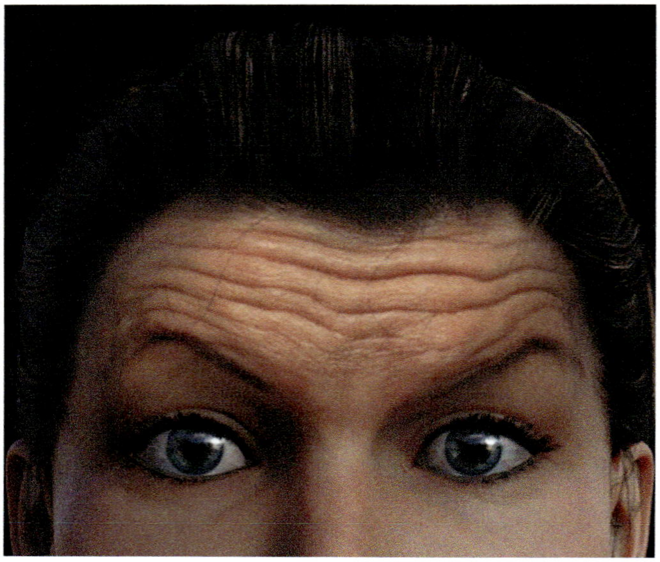

Figure 1.6 Narrow forehead, loss of skin elasticity, and lateral brow elevation compensating for excess upper eyelid skin. This patient is unsuitable for forehead toxin.

SKIN

Facial topography is an indicator of underlying anatomy as creases and wrinkles identify the course and location of vessels (see Figures 1.7 and 1.8).

Creases tend to form in fascial membranes between adjacent fat compartments and are associated with deep vessels while wrinkles are associated with more superficial vessels. The **corrugator crease** is a surface landmark for the **supratrochlear** vessels, which cross the supraorbital rim directly beneath. Thereafter, they travel beneath the corrugator and frontalis muscles to become superficial 1.5–2 cm above the supraorbital ridge. The **supraorbital crease** marks the position of the underlying supraorbital neurovascular bundle, which exits the skull through the supraorbital foramen/notch. In contrast to the supraorbital and supratrochlear vessels, the **central forehead vessel** is very superficial, lying directly beneath the skin, and marks a watershed area for perfusion. This contributes greatly to the risk of intravascular complications with filler injections in this region.

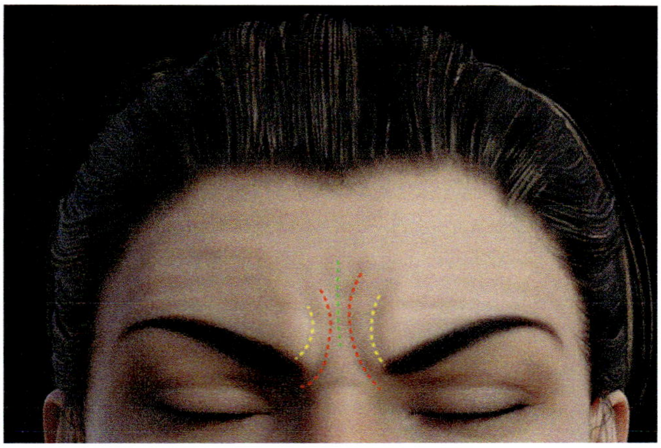

Figure 1.7 Topographical landmarks: yellow: corrugator/supraorbital crease; red: supratrochlear crease, green: crease overlying central forehead vessel.

The central forehead and scalp consists of 5 distinct layers, identified by the mnemonic **SCALP**.

S	Skin
C	Connective tissue
A	Aponeurosis
L	Loose areolar connective tissue
P	Pericranium

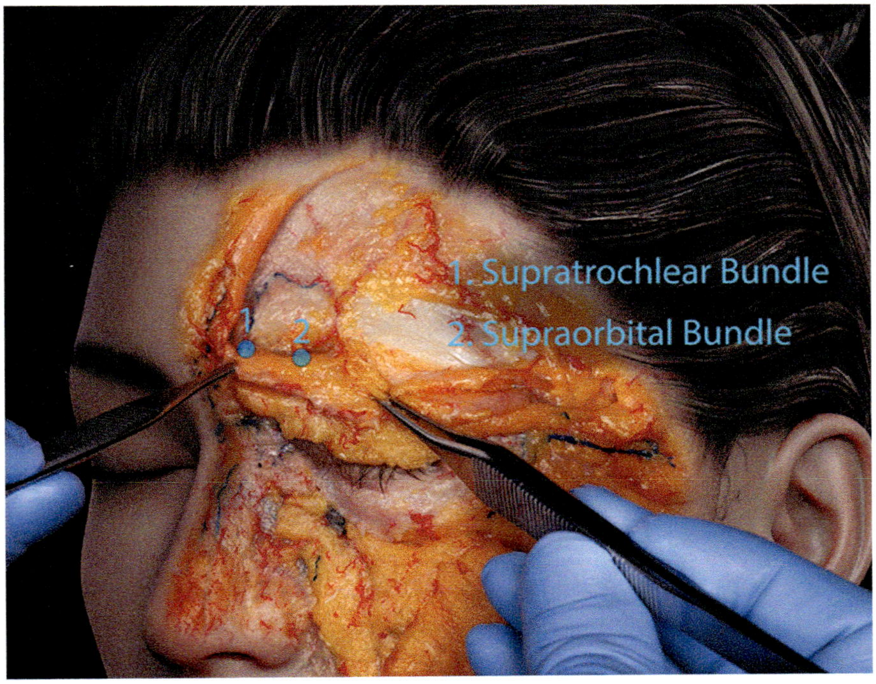

Figure 1.8 Supraorbital and supratrochlear vessels and nerves exiting bony foraminae at the orbital rim. Note the superficial fat compartments.

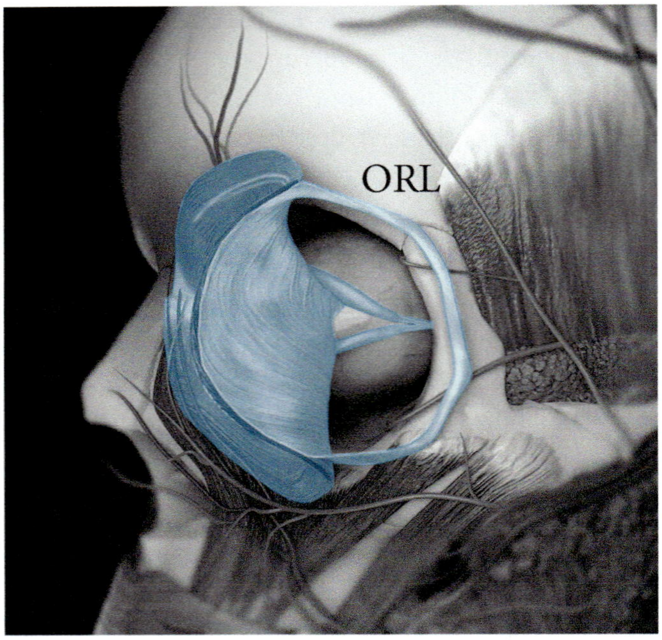

Figure 1.9 The orbital retaining ligament (ORL) inserts 2–3 mm above the orbital rim.

The well-vascularized skin of the forehead and scalp is thick, averaging 2381 μm in thickness, and contrasts sharply with the adjacent thin skin of the eyelid. It is important to note, however, that the average thickness of subcutaneous tissue in the glabellar area is ~2–4 mm, making the difference between "deep" and "superficial" injections negligible.

The galea aponeurosis, or epicranial aponeurosis, is the fibromuscular extension of the superficial muscolar aponeurotic system (SMAS), which encircles the entire skull. It splits to envelop the frontalis, occipitalis, procerus, and the periauricular muscles. The pericranium and overlying galea are connected by an avascular layer of loose connective tissue.

The **orbital retaining ligament** (ORL) inserts 2–3 mm above the orbital rim and forms the deep boundary between the forehead and the upper eyelid (Figure 1.9). The seal of this boundary is imperfect, thus injections placed directly at creases can travel along vessels and nerves to traverse anatomic compartments (e.g., along the supraorbital neurovascular bundle). Inadvertent

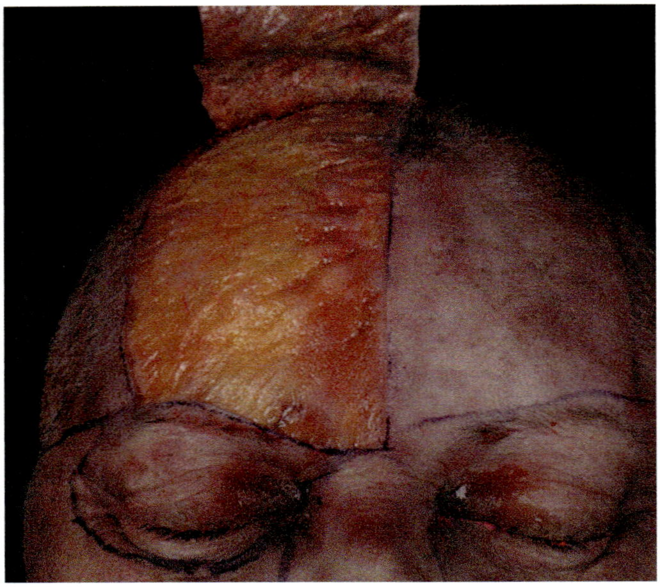

Figure 1.10 Cadaver with fat pads of the forehead exposed.

injection of toxin into the levator palpebrae superioris may cause lid ptosis; thus, injections should be meticulously placed above the ORL (Figure 1.10).

FAT

Subcutaneous fat occurs as discrete superficial and deep compartments that age at different rates, thus leading to irregularities in facial contour. Compartments are separated by delicate fascial septae that converge to form retaining ligaments. The glabella has distinct medial and lateral fat compartments. These are topographically marked by creases that serve as markers for underlying vessels (Figure 1.7). The galea fat pad envelops the corrugator and procerus muscles and aids as a gliding plane during animation. It lies deep to frontalis and extends superiorly for about 3 cm. The retro-orbicularis oculi fat (ROOF) is the deep fat compartment of the upper eyelid and brow, giving shape to the brow and to the upper eyelid. Volume loss contributes to deflation and descent of the tail of the brow (Figure 1.11).

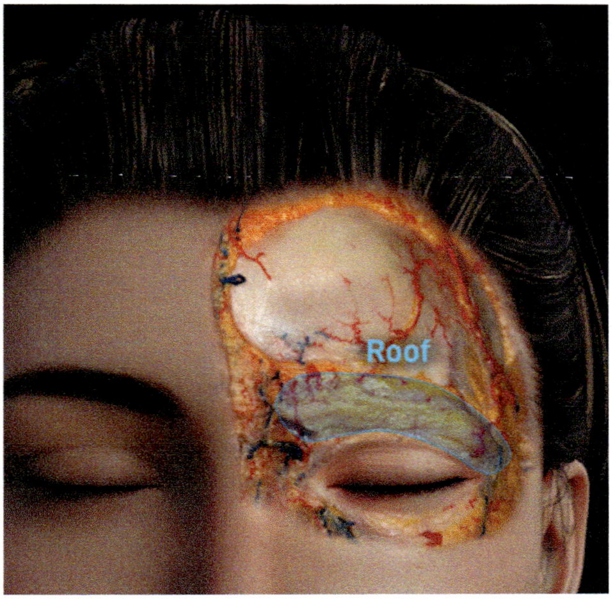

Figure 1.11 Schematic illustration of the ROOF, which gives support and shape to the brows.

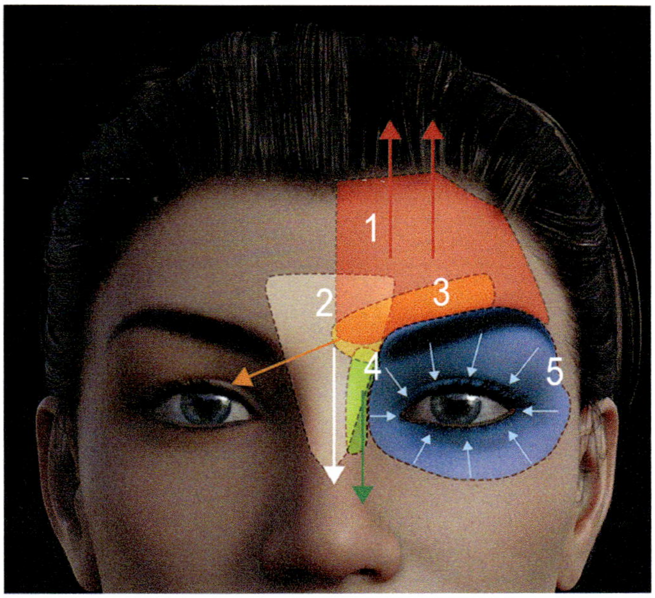

Figure 1.12 The balance of opposing brow elevators and depressors.

MUSCLE

Facial movements represent a dance of the muscles with opposing groups of elevators and depressors competing for dominance in an ongoing balance that evolves with age and volume depletion. Brow shape and location is influenced by the balance between these two groups (Figure 1.12).

ELEVATOR

1. Frontalis

DEPRESSORS

2. Procerus
3. Corrugator supercilii
4. Depressor supercilii
5. Orbicularis oculi

Facial muscles originate from the bone/superficial fascia, insert into the skin, and vectors run from insertion (mobile portion of the muscle) to origin (fixed portion of the muscle). Hyperkinetic lines form perpendicular to the direction of muscle action, indicating individual variations in muscle contraction patterns (Figure 1.13).

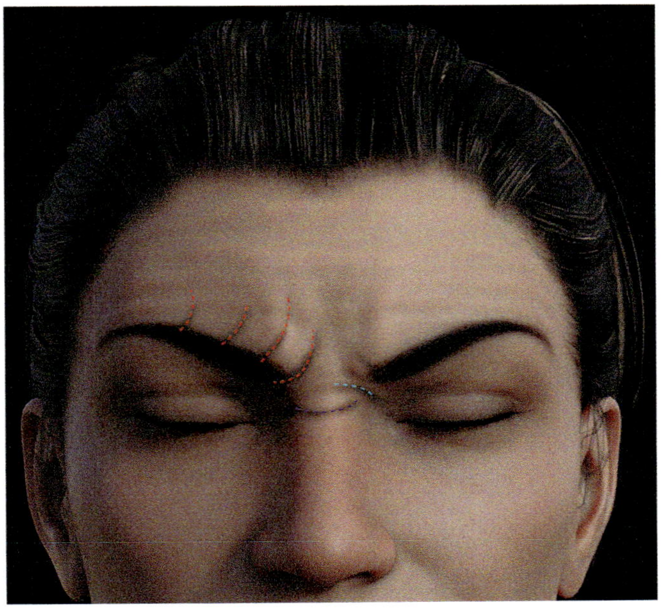

Figure 1.13 Asymmetrical muscle pattern, with lines forming perpendicular to the direction of muscle action. Toxin treatment should be tailored accordingly.

Brow Elevator (Frontalis)

Frontalis has a belly on either side of the forehead and comprises lateral, intermediate, and medial fibers (Table 1.1). Its fibers lie at a uniform but variable depth (~3–5 mm) beneath the skin. Because frontalis is wide and its two halves may contract independently, it can generate vertical, lateral, and angular movements of the brow. Vertical upward movements generate horizontal frontal lines (HFLs). Toxin treatment of frontalis may unmask underlying weakness of the levator palpebrae, causing overt eyelid ptosis. As frontalis is the main elevator of the brows and is counterbalanced by the glabellar complex, these opposing groups should ideally be treated in conjunction.

Four distinct morphological frontalis patterns have been identified, each effecting a unique dynamic pattern of parallel horizontal lines: type 1, 2, 3, and 4 (see Figures 1.14 through 1.17).

Brow Depressors (Procerus, Corrugator Supercilii, Orbicularis, Oculi, Depressor Supercilii)

The glabella represents a focal expressive area for undesirable emotions such as anger and impatience (Table 1.2). Because of diverse facial anatomy and animation patterns, tailored treatment strategies are mandatory for achieving natural results. Existing classifications of both muscle morphology and animation patterns are well worth studying as they help to refine analytical treatment strategies (Figures 1.18 and 1.19).

Procerus presents as a single morphological type with two small pyramidal muscles originating at two levels above the nasal bone. The superficial portion has been described as an hourglass shape, with the narrowest portion at the level of the medial canthal ligament. Procerus passes superiorly to insert into the dermis between the brows, depressing of the

Table 1.1 Muscle Profile of Forehead Elevator

FRONTALIS	Large, symmetrical, rectangular/fan-shaped muscle with no bony attachments extending vertically from scalp to eyebrows
Origin	Galea aponeurotica
Insertion	Superciliary skin, where it interdigitates with the brow depressors
Connections/interdigitations	
Superior	Epicranial aponeurosis
Inferior	Procerus, corrugator, orbicularis oculi, depressor supercilii
Medial	Depending on morphological type: contralateral frontalis belly/central aponeurosis
Lateral	Temporal crest; inferior fibers interdigitate with orbicularis oculi over zygomatic process
Innervation	
Motor	Temporal branch of facial nerve; enters undersurface of frontalis at temporal fusion line (TFL) where the frontal branch of the superficial temporal artery (STA) lies superior to the nerve
Sensory	Trigeminal nerve: supraorbital and supratrochlear nerves
Vascularization	Frontal branch of superficial temporal artery (STA), supraorbital artery, supratrochlear artery, lacrimal artery
Action	Inferior: elevates the brow
	Superior: causes descent of anterior hairline
Wrinkles	Transverse forehead wrinkles: 4 patterns (continuous, gull-wing, central, lateral)

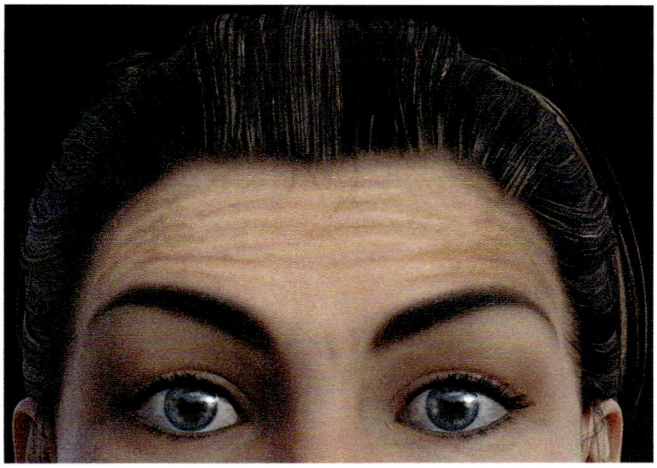

Figure 1.14 Forehead Pattern Type 1 (45%), Full form: Centrally confluent bellies causing straight lines across the entire forehead.

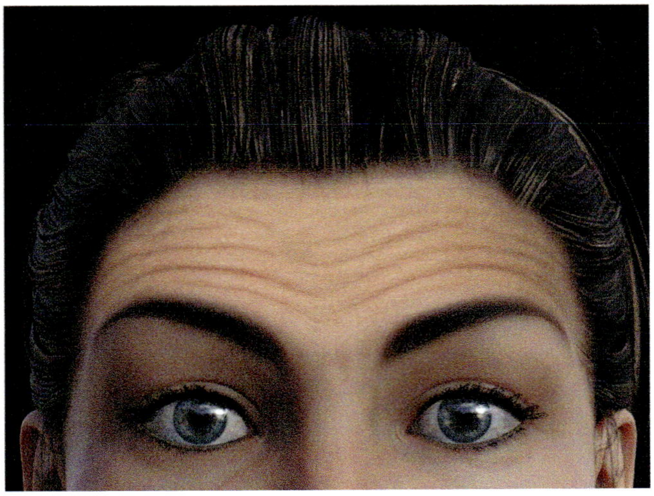

Figure 1.15 Type 2 (30%), V-shaped: Bellies separated medially by a V-shaped projection of aponeurotic galea, creating a gull-shaped line across the forehead.

lower forehead skin to create a midline horizontal crease at the nasal bridge.

Corrugator supercilii originates at the superomedial aspect of orbital rim along the nasal process of the frontal bone. It has transverse and oblique bellies. The latter may have a narrow rectangular or broader triangular shape. The two bellies course superolaterally from their origin, passing through

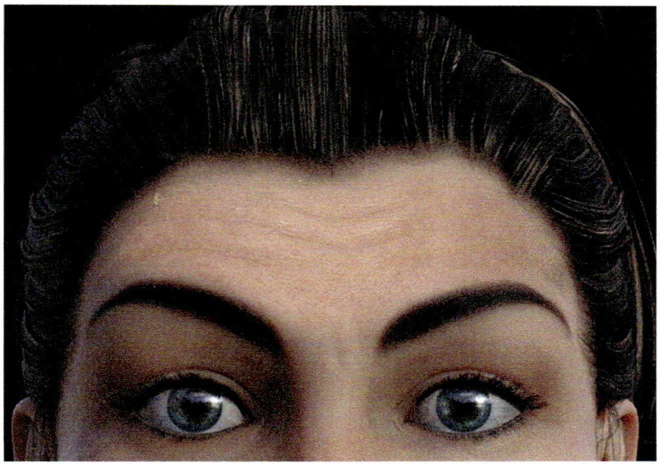

Figure 1.16 Type 3 (10%), Central: Bellies centrally joined, extending over the medial half of the orbital rims and causing a column of short lines over the central forehead.

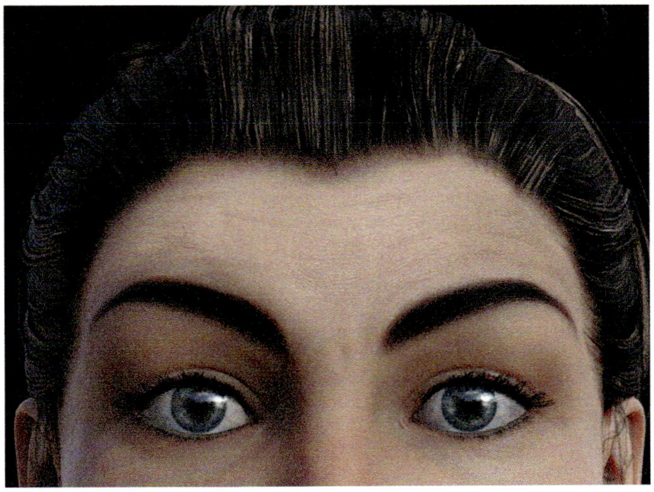

Figure 1.17 Type 4 (15%), Lateral: Bellies located over lateral half of orbital rim and separated medially by a vertical rectangular projection of aponeurotic galea, effect-ing a column of short lines on either side of the lateral forehead.

fibers of frontalis to reach the dermis at the midbrow. The superficial and deep branches of the supraorbital nerve are intimately related to corrugator supercilii at its origin. Corrugator supercilii approximates and depresses the brow. Over time, contraction of this muscle creates vertical rhytides at the brow level.

Table 1.2 Muscle Profile of Forehead Depressors

PROCERUS	Small pyramidal or hourglass-shaped muscle overlying the nasal bone
Origin	Superficial and deep layers
Deep	Few fibers from nasal bone near medial palpebral ligament
Superficial	Hourglass shape with narrowest part at level of medial palpebral ligament
Insertion	Lower forehead skin between brows on either side of the midline; merges with frontalis
Connections	May be indistinguishable from the superomedial fibers of orbicularis oculi
Superior	Frontalis
Lateral	Levator labii superioris aleque nasi (LLSAN), transverse part of nasalis
Inferior	Lateral fibers of nasalis
Innervation	
Motor	Facial nerve: temporal and lower zygomatic branches
Sensory	Trigeminus
Vascularization	Dorsal nasal artery, supra- and infratrochlear artery, anterior ethmoidal artery
Action	Brow depressor Two contraction patterns: Type 1 lowers lateral end of brow; Type 2 produces lateral eyelid crow's feet
Wrinkles	Horizontal rhytides over nasal radix
CORRUGATOR SUPERCILII	Comprises oblique and transverse bellies; there are 2 types of oblique belly: i) narrow vertical or ii) broad triangular Corrugator lies under the other brow muscles; the thickest portion is ~19 mm from nasion
Origin	Medially and deep along nasofrontal suture/superciliary arch of the frontal bone
Insertion	Highly variable lateral insertion in skin superior to middle of supraorbital margin
Connections	Orbicularis oculi and frontalis at medial brow; medial portion of depressor supercilii
Innervation	
Motor	Facial nerve: temporal branch
Sensory	Supraorbital nerve
Vascularization	Supra- and infratrochlear artery, supraorbital artery
Action	Inferior: approximation and depression of brows, creating vertical glabellar lines
Wrinkles	Vertical glabellar wrinkles on frowning
DEPRESSOR SUPERCILII (Figure 1.29)	Thin slip of muscle difficult to distinguish from medial fibers of o. oculi. It runs parallel to, but separate from, the vertical fibers of the procerus. Classified by some as corrugator supercilii Type 3.
Origin	Medial orbital rim near lacrimal bone
Insertion	Deep layer of medial head of brow, inferior to origin of corrugator supercilii
Connections	Medial orbicularis oculi
Innervation	
Motor	Facial nerve: temporal branch
Sensory	Trigeminus
Vascularization	Supra- and infratrochlear artery, supraorbital artery
Action	Inferior: eyebrow depressor
Wrinkles	Horizontal, lateral nasal

(*Continued*)

Table 1.2 (*Continued*) Muscle Profile of Forehead Depressors

ORBICULARIS OCULI	Encircles the eye and comprises pretarsal, septal and orbital portions
Origin	Medial orbital margin, medial palpebral ligament, anterior lacrimal crest
Insertion	Preseptal segment inserts into the dermis of the upper eyelid and brow
Connections/interdigitations	
Superior	Corrugator and frontalis
Medial	Medial canthal ligament
Lateral	Pretarsal portion fuses with lateral canthal tendon
Innervation	
Motor	Facial nerve: temporal and zygomatic branch
Sensory	Trigeminus
Vascularization	Facial artery, supraorbital artery, lacrimal artery, supra- and infratrochlear artery
Action	Inferior: thick orbital part closes eyelids tightly, thin palpebral part closes eyelids lightly
Wrinkles	Wrinkling on forehead from orbital part

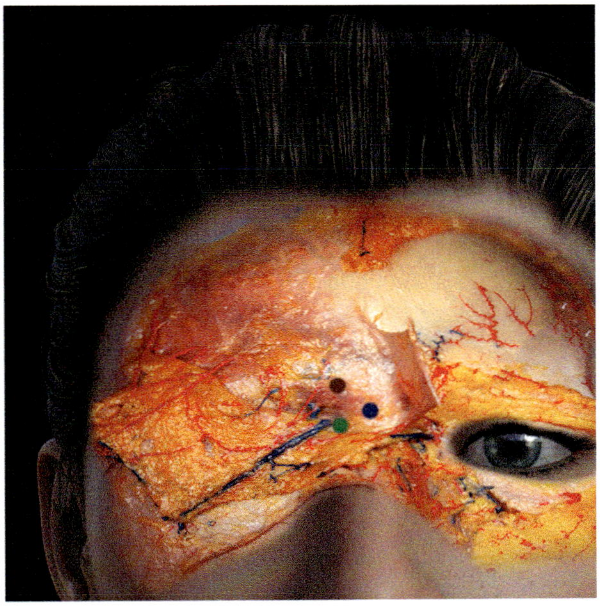

Figure 1.18 Blue dot: The procerus; green dot: depressor supercilii; brown dot: corrugator muscle.

There are six morphological corrugator muscle patterns (three symmetrical and three asymmetrical) pertaining to shape, dimension, and insertion on either side of the midline (see further Figures 1.20 through 1.24).

Type 1 (30%): Symmetrical; fan-shaped, with insertion along entire medial half of eyebrow, creating a hockey stick-shaped line over the medial brows (Figure 1.20).

Type 2 (20%): Symmetrical; rectangular form with insertion in the medial end of the eyebrow, creating parallel straight lines on the glabella (Figure 1.21).

Type 3 (5%): A narrow ribbon with insertion in the medial end of the eyebrow, creating a single vertical line; there is an asymmetrical variant (different shapes, sizes, and insertions on each side of the glabella).

Type 4 (25%): A fan-shaped form on one side and a rectangular form on the other, creating a hockey stick shape and parallel straight lines, respectively.

Type 5 (10%): A fan-shaped form on one side and a narrow ribbon on the other, creating a hockey stick-shaped line and single-straight line, respectively.

Type 6 (15%): A rectangular form on one side and a narrow ribbon on the contralateral side, creating several parallel straight lines on the glabella.

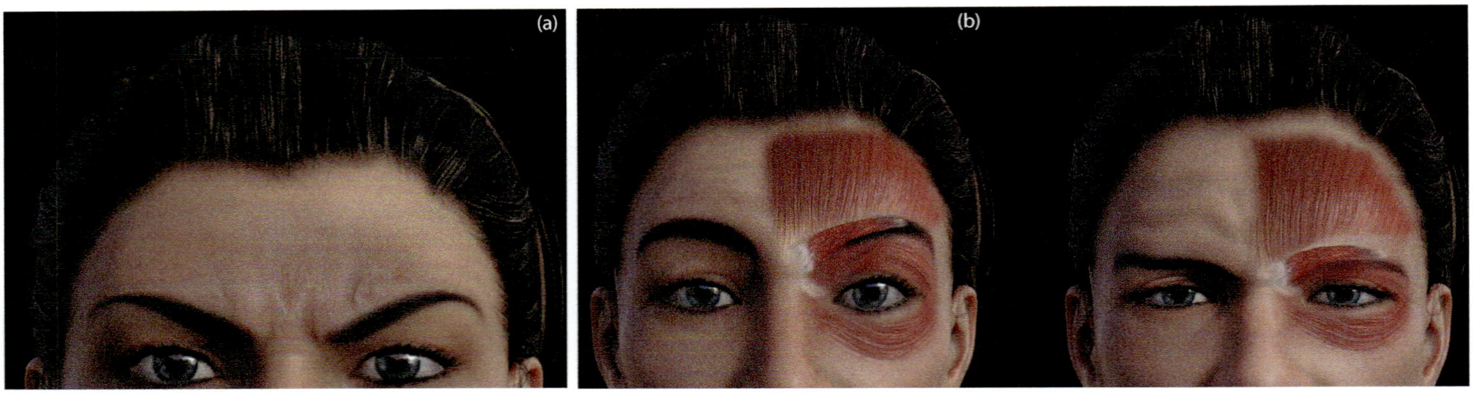

Figure 1.19 (a) Hockey-stick shaped corrugator insertion above left brow. (b) Brow asymmetry on frowning.

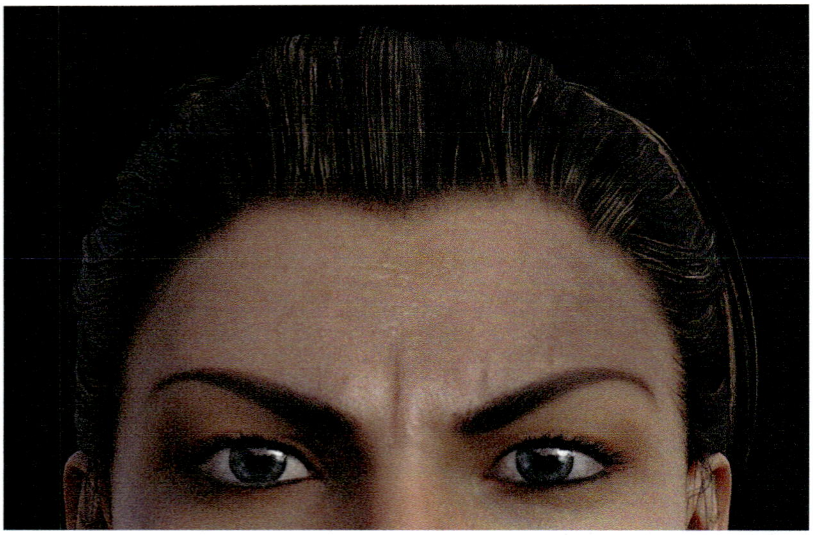

Figure 1.20 Vertical glabellar lines.

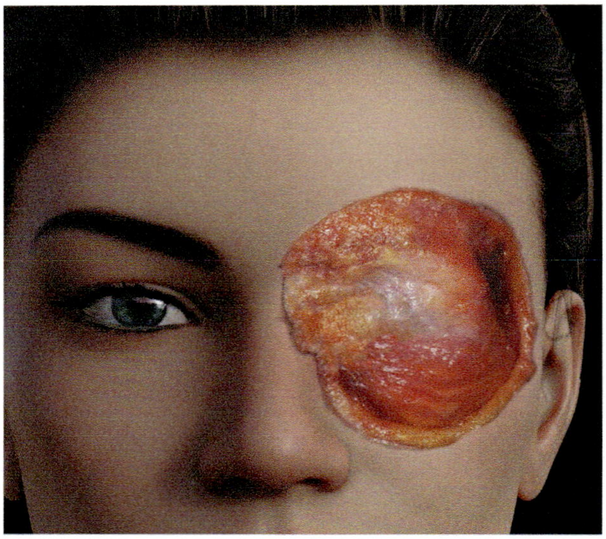

Figure 1.21 The sphincteric orbicularis oculi muscle.

Orbicularis oculi (Figure 1.21) arises from the frontal process of the maxilla and nasal process of the frontal bone running under the corrugator supracilii. Two patterns are identified:

Single Type I: The thicker peripheral fibers insert in the deep layer of the eyebrow lateral end, being responsible for its lowering.

Single Type II: The thinner central fibers insert in the deep layer of the palpebral skin, creating eyelid crow's feet.

Dynamic Contraction Patterns

Frontalis elevates the brows. Procerus and depressor supercilii cause depression of the brows while corrugator and orbicularis oculi (pars palpebralis) cause both depression and approximation. Glabellar contraction patterns have been classified according to the predominant movement. In patients with longer and more horizontal corrugators, the predominant movement may occur in two phases with initial

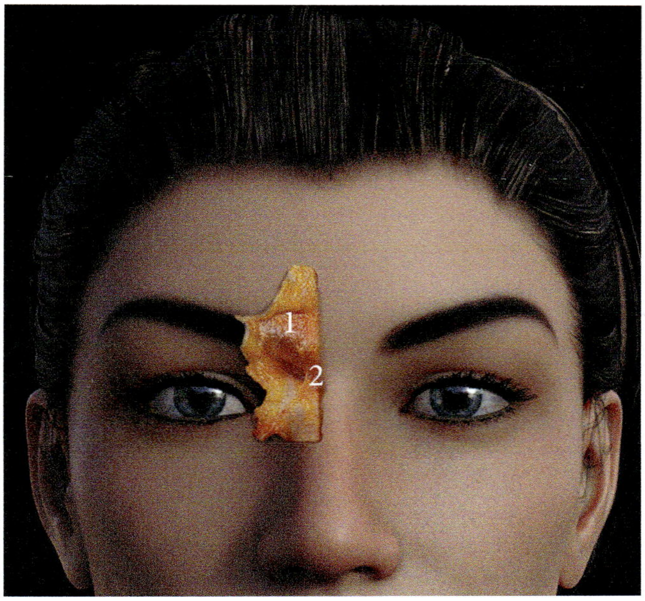

Figure 1.22 (1) Corrugator; (2) depressor supercilii.

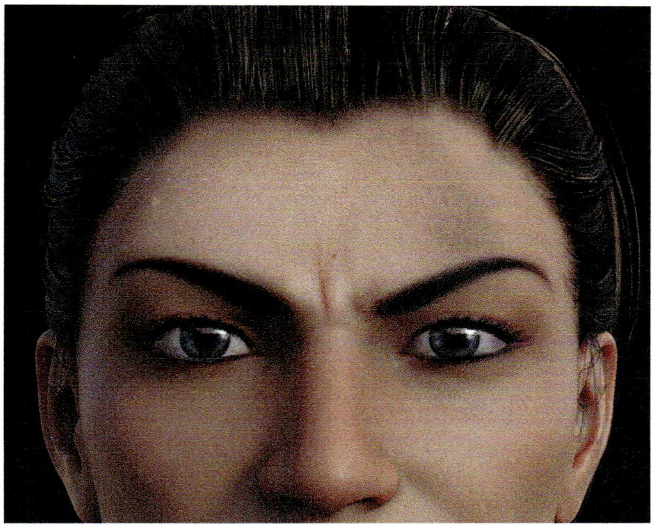

Figure 1.23 Glabellar U pattern of contraction, most commonly seen in women.

horizontal approximation (converging arrows) and then elevation (omega) or depression ("V"). The predominant pattern should be correctly identified for a tailored treatment approach.

U pattern (32%) (Figure 1.23): This is the most common pattern in women and third most common in men. Approximation and depression result in movement taking the form of the letter "U." The corrugator insertion is medial to the mid-pupillary line and eyebrows are more arched at rest. Procerus and corrugators are the dominant contributory muscles. The five-injection-site model is an effective approach.

"V" Pattern (24%) (Figure 1.24): This is the second most frequently seen pattern in women and the most common in men. The corrugator insertion is lateral to the mid-pupillary line and the eyebrow position is lower and more horizontal at rest. There is more wide-range approximation and depression, with important participation of the medial orbicularis. A seven-site model is the best approach, with higher doses required in procerus and the corrugators.

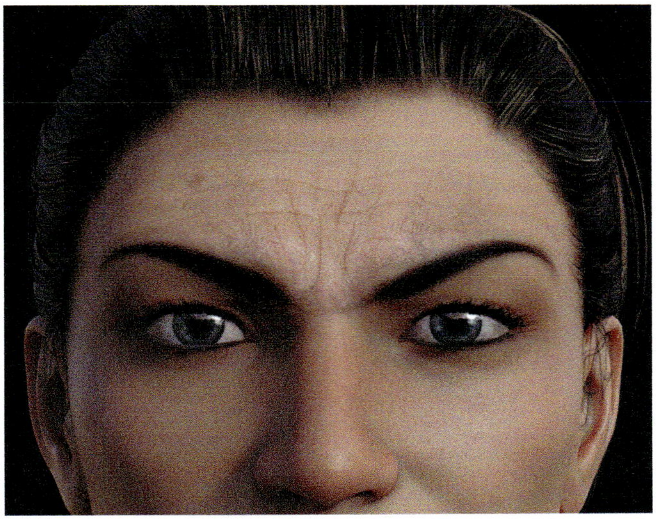

Figure 1.24 V pattern, most common pattern in men.

"Converging Arrows" Pattern (Figure 1.25): This pattern of "brow opposers" shows approximation with little or no brow depression or elevation. The resulting movement is horizontal approximation with balancing of forces between procerus and frontalis. The muscles involved are corrugators and the medial portion of the orbicularis. The injection technique should target corrugator, with minimal or no treatment of procerus and frontalis.

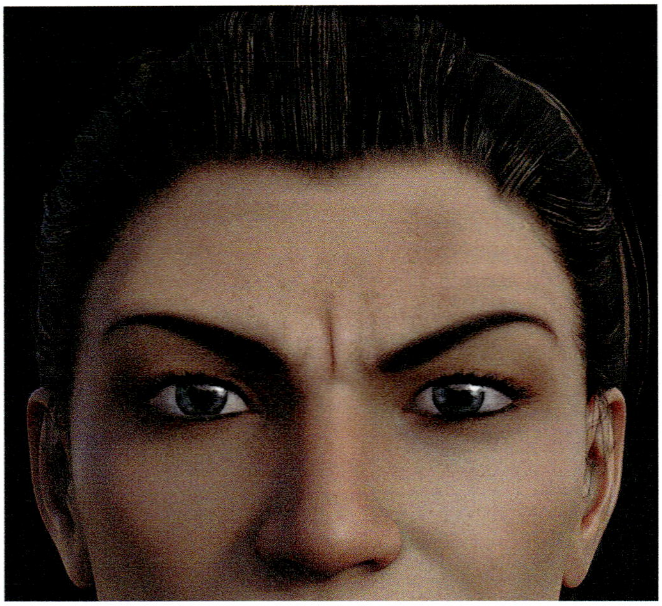

Figure 1.25 "Converging arrows" pattern, with mainly approximation and little brow depression.

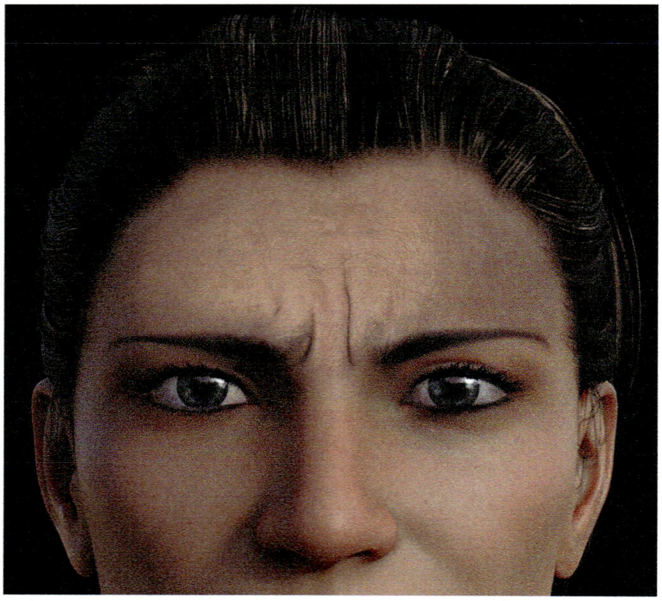

Figure 1.26 "Omega" pattern, with accompanying recruitment of frontalis and elevation of medial brows. Beware of unmasking brow ptosis with toxin treatment.

"Omega—Ω" Pattern (10.2%) (Figure 1.26): The predominant movements are approximation and elevation of the glabella, taking the form of the Greek letter omega. The dominant muscles are the corrugators, medial orbicularis, and frontalis, with little or no procerus contraction. The best approach would be to inject into the corrugators, orbicularis oculi pars palpebralis, and medial frontalis, with higher doses into the corrugators and orbicularis and lower doses into the frontalis sites. The procerus requires little or no treatment.

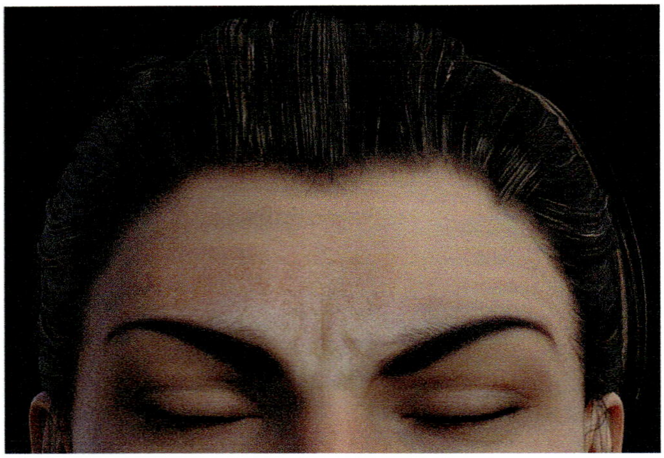

Figure 1.27 "Inverted-omega" pattern with approximation and depression of brows. These patients often have a wide intercanthal distance; beware of high toxin doses at medial corrugator points which could create a splayed appearance.

"Inverted-Omega—Ω" Pattern (8.4%) (Figure 1.27): The predominant movement is depression with little approximation, resembling an inverted omega. This pattern is more frequent in patients with a flat nose apex. Involved muscles are mainly procerus, depressor supercilii, medial orbicularis, oculi pars palpebralis, with less corrugator activity. Nasalis action may be contributory. Appropriate treatment would imply higher doses in procerus and depressor supercilii, with additional sites at the medial orbicularis oculi and nasalis muscles. A minimal dose may be optionally injected into the medial corrugators, with care being taken not to create an unnaturally splayed brow. Individuals with asymmetrical eyebrows show different patterns on either side and should be classified and treated accordingly.

VESSELS

The vasculature at the brow and glabella is initially deep but quickly transitions to the intramuscular and subcutaneous levels (Figure 1.28):

- The **supraorbital (SO) artery**, a branch of the ophthalmic artery, exits the orbit through the SO notch approximately 27 mm lateral to midline and underlies the SO crease. This point is generally just medial to a vertical line intersecting the medial limbus of the cornea. The artery most commonly pierces the frontalis 20–40 mm above the orbital rim and then surfaces in the subcutaneous tissue between 40 and 60 mm caudally. Vertical branches as low as 15–20 mm have been described. In addition to the dorsal nasal, supratrochlear (ST), and angular arteries, the SO artery sends branches that anastomose with the frontal branch of the superficial temporal artery, most often at the junction of the transverse inferior and middle third of the forehead.
- The **ST artery** exits the orbit ~17 mm from the midline and branches to anastomose with the angular, SO, and dorsal nasal arteries.

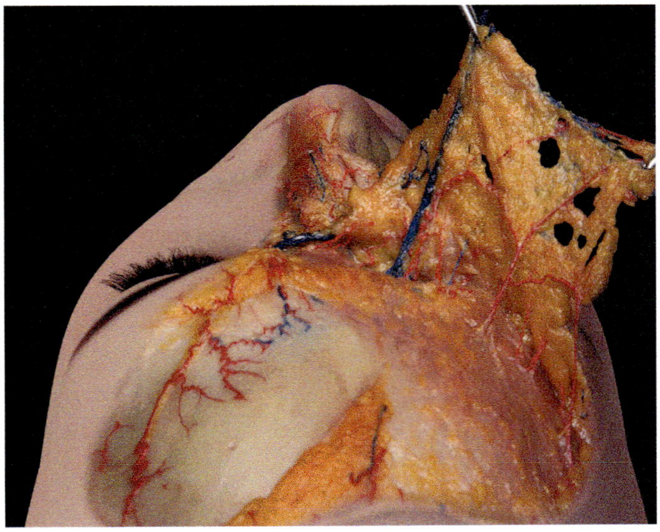

Figure 1.28 Supraorbital and supratrochlear vessels entering the forehead deep at the supraorbital rim before transitioning to the superficial plane.

- Branches from internal and external carotid vascular systems have several anastomoses in the forehead, posing a potential danger of ophthalmic and central thromboembolic complications (Figures 1.29 and 1.30).

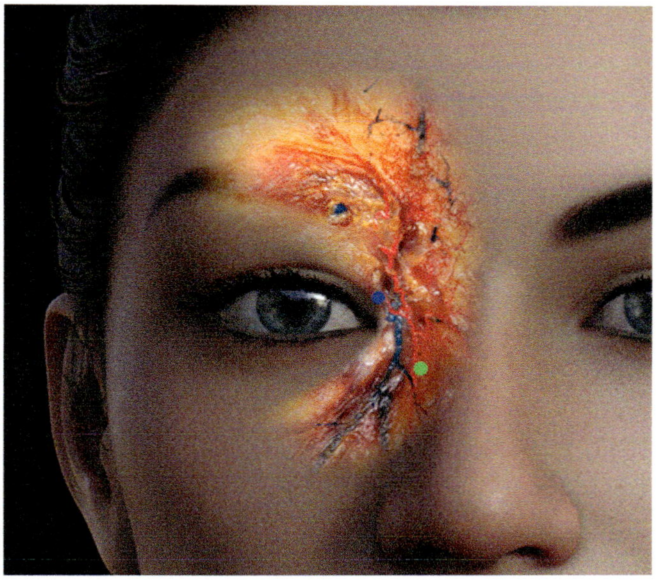

Figure 1.29 Danger areas: The periorbital internal (Blue)/external (green) carotid communications are potential routes for ophthalmic artery embolization.

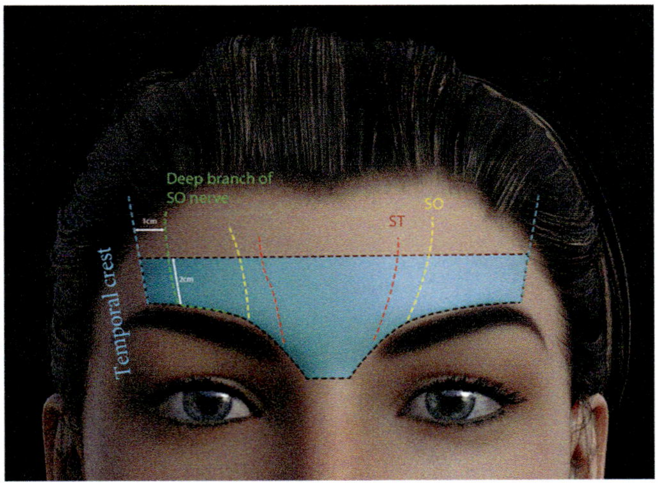

Figure 1.30 Topographical landmarks: Vessels underlie creases. In the lower 2.5 cm of the forehead, filler should be placed superficially to avoid vessels; above this line. Place fillers deep on the bone. ST = Supratrochlear, SO = Supraobital vessels.

- The **frontal branch of the superficial temporal artery (STA)** may anastomose with the ipsilateral ST artery. Superficial (needle or small-gauge cannula) injection of filler in this region should be avoided, as inadvertent intravascular injection can cause central retinal artery occlusion via retrograde embolization into the ophthalmic artery.
- In contrast to the SO and ST vessels, the **central forehead vessels** lie just beneath the skin in the lower forehead. To avoid intravascular complications, filler injections beneath this wrinkle should be meticulously placed in the superficial dermis. The glabella constitutes an area of watershed circulation and is the most common injection site leading to visual loss after intravascular embolization.

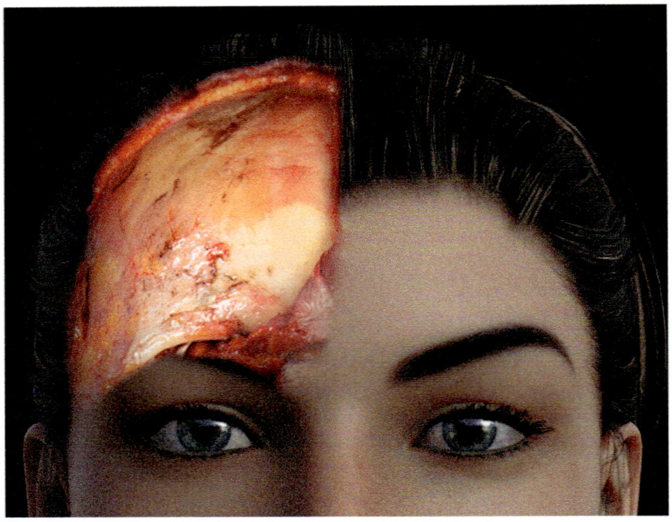

Figure 1.32 Squamous portion of the frontal bone, inferiorly joining the orbital, temporal and nasal bones. Note the supraorbital notch.

NERVES

The ophthalmic nerve V1 supplies the forehead via the supraorbital and supratrochlear nerves (Figure 1.31).

- The **supraorbital (SO) nerve** exits the superior orbital foramen/notch 23–27 mm from the midline in men and 22–25 mm from the midline in women and then runs under the frontalis fascia to innervate the anterolateral forehead and scalp. Branches may exit through separate foraminae. The **deep branch** usually runs superiorly between the galea and the periosteum of the forehead in the region 0.5–1.5 cm medial to the temporal fusion line.
- The **supratrochlear (ST) nerve** exits the orbit about 10 mm medial to the SO nerve and runs close to the periosteum under the corrugator and frontalis. Its branches supply the skin over the medial eyelid and lower medial forehead.

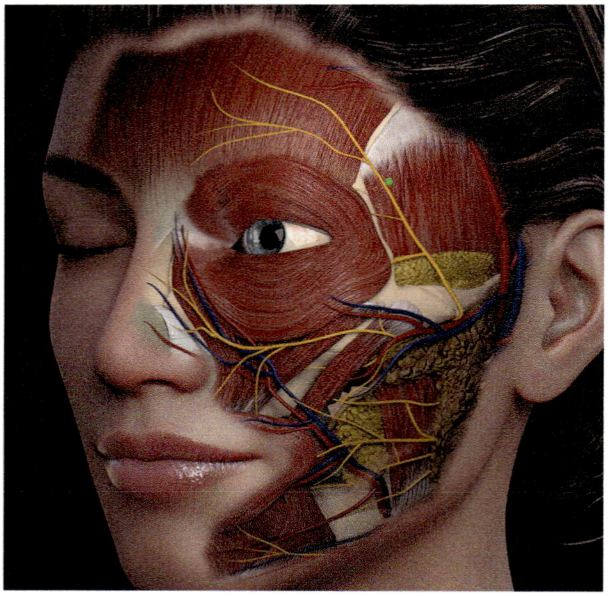

Figure 1.31 Forehead motor innervation. Green dot: temporal branch of the facial nerve.

The muscles of facial expression are innervated by branches of the **facial nerve (VII)** (Figure 1.32). The temporal branch enters frontalis about 2 cm above the brow, just below the anterior branch of the superficial temporal artery.

BONE

The facial skeleton provides areas of attachment for the muscles of facial expression. The squamous por-tion of the frontal bone forms the foundation of the forehead (Figure 1.32).

- Palpable bony landmarks include the **temporal crest** (temporal fusion line), **orbital rim**, and **orbital foramen**, which is often palpable above the level of the medial limbus. These important landmarks predict adjacent vital structures and are best palpated and marked before treatment.
- The **superciliary arches** form the bony ridges underlying the eyebrows.
- The **glabella**: Smooth midline bony elevation connecting the superciliary arches.
- The **nasion**: Craniometric midline point indicating the articulation between the frontal bone and paired nasal bones.
- The **supraorbital foramen** (or notch) and **frontal notch**: Found at the superior border of each orbit, transmitting, respectively, the supraorbital and supratrochlear nerves.

HOW I DO IT: BOTULINUM TOXIN

While the forehead and glabellar regions constitute the most frequently treated toxin areas, filler treatment in these areas mandates caution. Potential side effects such as skin necrosis and blindness make the forehead a challenging area for fillers. Anatomical danger zones should be consciously avoided and insightful knowledge of all soft tissue and skeletal structures, from superficial to deep, is essential. As vascular anatomy is extremely variable, estimating needle depth may be unpredictable, and vascular injuries are possible even after the best precautions. Vigilant technique, early recognition of vascular compromise and proactive management is thus vital. Analysis of both muscle morphology and dynamic function is mandatory. An integrated, pan-facial approach is advised, first using BoNT-A for excessive muscle movement and then restoring volume where applicable. When used in the same session, filler should be injected first with proper massage and, thereafter, botulinum toxin.

- Evaluate the brows for shape and symmetry both in repose and in animation.
- Choose age-appropriate goals and respect muscle laxity in older individuals.
- Understand and treat the muscle balance between elevator (frontalis) and depressors (corrugator, procerus, orbicularis oculi, depressor supercillii).
- Aim for modulation versus paralysis; analyze target muscle in the context of adjacent muscles as well as hard and soft tissues.
- Eyelid and brow ptosis may ensue if incorrect placement or injection depth is used.
- Reassess and adjust 1–2 weeks after treatment.
- Detailed comprehension of the location and depth of each glabellar muscle is vital for optimal placement of botulinum toxin. The use of 30–33G needles is recommended. Dosages are given as for onabotulinumtoxin-A.

Glabellar Toxin

See Figures 1.33 through 1.36.

- Place thumb on supraorbital rim to evaluate muscle strength and avoid migration into upper eyelid levator.
- Inject 2–3 mm above the ORL to prevent eyelid ptosis.
- Be careful not to inject too high in the corrugator points, thus inadvertently treating lower frontalis and inducing brow ptosis.
- Depth

Procerus	Mid-depth (insert 13 mm needle to half depth, angled upward)
Medial corrugator	Deep (insert needle to full depth, angled laterally upward)

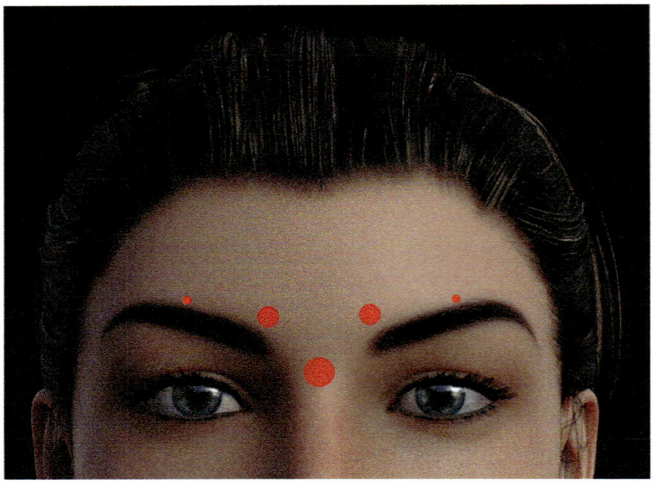

Figure 1.33 Standard 5 points of 4 U on the glabella. In the opposing arrow pattern, the procerus point may be omitted.

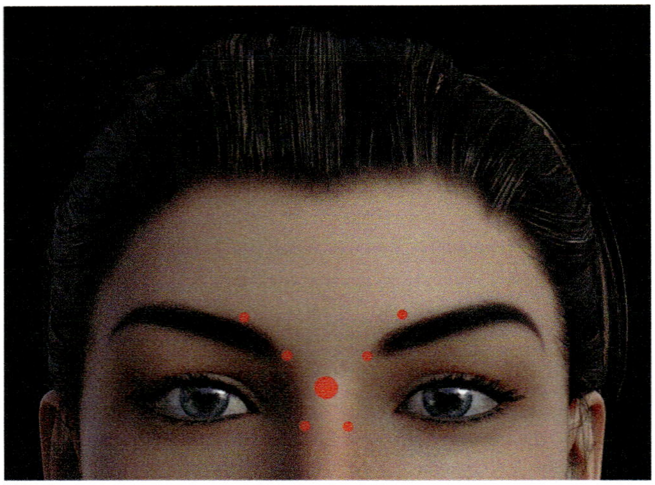

Figure 1.35 Standard 5 points of 4 U on the glabella plus 2 points of 1 U on LLSAN.

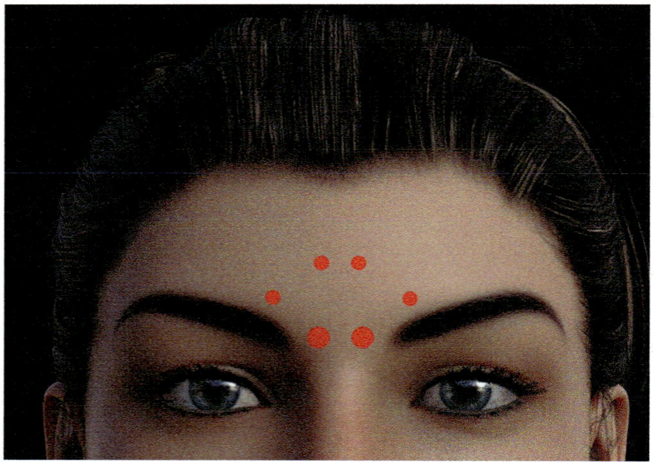

Figure 1.34 2 points of 4 U and 4 points of 2 U in the omega pattern.

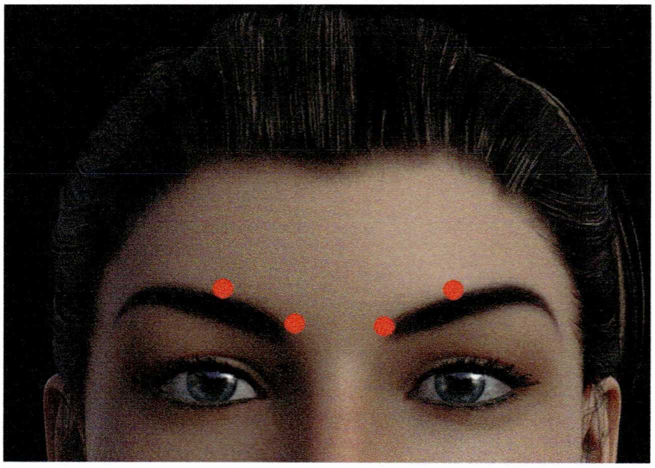

Figure 1.36 Opposing arrow pattern: 4 points of 2-4 U.

Lateral corrugator	Superficial (insert needle one-third its length, angled laterally upward)
Depressor supercilii	Mid-depth
Frontalis	Superficial intramuscular or intracutaneous (insert needle one-third of its length, angled laterally upward)

- Dose
  - The standard onabotulinum dose is 2–4 U/point over a 3–7 injection pattern.
  - Exact dosing should be tailored to individual muscle strength and pattern and may be higher in hyperkinetic and hypertonic muscles as well as in male patients.

CAUTION

- Inject above ORL to prevent toxin migration to upper eyelid levator.
- Protect orbital rim with finger of non-injecting hand.

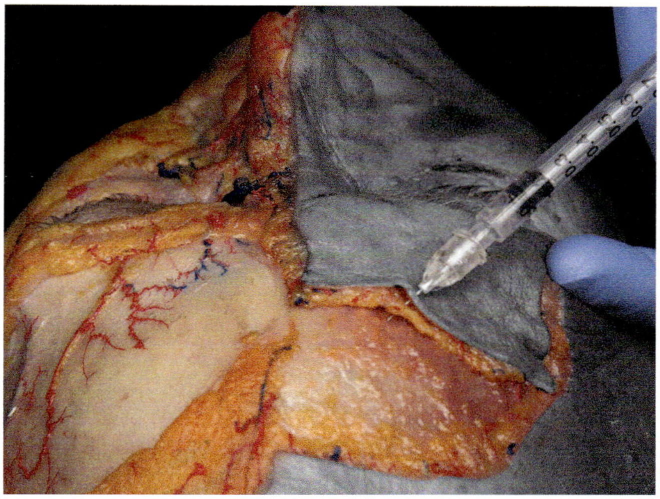

Figure 1.37 Botulinum toxin injected in the supramuscular plane.

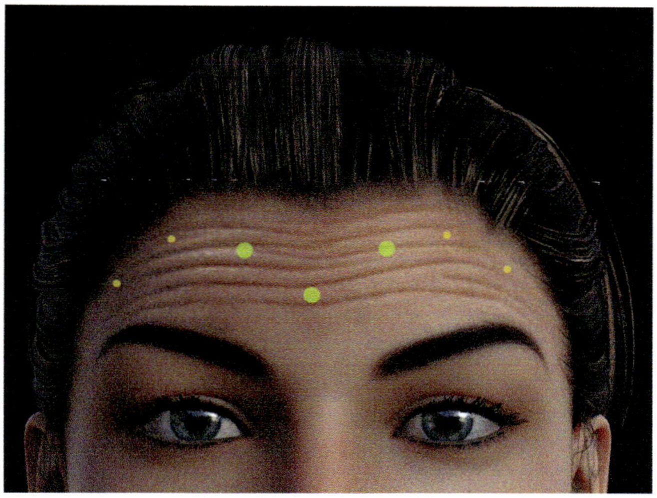

Figure 1.38 Forehead botulinum toxin in the full form pattern. Always tailor points to muscle pattern and strength.

Frontalis Toxin

- Injecting too low in the central forehead may cause medial brow ptosis and a tired look.
- Beware of treating the narrow forehead as brow ptosis may ensue.
- Injecting too low in the lateral brow (1–2 cm suprabrow) may unmask compensatory brow ptosis.
- Beware of unmasking compensatory brow ptosis in older patients.
- Intracutaneous injection limits magnitude of effect, thus reducing brow descent (Figure 1.38).
- Aim for a natural, gradual grading between the upper and the lower (untreated) forehead.
- Inject in the upper half of forehead and stay more than 1.5 cm above orbital rim in mid-pupillary line to avoid brow ptosis (Figure 1.39).
- Overcorrection of lateral brow elevation may unmask ptosis.
- Depth: Superficial intramuscular injection.
- Extend injection points far enough laterally to avoid excessive elevation of the lateral brow (Mephisto/Spock sign).
- The lateral two points are not always necessary and may require lower dosing.

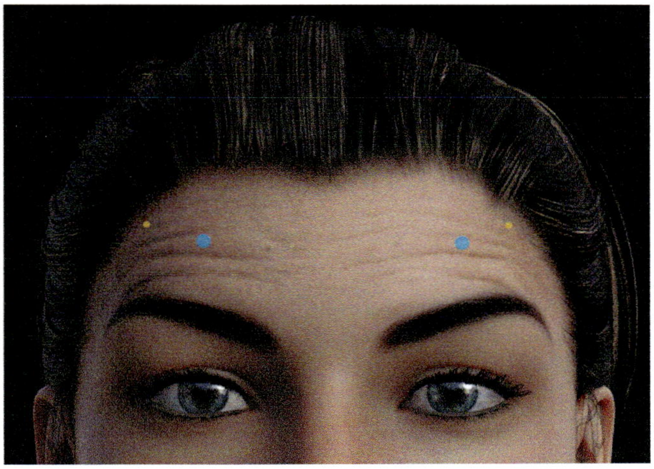

Figure 1.39 Forehead botulinum toxin in the lateral frontalis muscle extension.

- Treat the glabellar depressors and lateral canthal lines in conjunction with frontalis.
- Lateral hypokinetic muscle areas may not require treatment.
- Dose
    - 2–4U red of botulinum toxin per point (as per diagrams).
    - HFLs: 8–25 U (intramuscular or intracutaneous) (Figure 1.39).

- Lateral brow elevation: 0.5–1 U (intramuscular) (Figure 1.40).
- Medial brow elevation: 0.5–4 U (intramuscular) (Figure 1.41).

Microbotox (Figure 1.42) may be utilized to treat lower HFLs; use conservative doses and follow up at 1–2 weeks.

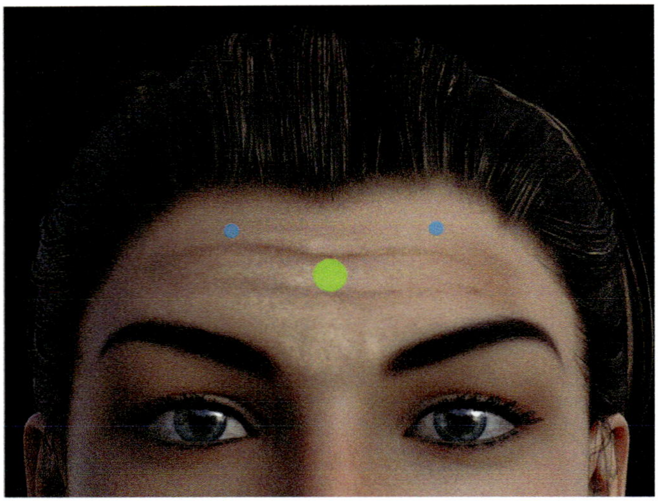

Figure 1.40 Forehead botulinum toxin in patient with central muscle pattern.

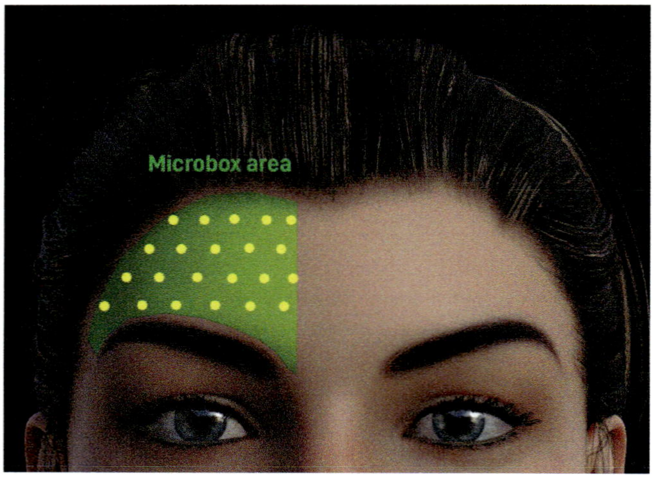

Figure 1.41 Microbotox: Dilution of 50 U with 2.5 mL of saline solution. The injection points of 0.05 U are spaced 1 cm apart.

Microbotox may be used to eradicate lateral brow frown lines without causing depression of the eyebrows; it requires careful preparation of the solution and a sensitive and refined injection technique.

Method	Draw up 24 U (0.6 mL of normal dilution); dilute to 1 mL with normal saline.
Dose	Entire forehead, including glabella and brows: 24–28 U.
	Lateral forehead alone: 16 U.
Technique	Multiple tiny intradermal blebs or superficial muscular injections spread over the area.
Effect	Weakening of superficial muscles attached to the undersurface of the skin. There is atrophy of sebaceous glands.
Duration of action	2–3 months.

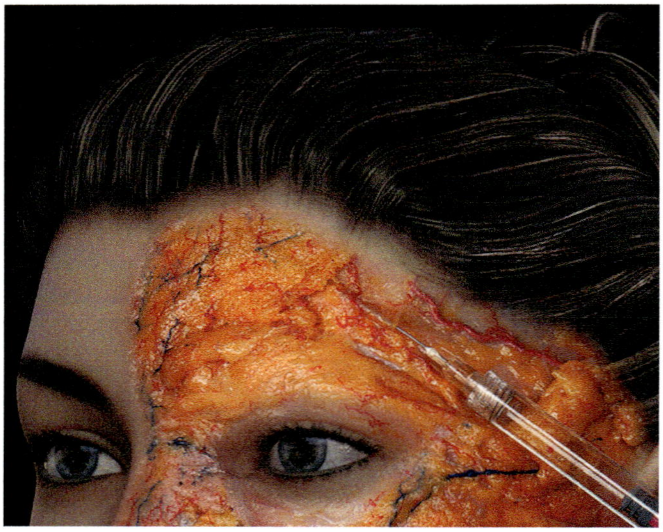

Figure 1.42 Forehead filler may be done with the cannula entering just above the tendon's fusion and with a 38 mm or a 50 mm 25G cannula. A 27G or 30G needle can also be used deep to bone. Unduly superficial placement may cause a "sunray appearance".

HOW I DO IT: FILLERS

Central Lower Forehead

- At the level of the supraorbital rims, vessels are initially deep, transitioning to the intramuscular and subcutaneous level approximately 2 cm above the orbital rims (Figure 1.43).
- In the 1.5–2 cm directly above the supraorbital rim, placement with needles should preferably be in the superficial plane (deep injections in the horizontal zone extending between the temporal fusion lines approach the position and depth of underlying vessels and are ideally only to be undertaken by experienced injectors).
- A deep branch of the supraorbital nerve runs caudally beneath the frontalis muscle approximately 1 cm medial to the temporal crest. The use of sharp needles in this area is cautioned against and cannulae are advised.
- Glabellar area: The central forehead artery lies just beneath the skin, so extreme caution should be exercised in this watershed perfusion area as this is the most common injection site leading to visual loss after intravascular embolization.

Central Upper Forehead

For higher than 2 cm above the supraorbital rim:

- Deep, subgaleal placement is advised to avoid the more-superficially placed vessels (Figures 1.44 and 1.45).

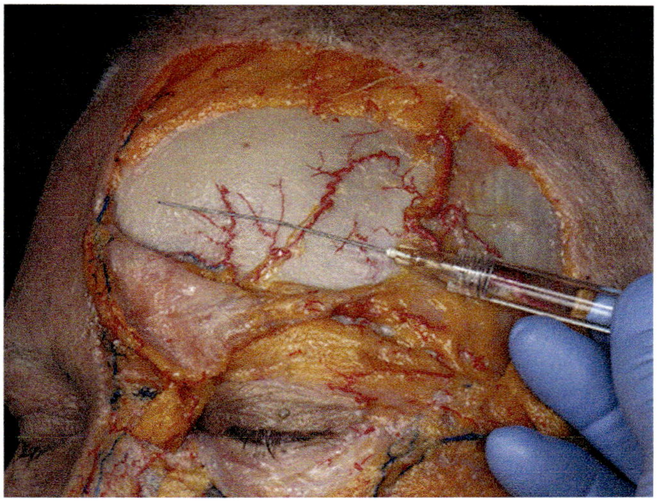

Figure 1.44 Frontal bone exposed to evaluate the cannula depth.

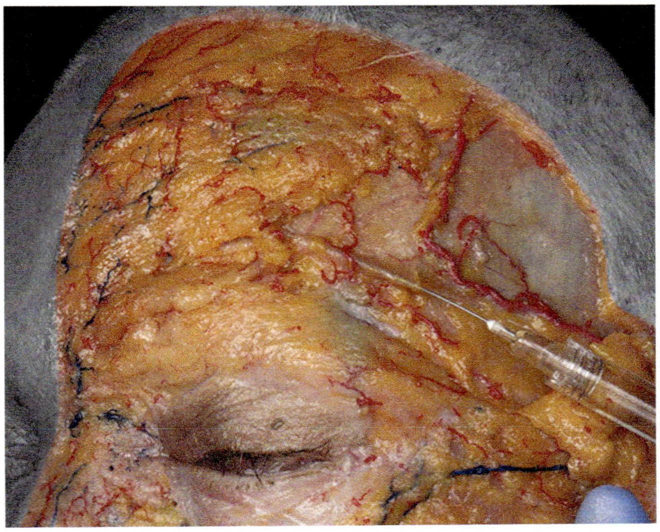

Figure 1.43 Cannula must be on the subgaleal plane touching the bone.

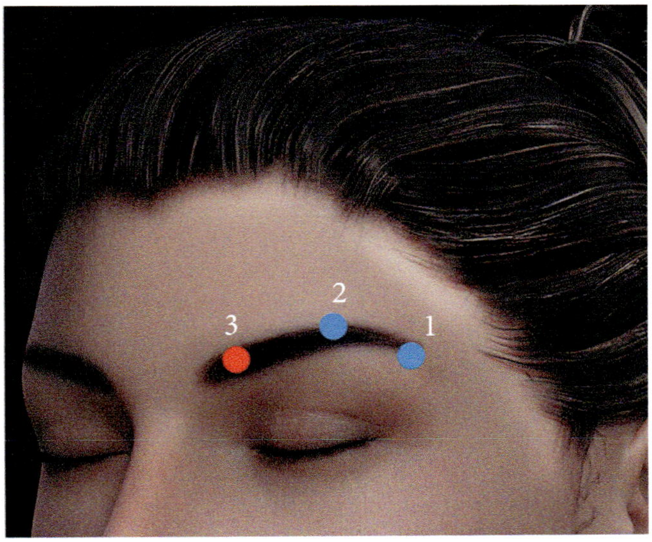

Figure 1.45 Brow reshaping (filler) points: Area 3 denotes a danger area for intravascular injection.

- Safer placement may be effected by injecting on the bone at a 45° angle and keeping the needle bevel down.
- Subgaleal placement effects a round mound of product, while supragaleal placement effects a linear configuration, which may extend caudally.

For horizontal forehead lines in the upper forehead, fillers should be placed in the superficial or mid-der-mis as vessels run in the superficial plane. Use of a low G′ product is advised.

CONTOURING OF CENTRAL FOREHEAD

Target: Subgaleal plane/bone (Figure 1.37)

Device: Needle (or cannula)

Product: Low G′ product

Technique:

- Place needle tip on the bone beneath the galea to access avascular plane (Figure 1.37).
- Face needle bevel down at 45° to minimize bevel distance from subgaleal plane.
- Inject very slowly using a supraperiosteal bolus injection, and inject deeply to avoid the supraorbital and supratrochlear neurovascular bundles.
- Aspiration is mandatory before each injection.
- Raise a round papule.
- Linear product spread denotes supragaleal placement in the more dangerous vascular plane.
- Lateral points: Inject deep; avoid temporal vessels and nerves.
- Central points: Inject deep; avoid supraorbital and supratrochlear nerves.
- Massage carefully.

CAUTION

- Place deep injections at least 2 cm above the eyebrow to avoid deep vessels and nerves.
- Avoid the supratrochlear and supraorbital vessels, as well as the transverse frontal branch of the superficial temporal artery.

Superficial Forehead Lines

Use intradermal or directly subdermal injection in microdroplet technique.

CAUTION

- The central forehead vessel is very superficial.
- The distance between bone and skin in glabella is only 2–4 mm.

Eyebrow Reshaping

Fillers may improve contour and volume and elevate the tail of the brow in the three points described (Figure 1.45).

At (1), use a very slow supraperiosteal bolus technique with an intermediate G′ hyaluronic acid (HA) and a 30G needle or a 25G 38 mm cannula to reflate the ROOF. Massage upward to shape; at the more medial points (2) and (3), use 25G 38 mm cannula in the subcutaneous plane, with meticulous avoidance of underlying vasculature (Figures 1.46 and 1.47).

- Place finger on orbital rim and protect to avoid migration of the filler into the upper eyelid.
- At point (2), a more medial injection should be used than in (1) while avoiding the supraorbital foramen; in the “A-frame” deformity, inject slowly using a 25G 38 mm cannula (Figure 1.48).

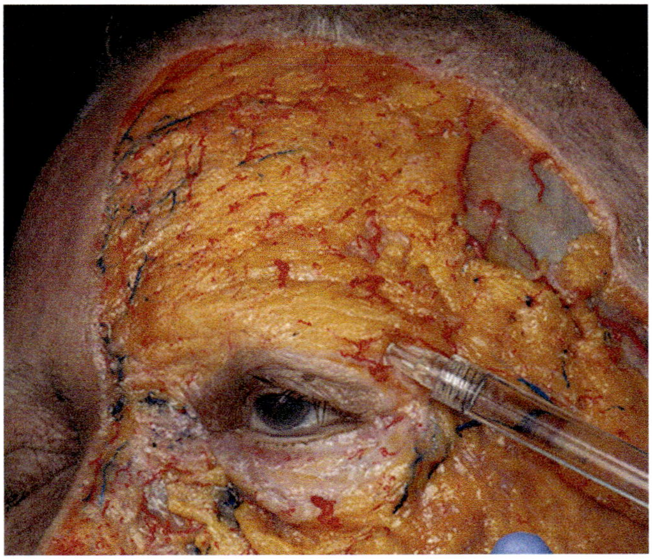

Figure 1.46 **Lateral brow**: Insert needle or cannula deep in the ROOF, 3 mm above the bony margin.

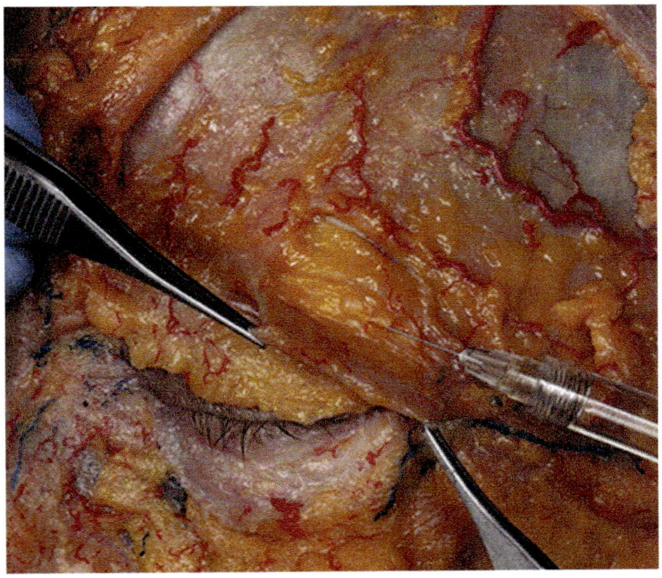

Figure 1.47 ROOF exposed showing the injected HA.

Eyebrow Area	Placement	Device
i. Tail	Bone	Needle or cannula
ii. Central	Bone or fat pad	Cannula
iii. Head	Fat pad; danger area: inject lateral to SO foramen	Cannula

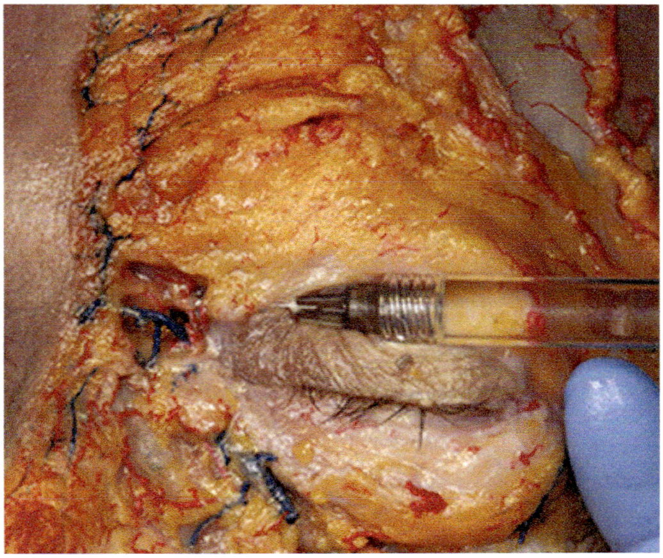

Figure 1.48 Danger area in "A-frame deformity" correction with the ophthalmic artery exposed and the needle in the most superficial plane.

COMPLICATIONS

For general complications and the concept of "safety by depth," see Chapter G.

Seckel divided the face into seven functional danger zones [1]; the forehead region includes danger zones 2 and 5 (Figure 1.49).

Toxin Safety Considerations

- Placing the medial corrugator points too high on the forehead will affect inferior frontalis fibers and cause medial brow ptosis.
- Placing the lateral corrugator points too low (inferior to the orbital retaining ligament) or too deep carries the risk of toxin migration into the levator palpebrae superioris, thus causing eyelid ptosis. Eyelid ptosis may be treated by the use of apraclonidine eyedrops, which stimulate the adrenergic eyelid levator, Müller's muscle.

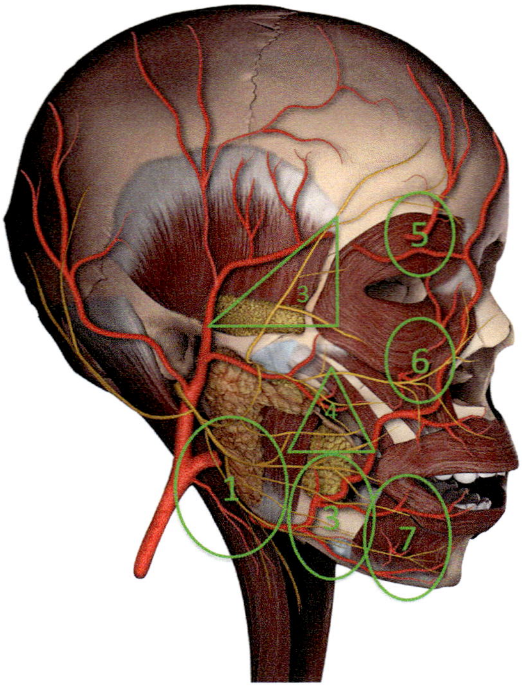

Figure 1.49 Seckel danger zones.

- Beware of treating compensatory lines in the lower half of the forehead as this may unmask the underlying problem (e.g. ptotic brows) to cause overt descent of the brows.
- Routinely monitor patients 1–2 weeks after glabellar toxin treatment to exclude or correct a possible Mephisto look.
- Place frontalis toxin points according to individual frontalis muscle anatomy.

Filler Safety Considerations

- The distance between glabellar bone and skin is 2–4 mm, making this a high-risk area for vascular compromise.
- The glabella poses the highest risk for visual compromise from inadvertent intravascular injection.
- In the lower ~2 cm of the forehead, vessels lie deep on bone, coursing to a more superficial position in the upper forehead (Figures 1.50 and 1.51). Filler injections in this area should be done with the utmost caution and only with insightful knowledge of vascular anatomy.
- Inject the upper forehead in the deep, subgaleal plane while angling the needle bevel at 45°, facing downward. A perpendicular needle position risks bevel position in the supragaleal plane with the concomitant risk of intravascular placement or vertical filler tracts visible beneath the skin.

CAUTION

- The central forehead vein, when present, runs just beneath the glabellar skin surface in the lower forehead, making this an extremely high-risk area for vascular compromise [2].

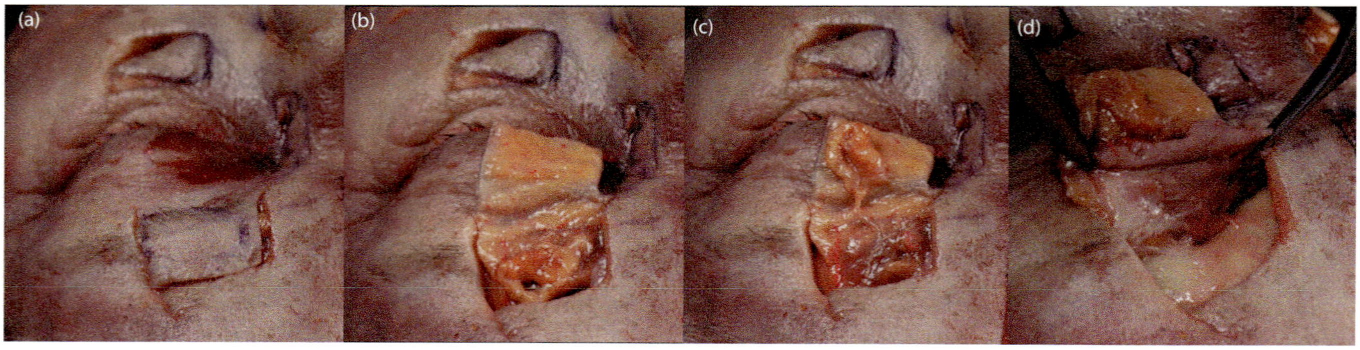

Figure 1.50 Danger area layer by layer of supratrochlear and supraorbital vessels: (a) skin is elevated; (b) fat is elevated; (c) muscle is elevated; (d) the vessels emerge from the bone.

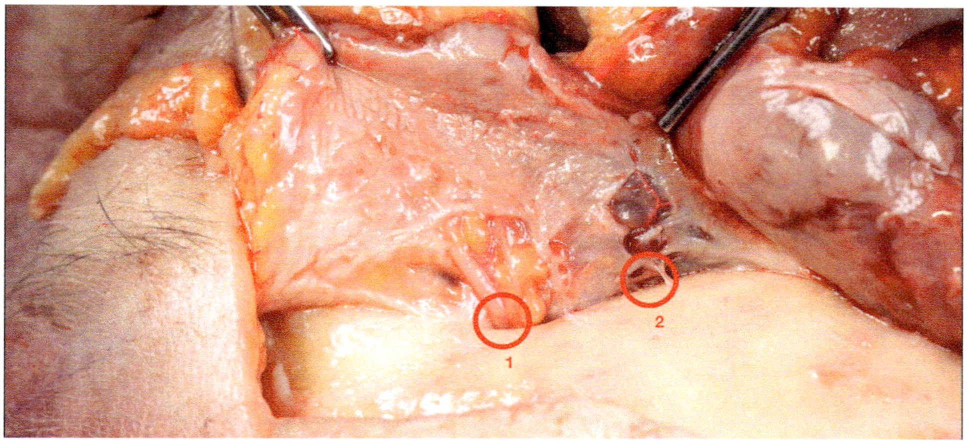

Figure 1.51 Bone exposure of the supratrochlear and supraorbital vessels.

References

1. Seckel B. *Facial Danger Zones*, 2nd ed. *Thieme*; 2010.
2. Pessa J & Rohrich RJ. Facial Topography: Clinical Anatomy of the Face. *Thieme*; 2014.

Further Reading

Braz AV & Sakuma TH. *Surg Cosmet Dermatol.* 2010;2(3):191–4.

Coleman SR & Grover R. *Aesthet Surg J.* 2006; 26(1):S4–S9.

De Almeida A et al. *Dermatol Surg.* 2012;38: 1506–15.

Kim HJ et al. *Clinical Anatomy of the Face for Filler and Botulinum Toxin Injection.* Singapore: Springer; 2016 May 17.

Lamilla GC et al. *Anatomy & botulinumtoxin injections.* Paris, France: Expert 2 Expert, 2015.

Maio MD et al. *Plastic Reconstr Sur.* 2017;140(2): 265–76.

Rohrich RJ & Pessa JE. *Plast Reconstr Surg.* 2012; 129(5S):31–9.

Scheuer JF et al. *Plast Reconstr Surg.* 2017;139(1): 50–8.

Sundaram H et al. *Plastic Reconstr Sur.* 2015;137(3): 518–29.

Sykes JM et al. *Plast Reconstr Surg.* 2015; 136(5S):204–17.

Yang H & Kim H. *Surg Radiol Anat.* 2013;35(9): 817–21.

2 TEMPORAL REGION AND LATERAL BROW

Krishan Mohan Kapoor, Alberto Marchetti, Hervé Raspaldo, Shino Bay Aguilera, Natalia Manturova, and Dario Bertossi

INTRODUCTION

Facial shape is integral to facial beauty, with an oval face being considered youthful, healthy, and attractive by individuals of all ethnicities. A smooth, slightly convex temporal contour with inconspicuous anterior bony margins and smooth transitions from the forehead through the temples and cheekbones is considered the ideal. There is, however, considerable ethnic variation in the awareness of this region, with great treatment demand from an early age in the Asian population contrasting sharply to non-Asian populations where the temporal region has, until recently, often been neglected. Other than contributing to facial proportion, the temporal fossa also supports the tail of the brow. The fossa may be likened to a swimming pool with a superior shallow and zygomatic deep end. It contains the superior aspect of the temporalis muscle and its layered fascia, the superficial temporal artery and vein, and the auriculotemporal nerve (V3) [1]. The anterior part of the temporal fossa houses the lateral orbital fat pad in the superficial plane, while the posterior part is covered by the lateral temporal-cheek fat pad.

BOUNDARIES AND LAYERS

- Anterosuperior: Curved superior temporal line, periorbital septum, and lateral brow thickening
- Anteroinferior: Frontal process of the zygomatic bone
- Inferior: Zygomatic arch
- Posterior: Temporal hairline

The temple transitions to the forehead at the superior temporal line (region of the conjoined tendon) and transitions to the midface inferiorly at the zygomatic arch (Figure 2.1).

The temple is an anatomically complex region, with currently a lack of consistent nomenclature in the literature. However, from superficial to deep, the horizontal tissue layers may be described as the following:

1. Skin (Figure 2.2)
2. Subcutaneous tissue (Figure 2.3)
3. Superficial temporal fascia (Figure 2.4)
4. Loose areolar tissue and deep fatty layer

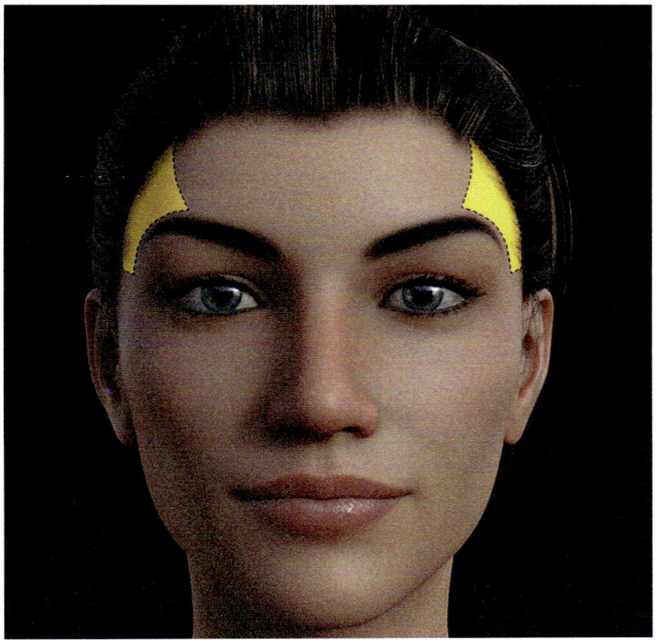

Figure 2.1 The temporal region extends from the temporal crest to the zygomatic arch. The orbital margin forms the anterior and hairline the posterior limit.

5. Superficial layer of deep temporal fascia (Figure 2.5)
6. Superficial temporal fat pad
7. Deep layer of deep temporal fascia (Figure 2.6)
8. Deep temporal fat pad (temporal extension of buccal fat pad)
9. Temporalis muscle (Figure 2.7)

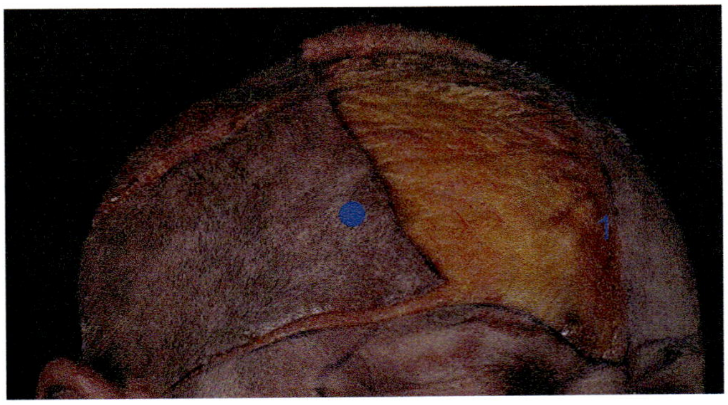

Figure 2.2 The anterior temporal skin (1) is thin, mobile and hairless, while the posterior aspect (blue dot) is thick, less mobile, highly vascularized, and has abundant hair. The temporal skin is tightly adherent to the superficial fat layer.

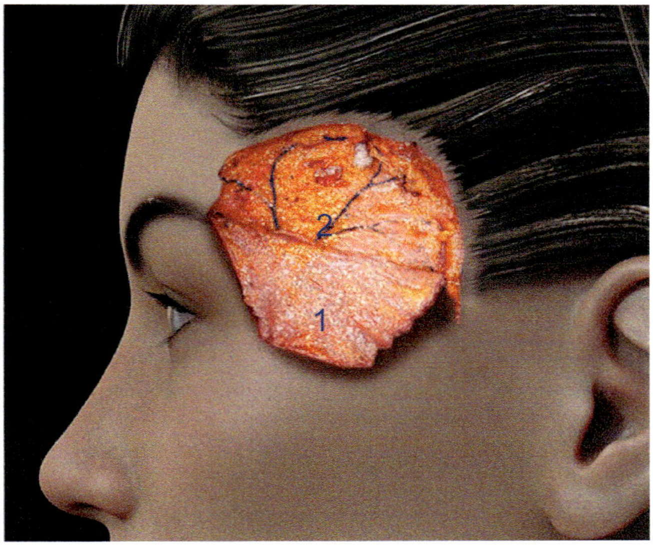

Figure 2.3 The subcutaneous fat (2) lies between the skin (1) and temporoparietal fascia, and forming a scant layer containing the hair follicles of the scalp.

10. Periosteum
11. Bone (Figure 2.8)

AGING

With aging, the upper part of face becomes more concave, the hairline starts to recede and cutaneous thinning and wrinkling leads to prominence of underlying vessels (Figure 2.9).

The bony margins of the zygomatic arch, temporal line and lateral orbital rim become more prominent, and narrowing of the upper face contrasts adversely with high cheekbones or a fuller midface. Volume loss in all the temporal layers may contribute to temporal hollowing, thus contributing significantly to the manifestation of both aging and disease.

Weight loss, inhibition of skeletal growth and soft tissue or bone injury may also cause volumetric loss of the temporal fat compartments. With temporal hollowing (Figure 2.10), the tail of the brow loses support, thus contributing to a tired and saggy appearance.

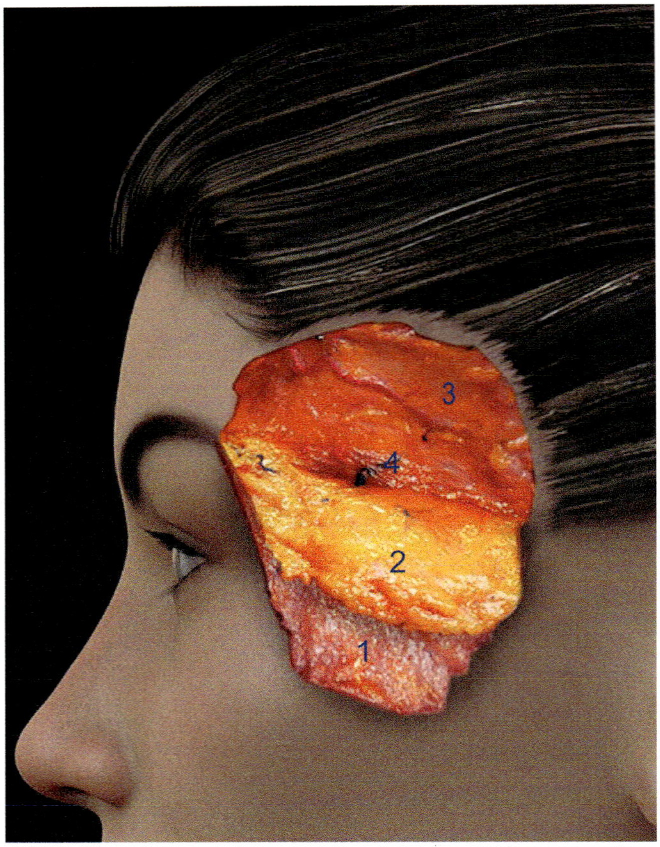

Figure 2.4 The superficial temporal fascia (3) lies just beneath the skin and superficial fat. It is the direct continuation of the SMAS above the zygomatic arch and is closely related to the superficial temporal artery and the frontal branch of the facial nerve. The superficial temporal fascia consists of highly vascular connective tissue which can be dissected as a distinct layer.

SKIN

The anterior temporal skin is thin, mobile and hairless, while the posterior aspect is thick, less mobile, highly vascularized, and has abundant hair (Figure 2.11). Temporal skin is tightly adherent to the superficial fat layer and prone to actinic damage and dyspigmentation. A recent study described an unexpectedly high incidence of non-melanoma skin cancer (NMSC) along the course of frontotemporal arterial branches, with pulsatile arterial blood flow possibly being factorial in determining the precise localization of NMSC, in addition to ultraviolet (UV) exposure. Physicians should be vigilant as to the possibility of cutaneous malignancies while performing aesthetic facial assessments [2].

FAT

The youthful temple is characterized by fullness of four temporal fat layers [3]. These are highly compartmentalized and develop distinct age-related changes in both volume and position. While all the structures in the temporal hollow may contribute to temporal hollowing, loss in different layers results in distinct contour changes. Loss of the deep temporal fat pad is pathognomonic, causing increased prominence of the lateral orbital rim and zygomatic arch. The 4 temporal fat compartments may be divided into two superficial fat compartments-lateral temporal-cheek fat compartment and lateral orbital fat compartment—in the subcutaneous layer, and two deeper compartments—the upper and lower temporal compartment—in the loose areolar tissue layer. A recent study by Cotofana et al. (2019) has raised the hypothesis that the zygomatic arch functions as a boundary between the two superficial temporal compartments and the midfacial fat compartments, causing these to be discrete entities.

The subcutaneous fat (Figure 2.12) is a scant layer containing hair follicles and lying between the skin and superficial fascia, whilst the superficial fat (temporal layer 4):

- Lies between the superficial and deep layer of the deep temporal fascia.
- Is a loose areolar connective tissue plane often utilized for filling with cannula.
- Is divided into a superoposterior (temporal) and inferoanterior (orbital) portion by the inferior temporal septum [4].

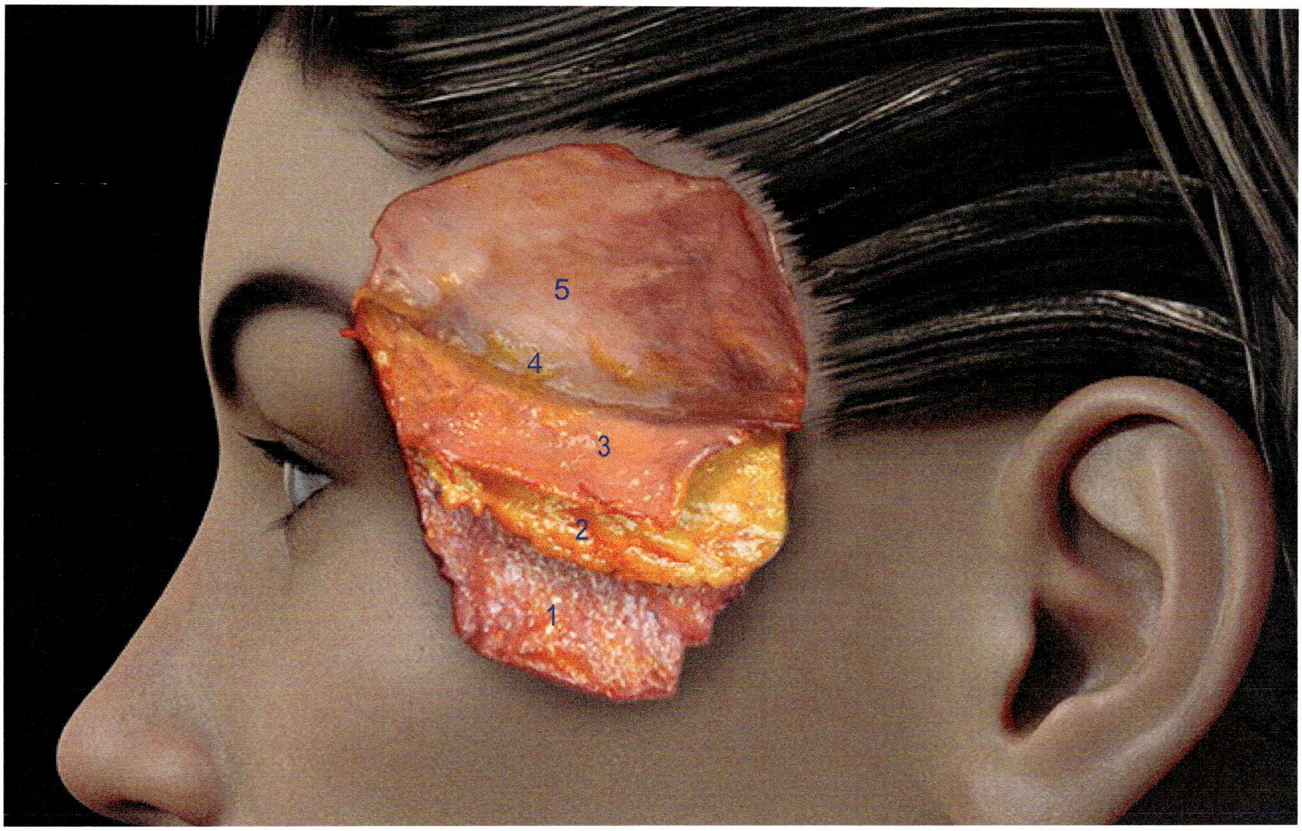

Figure 2.5 The deep temporal fascia (DTF) (5) is a thick layer of aponeurotic tissue directly covering the temporalis muscle and extends from the temporal crest to the zygomatic arch. The DTF splits into a superficial and deep layer before reaching the zygomatic arch and encloses the superficial temporal fat pad. The superficial layer of the DTF is visible over the muscle, with the superficial temporal fascia deflected; (4) denotes loose areolar tissue layer.

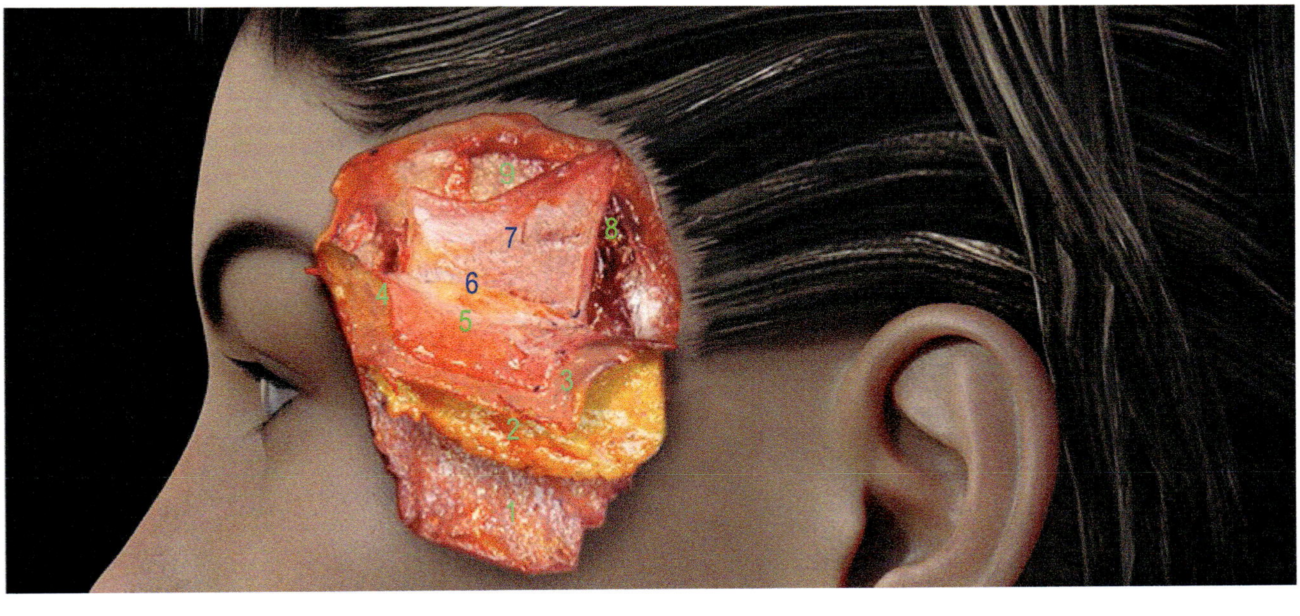

Figure 2.6 The deep layer of the DTF (7) is shown just above the temporalis muscle (8), whilst the superficial layer of DTF is reflected.

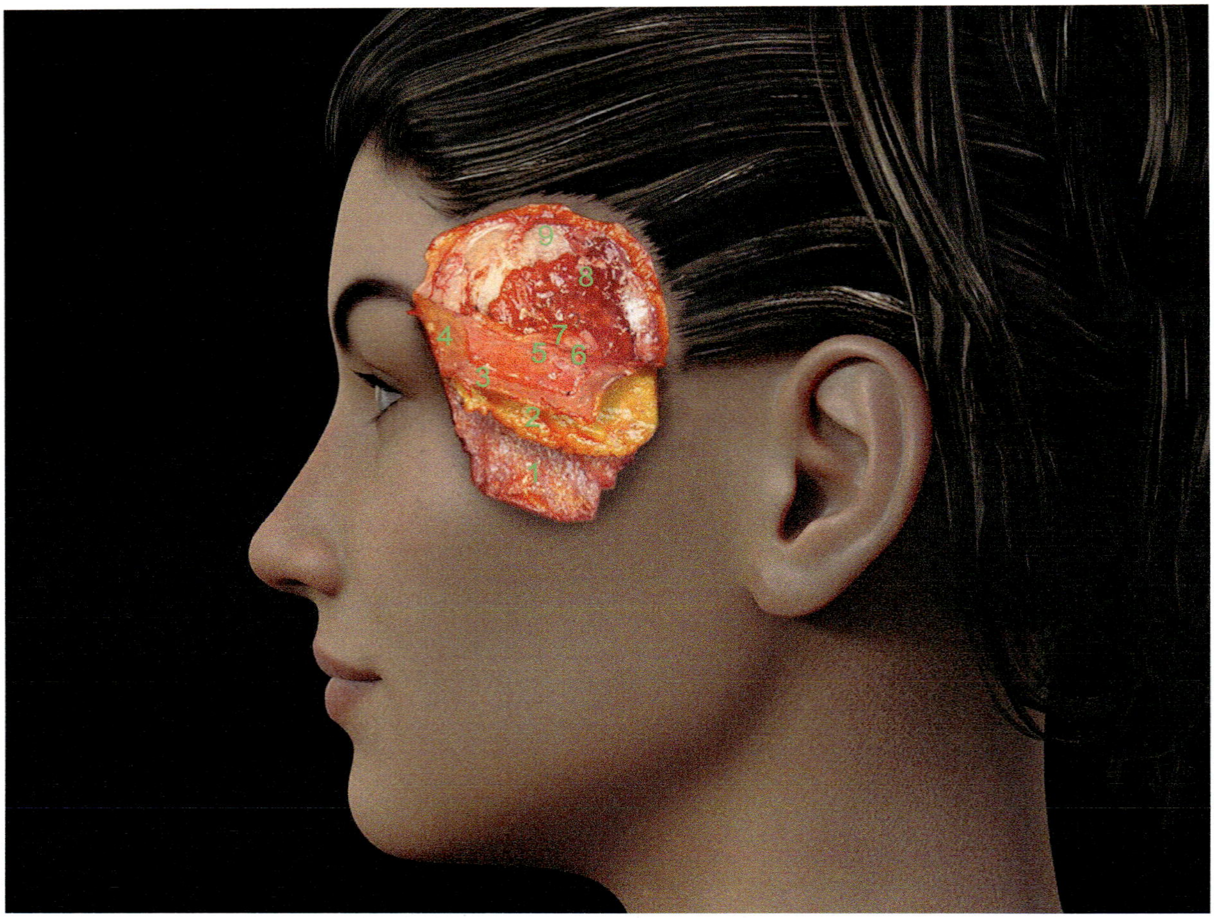

Figure 2.7 Temporalis muscle (8) is shown between bone (9) and the deep temporal fascia (7).

The temporal compartment is larger and substantially avascular.

The orbital compartment is smaller and crossed by both the frontal branch of the facial nerve and the sentinel vein.

- Connected to the SOOF and ROOF, respectively, through the temporal tunnel and the superior interval [5].

Deep temporal fat (temporal layer 8)

- Lies between the deep temporal fascia and the temporal muscle.
- Comprises the temporal extension of the Bichat's fat pad or buccal fat pad [7].

The buccal fat pad is the deep fat pad of the cheek which facilitates sliding of the masticatory muscles

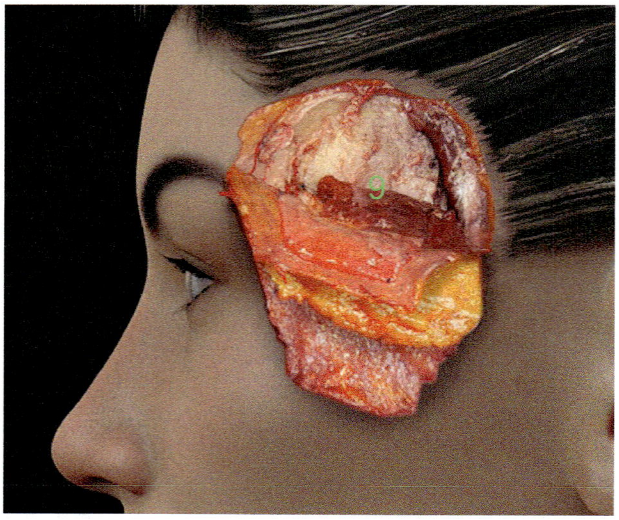

Figure 2.8 The bone (9) forms the deepest layer of the temporal fossa, with the pterion representing the confluence of the greater wing of the sphenoid, squamous portion of the temporal bone, frontal bone, and parietal bone.

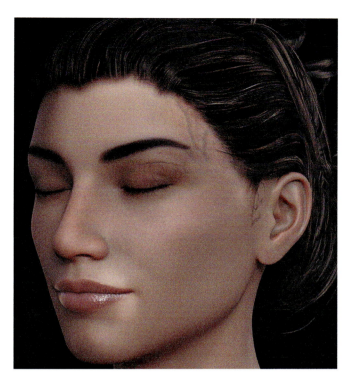

Figure 2.9 The effects of aging include: hairline recession, cutaneous thinning and wrinkling, prominence of underlying vessels (see superficial temporal vein), and greater visibility of the orbital margin and temporal crest due to volume loss in all temporal layers.

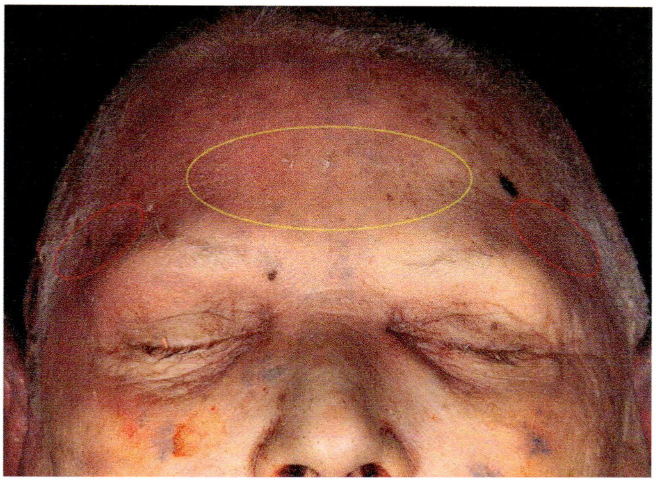

Figure 2.10 With aging there is hollowing of the forehead, suprabrow area and temples. The tail of the eyebrow loses support and moves downwards, causing a tired, sad appearance with excess skin visible in the upper eyelid.

and has three extensions: buccal, pterygoid, and temporal.

- The temporal extension passes below the zygomatic arch to end between the deep temporal fascia and the temporal muscle [3].
- HA filler placed in this compartment may migrate to the cheek [6].

RETAINING LIGAMENTS

The retinacular ligaments of the temple (Figure 2.13) were first described by Moss et al. [4] and comprise the:

- Superior temporal septum which
  - Has an arched shape.
  - Connects the temporoparietal fascia to the bone of the temporal crest.
  - Ends medially in the temporal ligamentous adhesion (TLA).
- Inferior temporal septum which
  - Crosses the temporal fossa obliquely to connect the TLA to the acoustic meatus.
  - Divides the temporoparietal fat pad into a temporal and orbital compartment.

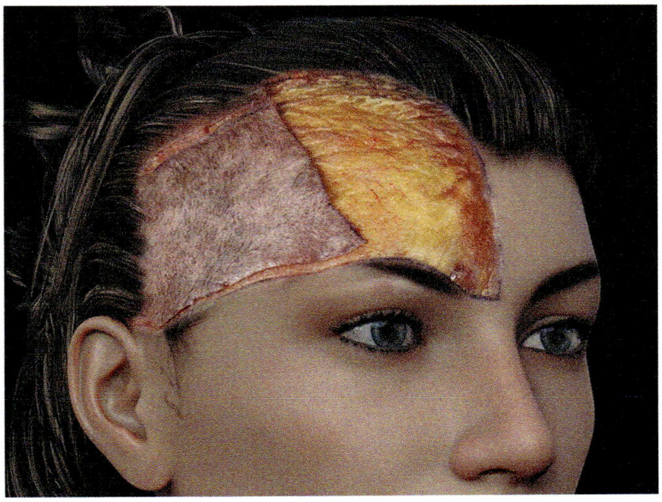

Figure 2.11 Temporal skin in this specimen is thin, and the vessels can be seen in transparency.

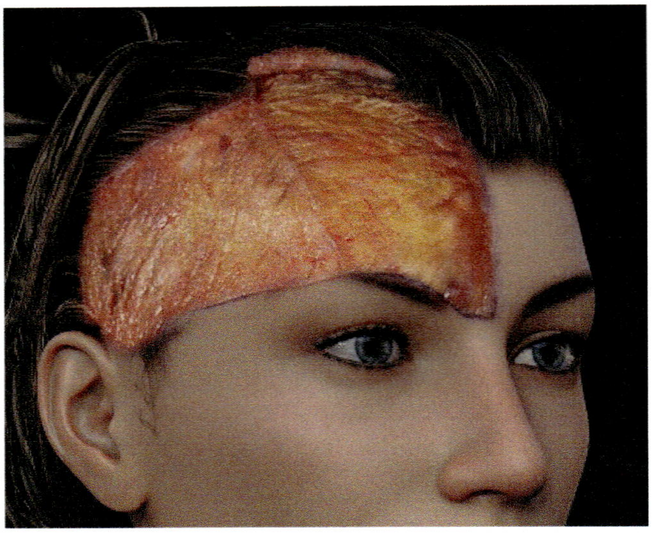

Figure 2.12 The superficial temporal fat lies over the zygomatic arch, between the superficial and deep layer of the deep temporal fascia. The volume of this fat pad is variable. When the canula penetrates the superficial layer of the deep fascia, a pop can be heard. Note that the middle temporal artery runs in this layer.

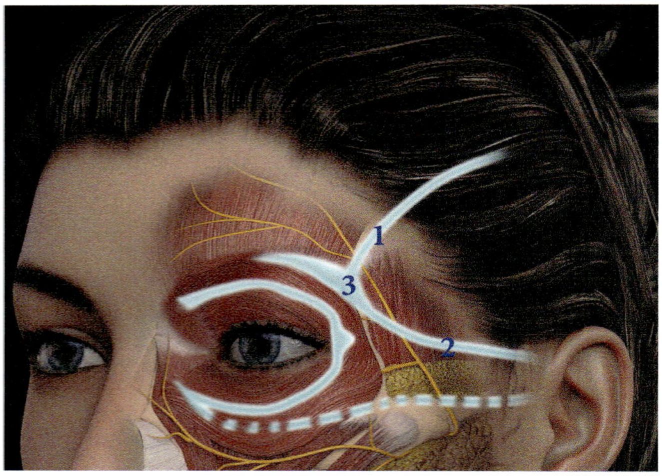

Figure 2.13 The retinacular ligaments of the temple: Superior temporal septum (1) is the upper limit of the temporal fossa. This is a fusion zone between bone and superficial fascia. The inferior temporal septum (2) crosses the temporal fossa obliquely to connect the TLA (3) to the acoustic meatus and divides the temporoparietal fat pad into temporal and orbital compartments.

  - Is an important landmark for the frontal branch of the facial nerve and the anterior branch of the superficial temporal artery.
- Temporal ligamentous adhesion (TLA) [5] which
  - Is a triangular ligamentous region positioned in the anterior part of the temporal crest.
  - Represents the merging point of the superior temporal septum, the inferior temporal septum, and the supraorbital ligamentous adhesion [8].

FASCIA

Superficial Temporal Fascia/ Temporoparietal Fascia (TPF)

- Lies just beneath skin and superficial fat
- Merges with the galea aponeurotica at the temporal crest
- Is the direct continuation of the SMAS above the zygomatic arch
- Consists of highly vascular connective tissue, which can be dissected as a distinct layer
- Is closely related to the superficial temporal artery and the frontal branch of the facial nerve running inside or just beneath the TPF
- Divides the subcutaneous fat from the temporoparietal fat and loose areolar tissue [9]

Deep Temporal Fascia

- A thick layer of aponeurotic tissue directly covering the temporalis muscle
- Extends from the temporal crest to the zygomatic arch as a direct continuation of the cranial periosteum
- Splits into a superficial and deep layer before reaching the zygomatic arch
- Encloses the superficial temporal fat pad, middle temporal artery, and vein [6]

MUSCLE

The temporalis muscle (Figure 2.14) is a large, fan-shaped masticatory muscle covering the lateral aspect of the cranium. At its origin, it is tightly adherent to the temporal line, while its tendinous portion passes beneath the zygomatic process to insert into the coronoid process of the mandible. It may be divided into anterior, middle, and posterior regions. As a masticatory muscle, it is capable of generating great contractile strength. The temporalis tendon extends from its insertion at the upper anterior border and inner surface of the coronoid process and mandibular ramus to approximately 45 mm superior to the zygomatic arch. When treating the temporalis muscle with botulinum toxin for headache or bruxism, injections need to be placed into the muscular portion of temporalis for maximal efficacy.

Understanding this anatomy is of great clinical importance, as toxin placement in the tendon is highly ineffective [10,11].

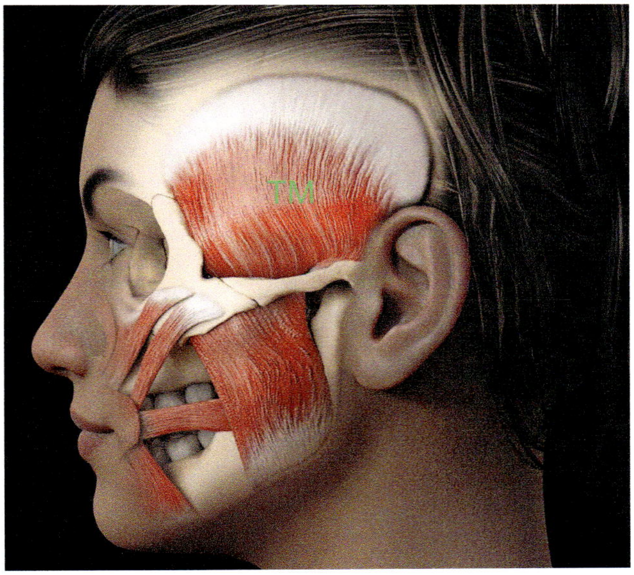

Figure 2.14 The temporalis muscle (TM) is a large, fan-shaped masticatory muscle. It originates from the temporal bone (temporalis crest) and its tendinous portion passes beneath the zygomatic process to insert into the coronoid process of the mandible.

The temporalis tendon disperses at the posterior border and can accordingly be divided into three types according to insertion (Figure 2.22).

1. Just anterior to L2
2. Between L2 and L3
3. Between L3 and L4

The temporalis muscle receives its vascular supply from the anterior and posterior deep temporal arteries arising from the maxillary artery; vessels anastomose with branches of the middle temporal artery which arises from the superficial temporal artery.

Neural innervation is from the deep temporal nerves arising from the mandibular nerve:

- All the branches of the deep temporal nerve traverse the temporal tendon, only branching after entering the temporalis muscle.
- The anterior branch runs through the anterior fibers which provide upward elevation of the mandible.
- The posterior branch traverses its posterior fibers which provide backward elevation of the mandible.
- The middle branch runs through the middle fibers.
- The temporal fascia splits into two fascial layers enclosing a fat pad at approximately 1.5 cm superior to the zygomatic arch. The muscle lies deep to this divided layer.
- The muscle is thickest before its insertion on the coronoid process of mandible.

VASCULARIZATION

Superficial Temporal Artery

The external carotid artery divides into the maxillary artery and superficial temporal artery (STA). The STA (Figures 2.15 and 2.16):

- Is the smaller branch, directionally appearing to be a continuation of external carotid artery.
- Is the primary arterial supply to the temporal fossa.

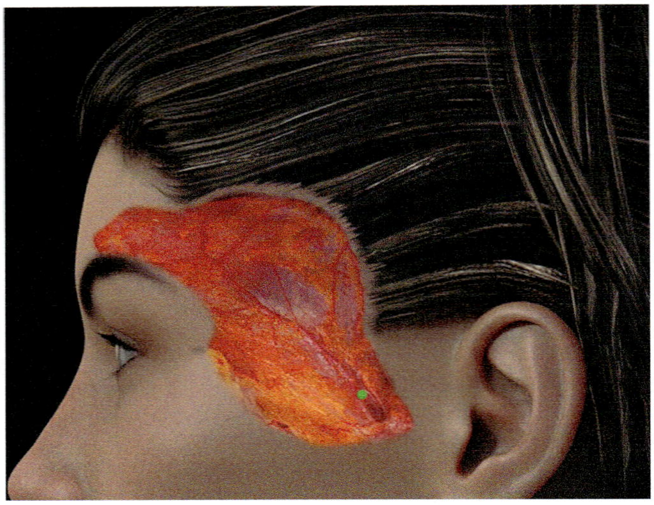

Figure 2.15 The STA (green dot) is palpable and frequently visible as a pulsation. This is an important safety aid during aesthetic medicine treatments.

- Begins in the parotid gland tissue, just behind the neck of the mandible, and passes superficial to the zygomatic arch.
- Gives off the transverse facial artery (just before leaving the parotid) which
  - Runs anteriorly through the substance of the gland
  - Travels between the lower border of the zygomatic arch and parotid duct
  - Communicates with the facial artery and infraorbital artery during its course.
- STA continues its upward course and, at a variable distance from the zygomatic arch, divides into the frontal and parietal branch.
- The parietal branch of the STA:
  - Curves posteriorly to run on superficial temporal fossa and
  - Communicates with posterior auricular, occipital artery, and its fellow from the other side.
- The frontal branch of the STA:
  - Runs within the superficial temporal fascia and takes an anterior, tortuous course to run on the galeal layer [12].
  - May communicate with the ipsilateral supraorbital and supratrochlear artery and its contralateral artery.

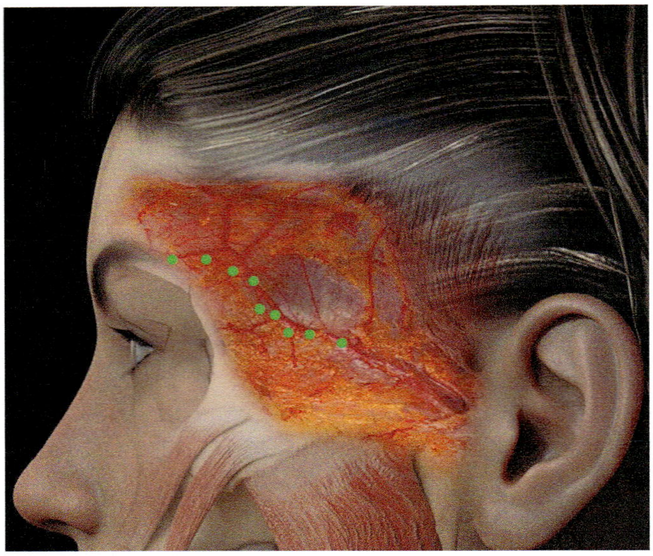

Figure 2.16 The frontal branch of the STA runs within the superficial temporal fascia, takes an anterior tortuous course, and communicates with the ipsilateral supraorbital and supratrochlear arteries.

  - Is palpable and frequently visible as a pulsation.
  - Is an important safety aid during aesthetic medicine treatments.

Middle Temporal Artery

During its course, the STA gives off the middle temporal artery just above the zygomatic arch:

- It perforates the deep temporal fascia, giving branches to the temporalis muscle.
- The zygomatico-orbital branch runs between the two layers of deep temporal fascia, parallel to the zygomatic arch, to the lateral orbital angle.

Deep Temporal Arteries

The anterior and posterior branches of the deep temporal artery travel with the middle temporal artery, deep in the temporalis muscle, diminishing in diameter on their upward journey.

- The middle part of the maxillary artery gives rise to the anterior and posterior deep temporal arteries, which run cranially between the temporalis muscle and the pericranium.
- These branches supply the temporalis muscle and anastomose with the branches of the middle temporal artery from the superficial temporal artery.
- The anterior deep temporal artery communicates with the branches of the lacrimal artery through small branches that perforate the greater wing of the sphenoid and zygomatic bones.

Superficial Temporal Vein

The superficial temporal vein drains a widespread region of the scalp. It:

- Joins with the corresponding vein of the contralateral side, and with the supratrochlear, supraorbital, posterior auricular, and occipital veins.
- Has a variable number of branches in the scalp.
- Runs independently from the frontal and parietal branches of the superficial temporal artery, except for its proximal portion.
- Crosses the zygomatic arch, unites with the maxillary vein inside the parotid gland, and forms the retromandibular vein.
- Receives blood from the parotid veins, articular veins from the temporomandibular joint, anterior auricular veins, and the transverse facial vein.

Middle Temporal Vein (MTV)

The MTV runs approximately 1 cm above and parallel to the zygomatic arch, buried in the superficial temporal fat pad, and travels between the superficial and deep layers of the deep temporal fascia. It (Figure 2.17):

- Is an important blood vessel in the temporal fossa.
- Drains blood from the temporal muscle and deep aspect of the temporal fossa.

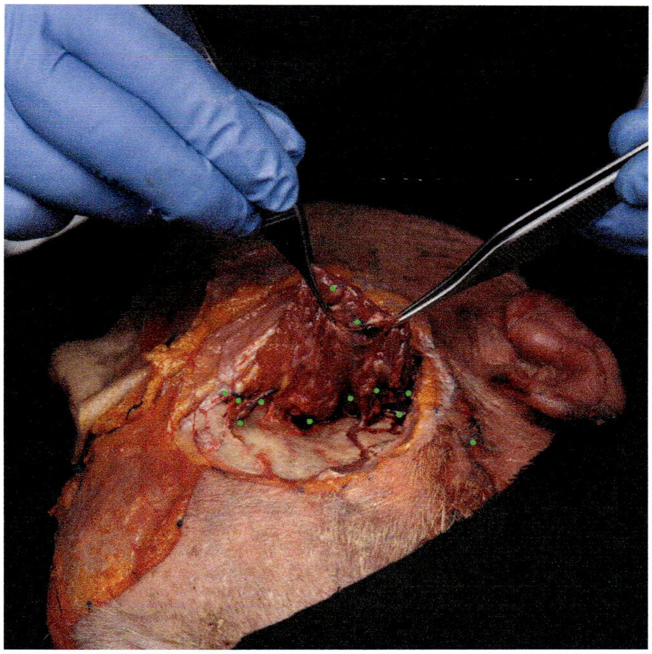

Figure 2.17 Note the large venous network visible within the thickness of the muscle and anteriorly the connection with the sentinel vein.

- Receives a communicating vessel from the supraorbital vein.
- Travels between the two layers of deep temporal fascia.
- Joins the superficial temporal vein just at or below the level of the zygomatic arch.

Zygomaticotemporal Veins

Generally, there are two veins, of which the major is called the "sentinel vein." These veins:

- Are communicating vessels between the deep and superficial venous circle.
- Travel with the zygomaticotemporal nerve.
- Run inside the orbital portion of the temporoparietal fat pad, inferior and medially to the inferior temporal septum.

The **sentinel vein** (medial zygomaticotemporal vein; Figure 2.18) is found in the superficial temporal fat pad lateral to the lateral orbital rim. It passes from the subcutaneous layer through the

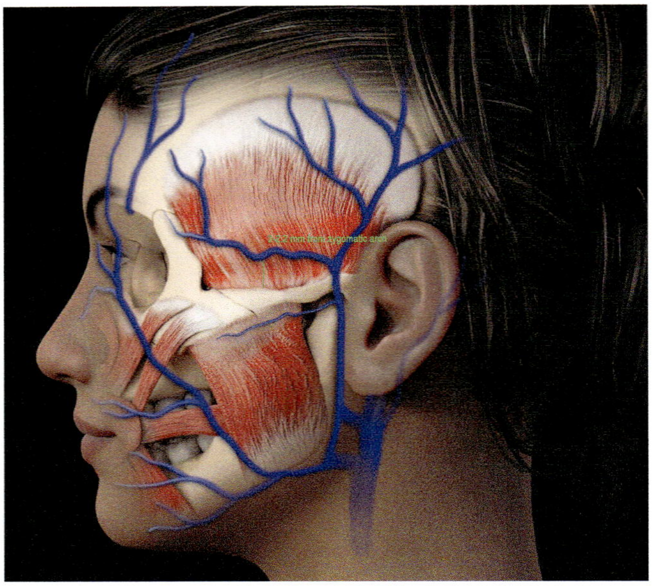

Figure 2.18 The sentinel vein (medial zygomaticotemporal vein) runs in the superficial temporal fat pad lateral to the lateral orbital rim and may be visible 2–2.2 cm from zygomatic arch (upper margin) 1.5 cm above and lateral to the external margin of the eye. It is important to avoid this vessel as it can bleed profusely if punctured.

superficial temporal fascia and then perforates the superficial layer of the deep temporal fascia to join in the middle temporal vein [13].
  - It may be visible in the recumbent patient in a position 1.5 cm above and lateral to the external margin of the eye.
  - May bleed profusely when punctured.
  - Is a landmark for the frontal branch of the facial nerve, which is located 1 cm behind it.
- Several perforator vessels (on average 2.6 with a range of 1–6) traverse the superficial temporal fascia layer, loose areolar tissue layer, and superficial layer of the deep temporal fascia, originating from or joining in the middle temporal vessels. The highest density of perforators is located at the junction of the zygomatic arch and lateral orbital rim (24 mm on average, range 18–32 mm) cranial to the anterior half of the zygomatic arch.
- The superficial venous plexus may be better visualized under good lighting or upon having the patient do the Valsalva maneuver or tilt their head forward.

INNERVATION

Sensory: Branches of the mandibular portion of the trigeminal nerve (cranial nerve V).

Motor: 2–4 temporal branches of the facial nerve cross the zygomatic arch obliquely one fingerbreadth behind the posterior margin of the zygomatic process of the frontal bone, running caudally parallel to the frontal branch of the superficial temporal artery (Figure 2.19).

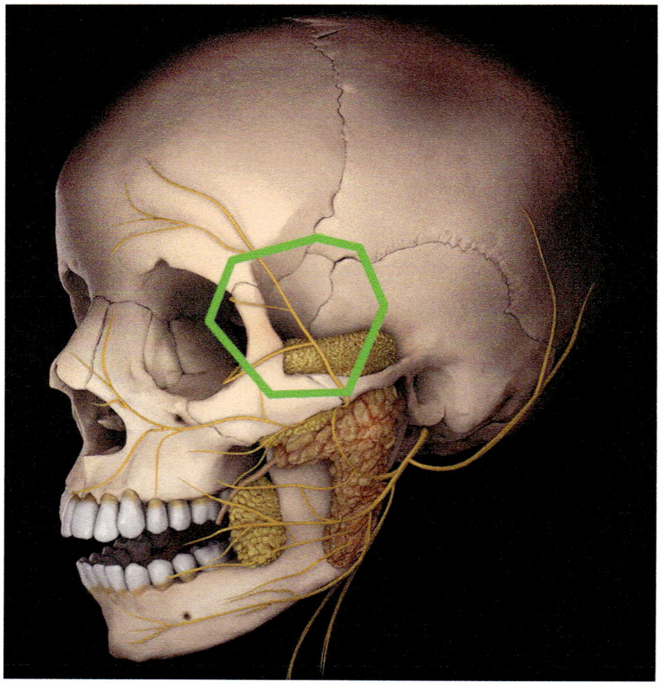

Figure 2.19 Branches of the facial nerve (note the course of the frontal branch through the temporal fossa).

Frontal Branch of the Facial Nerve

The facial nerve divides within the parotid gland into frontal, zygomatic, buccal, mandibular and cervical branches [14].

- The frontal branch crosses the temporal fossa to innervate the frontalis muscle.
- Frontal nerve injury causes paralysis of the ipsilateral frontal muscle, having important implications in facelift surgery.
- The course of the frontal branch can be approximated by a line extending from 0.5 cm below the external acoustic meatus to 1.5 cm superior to the orbital rim.
- The nerve is tightly adherent to bone at the zygomatic arch and subsequently travels upward to the loose areolar connective tissue just below the temporoparietal fascia.
- The inferior temporal septum is an important anatomical landmark of the frontal branch [15].

Zygomaticotemporal Nerve (ZTN)

The ZTN:

- Is one of the two terminal branches of the zygomatic nerve, which is a branch of the maxillary division of the trigeminal nerve (V2).
- The zygomatic nerve:
    - Enters the orbit via the inferior orbital fissure.
    - Travels along the lateral orbital wall.
    - Divides into the zygomaticofacial nerve (ZFN) and ZTN.
- The ZTN provides sensation to the temporal skin and parasympathetic innervation to the lacrimal gland.
- The ZTN exits the lateral orbit via a bony canal and emerges in the temporal fossa via a bony foramen, the localization of which has considerable ethnic variation.
- After exiting the orbit, the ZTN enters the deep aspect of the temporalis muscle or travels between the temporal periosteum and the temporalis muscle before piercing the deep temporal fascia.
- Injury of the ZTN may cause temporary paresthesia and anesthesia in the temporal region.

Auriculotemporal Nerve (ATN)

The ATN:

- Is a branch of the mandibular division of the trigeminal nerve V3.
- Is the sensory nerve providing sensation to the tragus, anterior ear, and posterior temporal region.
- Carries autonomic nervous fibers to the scalp and the parotid gland.
- Emerges within the superficial parotid gland, travels cranially within the temporoparietal fascia, and crosses the posterior aspect of the zygomatic arch.
- Runs parallel and lateral to the STA as it runs cephalad.
- Becomes more superficial in the upper temple, lying superficial to the temporoparietal fascia.

The course of the frontal branch can be approximated by a line extending from 0.5 cm below the external acoustic meatus to 1.5 cm superior to the orbital rim.

The frontal branch crosses the temporal fossa to innervate the frontalis muscle, and nerve injury causes paralysis of the ipsilateral frontal muscle.

BONE

The temporal region is highly variable in both morphology and stability and undergoes bone loss with age. Although this loss is not as profound as in areas such as the mandible, maxilla and orbit, it may contribute to temporal hollowing (Figure 2.20).

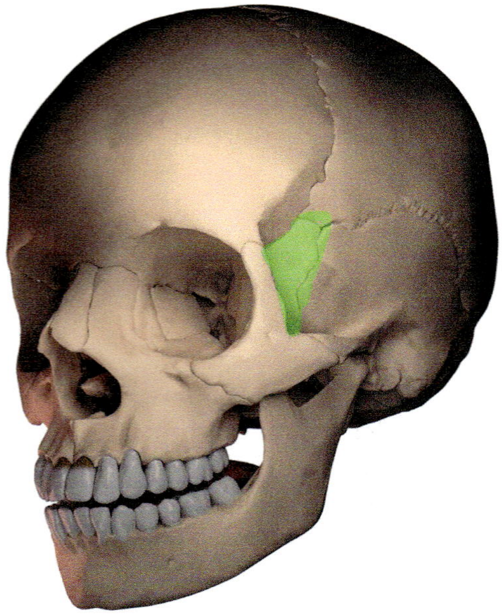

Figure 2.20 The temporal bone undergoes reabsorption with aging. The thinnest section is the pterion (green), where bone thickness varies from 0.9 mm to 13 mm.

The pterion is the H-shaped formation marking the union of four cranial bones:

- Greater wing of the sphenoid bone
- Squamous portion of the temporal bone
- Frontal bone
- Parietal bone

This is the thinnest part of the skull and receives its name from the Greek root *pterion*, meaning wing (said to represent the point where Hermes' wings were attached to his head). It lies superior to the zygomatic arch, posterior to the frontozygomatic suture, and overlies the anterior branch of the middle meningeal artery. The pterion is one of the craniometric points for radiological or anthropological skull measurement.

A recent publication states that bone thickness in this region varies from 0.9 mm to 13 mm [16].

HOW I DO IT: BOTULINUM TOXIN

- The temporalis tendon is fan-shaped, with the most distant tendinous point located 45 mm from the zygomatic arch. The BoNT-A injection site into the temporalis muscle should be at least 45 mm from the zygomatic arch as injections into the tendon are ineffective (Figure 2.21) [10].
- Sihler's staining shows that the nerve endings sensitive to BoNT-A action are densely dispersed within the temporalis muscle, proving the muscular region to be an effective site for BoNT-A injections.
- For identification of the temporalis muscle, place the second finger on the inferior margin of the zygomatic arch. The tip of the thumb will then be located approximately 45 mm from the zygomatic arch, making it easy to identify the temporalis muscle and thus the effective injection site for BoNT-A.
- For optimal clinical effect, mid-temporal toxin injections need to be given in the muscle and least 45 mm above the zygomatic arch to avoid injecting into the tendon [17].
- Up to 20 U of onabotulinum toxin may be given in 3–4 areas according to muscle activity and clinical need.
- Depending on clinical indication, both superficial and deep injections may be necessary.
- Superficial injections are performed in the thinner upper regions of the muscle in a fan shape [11], with up to 20 U of onabotulinum toxin being distributed over 3–4 points.
- The temporalis muscle may be injected 1 cm behind the hairline to avoid frontalis muscle paresis, then a further 1 cm behind it. Injections should preferably be applied at painful "trigger points" (Figure 2.22) [18].

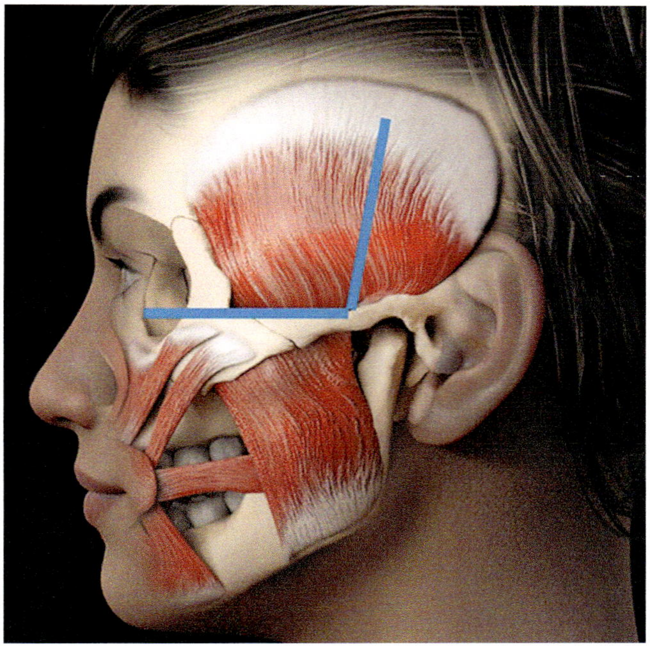

Figure 2.21 The finger technique to identify the temporal muscle. For optimal clinical effect, mid-temporal toxin injections should be performed in the muscle at least 45 mm above the zygomatic arch to avoid injecting into the tendon where efficacy is suboptimal.

Anatomical considerations when doing deeper injections include:

- The superficial temporal fascia splits into two fascial layers enclosing a fat pad at approximately 1.5 cm superior to the zygomatic arch. The muscle lies deep to this divided layer.
- The muscle is thickest before insertion on the coronoid process of mandible.

HOW I DO IT: FILLERS

- Mark the temporal fusion line, remembering that it may be most palpable at the level of the eyebrow. Meticulously mark the lateral orbital rim and superior border of the zygomatic arch.
- Palpate and mark arterial pulsation (e.g., ascending STA).
- Mark venous structures.
- Mark the desired treatment area 1 cm up from the inferior border of the fusion line and 1 cm lateral (Swift point) over the shallow superomedial aspect of the temporal rectangle (Figures 2.23–2.25) [19].

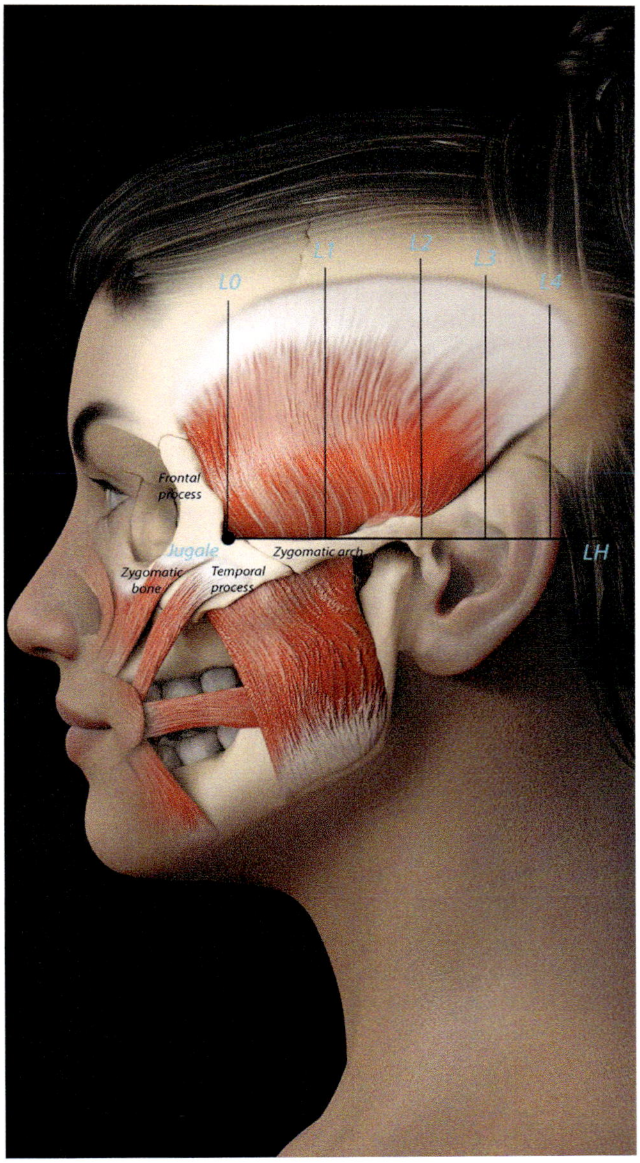

Figure 2.22 The temporalis muscle may be injected 1 cm behind the hairline to avoid frontalis muscle paresis, then 1 cm behind it. Injections should preferably be applied at "trigger points."

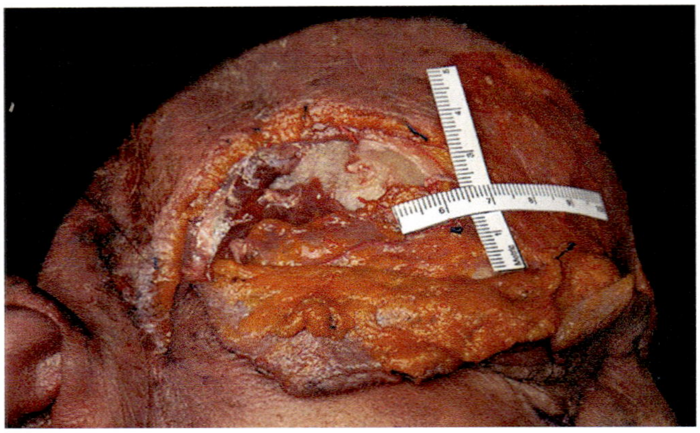

Figure 2.23 The Swift point coincides with the shallow zone of the temporal fossa. Injections in this area also directly affect the position of the eyebrow tail.

- In this relatively avascular area, the muscle fibers are less dense and vessels are of smaller diameter [20].
- Cleanse meticulously with chlorhexidine, alcohol, or alternative, being vigilant against dripping chlorhexidine into the eyes with possible corneal damage.
- Inject with a needle onto bone, ensuring that the tip remains on bone during the entire injection; be aware of bevel position (preferably down).
- Having the patient open their mouth releases temporalis tension and may diminish injection discomfort.
- Aspirate for at least 5–7 seconds, while understanding that a negative aspiration does not always safeguard against inadvertent intravascular placement.
- Release plunger pressure and wait a few seconds to check for reflux.
- Inject VERY SLOWLY, while constantly monitoring for undue pain or blanching in watershed vascular areas.
- Placing an index finger behind the injection point diminishes posterior product migration, thus encouraging circumferential and downward product flow.
- The use of 0.3–0.7 mL of cohesive HA product generally gives adequate correction.
- Maintain gentle pressure for 20–40 seconds upon needle withdrawal in order to minimize possible delayed ecchymoses.
- Filler injection can be done also onto superficial fat pad with low G′ HA and 25G 38 mm cannula (Figure 2.26), or into the deep part of the temporoparietal fascia (Figure 2.26).

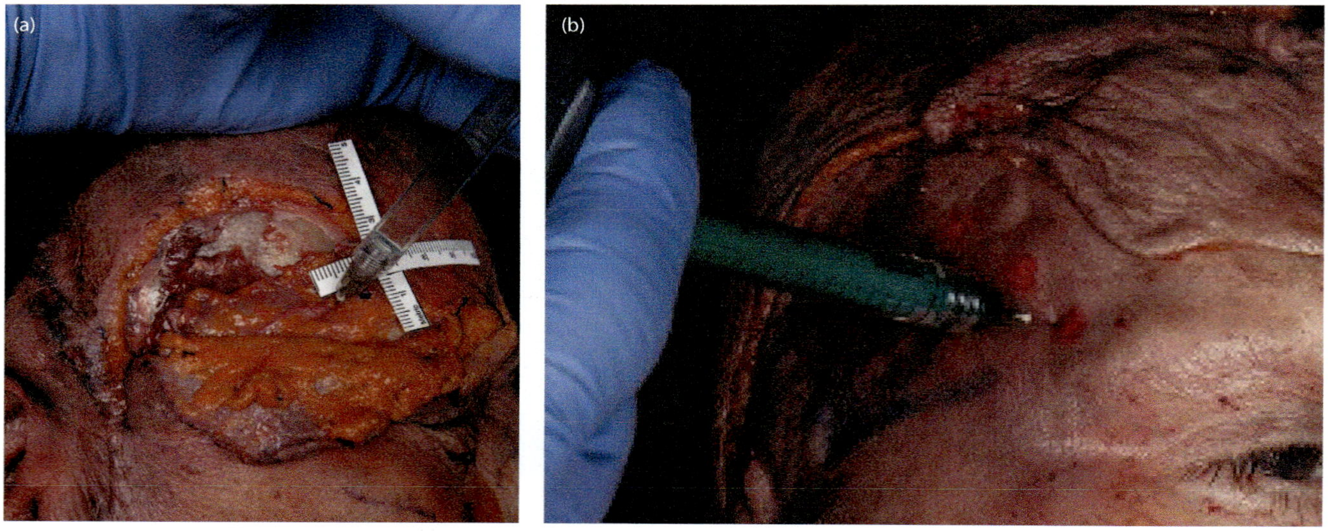

Figure 2.24 (a) The Swift point (indicated) is considered to be a safe point due to the absence of large caliber vessels. (b) Injections should be performed perpendicularly and with the tip of the needle in close contact with the bone.

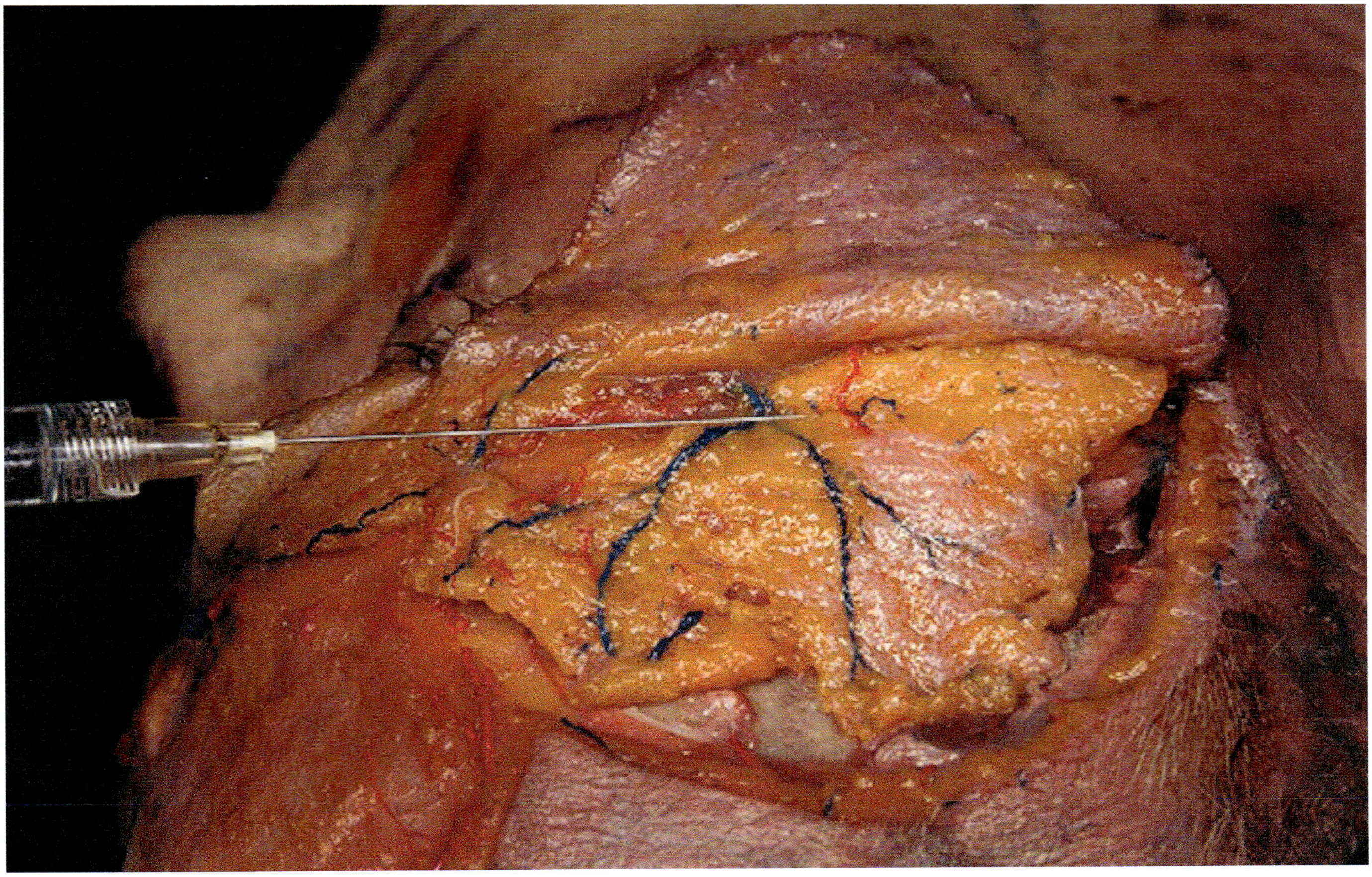

Figure 2.25 Cannula technique for superficial filling of the temporal fossa. A low G′ filler is distributed in a fan pattern in the fat layer 2 just below the skin. Although no large vessels are evident, a rich venous plexus may cause bruising. The filler must be thoroughly massaged to avoid irregularities.

COMPLICATIONS

For general complications and the concept of "safety by depth," see Chapter G. Seckel divided the face into seven functional danger zones [21]; the temporal region includes danger zone 2 (Figure 2.27a and b).

Toxin Safety Considerations

- Initial headache may result.
- Temporal hollowing/atrophy may ensue after the use of high doses of botulinum toxin

Filler Safety Considerations

- Intravascular injection into the superficial temporal arterial system may cause retrograde flow into the ophthalmic system with consequent retinal artery obstruction [22,23].
- Injection into the middle temporal vein may cause ipsilateral necrosis of the palate or pulmonary embolism [24].
- Venous congestion may ensue after high-volume injection or product placement in the superficial plane [25].
- Late ecchymoses may present despite not being immediately visible.

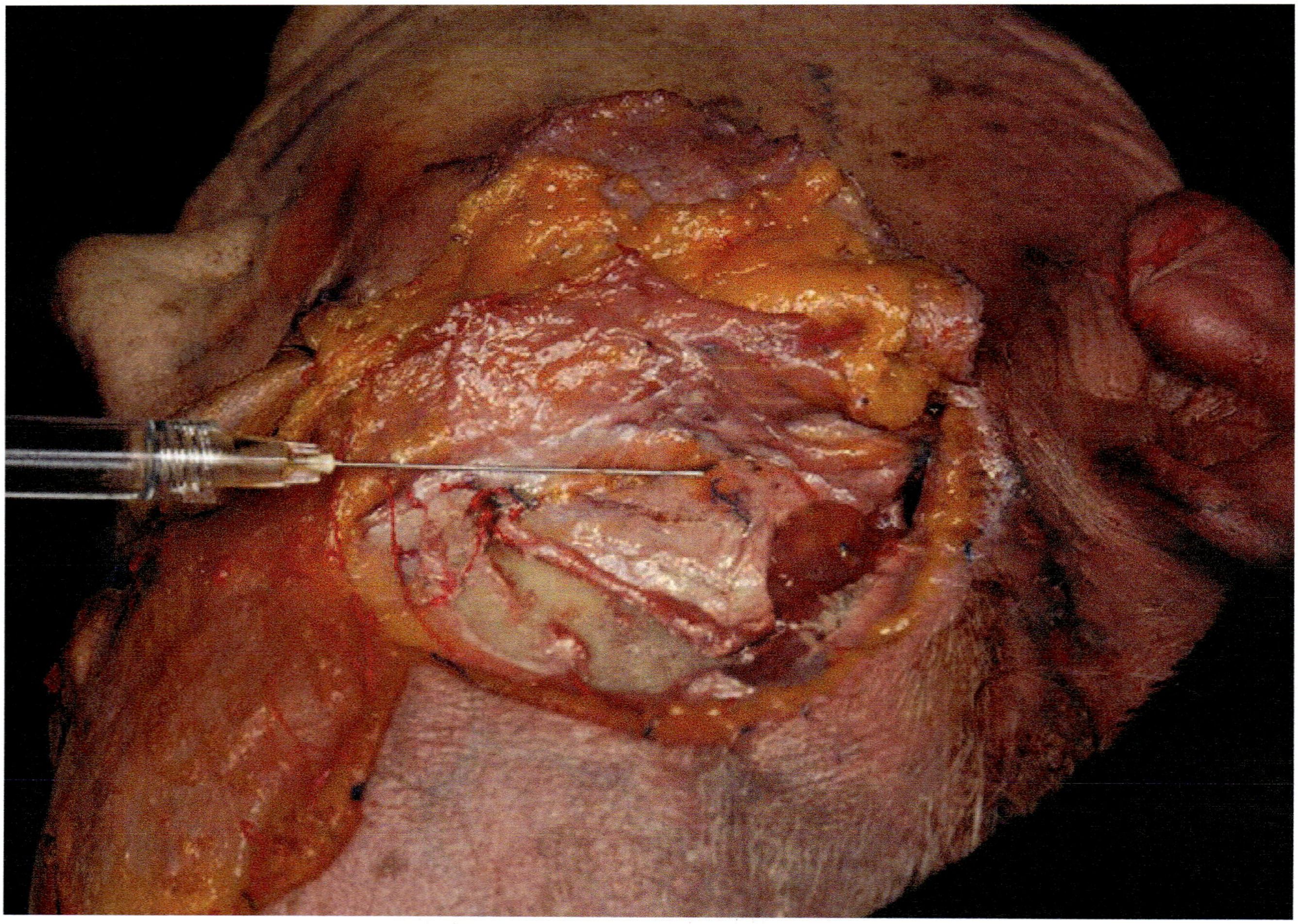

Figure 2.26 The filler may also be distributed via cannula in the connective areolar layer 4, just below the superficial temporal fascia. The cannula is visible just above the deep temporal fascia (layer 5). The superficial temporal fascia is reflected and the superficial temporal artery is seen in its thickness.

- Intracranial injection and filler deposition after penetration of pterion [16].
- Migration into buccal fat pad after injection into deep temporal fat pad.
- Headaches (lasting hours to days) due to rapid expansion of the deep temporal fascia [26].

TOP 10 TIPS

1. Temporal filling is indicated when the brow "disappears around the corner."
2. Overfilling may cause masculinization in female subjects; preferably undercorrect and re-treat when indicated.
3. Using good lighting, the Valsalva maneuver or tapping helps to localize and mark venous structures before treatment.
4. Ask the patient to open their mouth during injection in order to relax the temporalis muscle and reduce discomfort during injection.
5. Inject in the upper "shallow end" of the temporal fossa to ensure needle position below vessel and on bone.
6. Placing an index finger behind the injection point diminishes posterior product migration, thus encouraging circumferential and downward product flow.
7. Compress for 20–40 seconds upon withdrawal of needle to minimize late bruising.

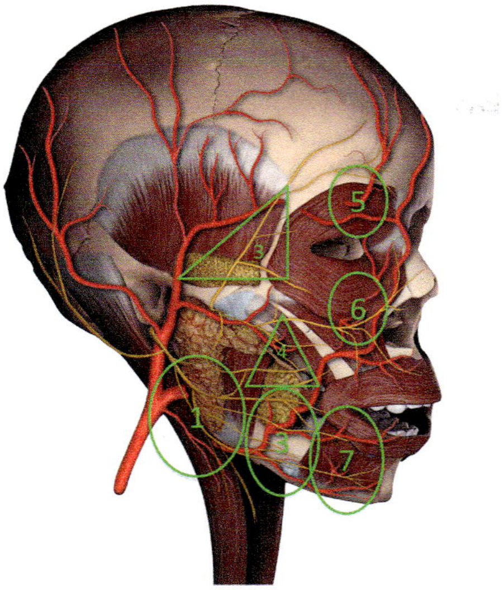

Figure 2.27a Danger areas.

8. Cannula injection in the more superficial plane requires less product but is more prone to venous congestion.
9. When using a cannula, inject perpendicular to the direction of vessels.
10. The anterior branch of the deep temporal artery runs 1.8 cm posterior to and parallel to the orbital rim, while the middle temporal vein runs 1 cm above and parallel to the zygomatic arch.

THE SUPRABROW

During the aging process, youthful contours are lost, and the suprabrow region becomes concave and more prominent. Reflation of this area thus leads to

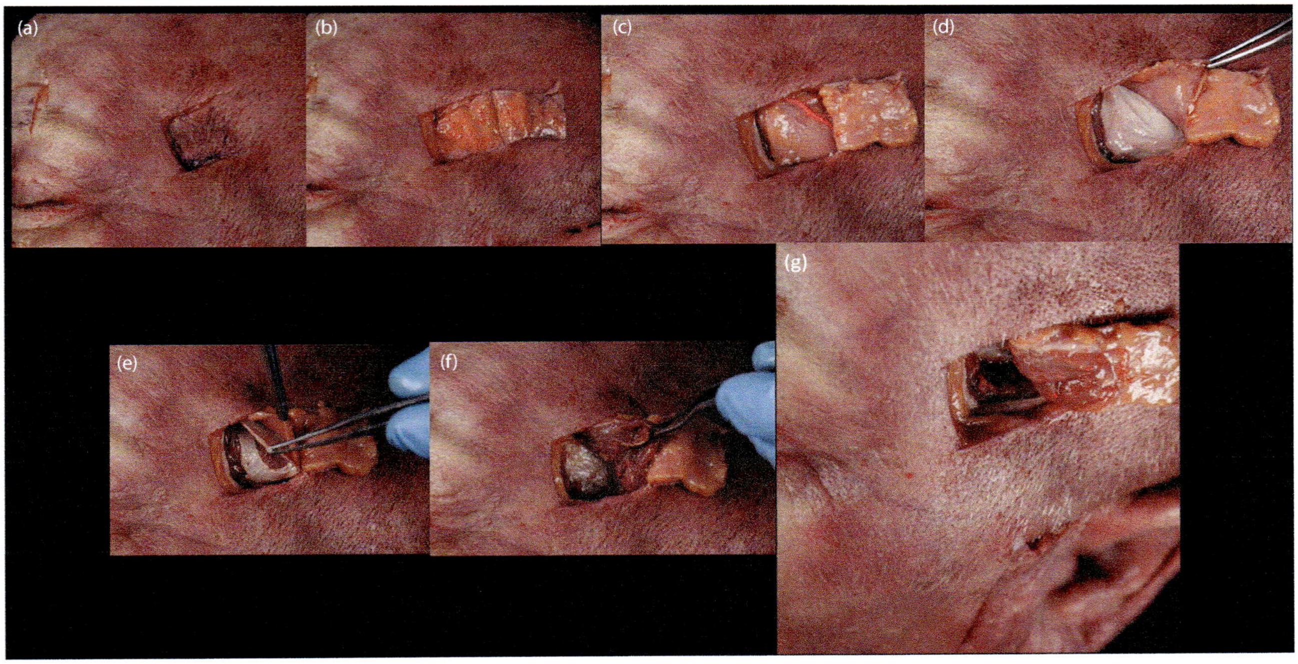

Figure 2.27b The temporal danger region is exposed in layers. (a) Skin. (b) In this specimen, the subcutaneous fat is very scant and the superficial temporal artery, injected with red latex, can be seen in transparency. (c) The superficial temporal fascia has been reflected and the superficial temporal artery is clearly seen. This vessel is anastomosed with the supraorbital artery of the same side and intravascular injection can lead to blindness due to anterior embolization. (d) The superficial layer of the deep temporal fascia is raised by the forceps. The deep temporal fascia is made of a dense connective tissue and is much more resistant than the superficial temporal fascia. (e) Both layers of the deep temporal fascia are visible, lifted by forceps, with the temporal muscle below. (f) With the temporal muscle raised from bone, numerous vessels are visible in the thickness and on the deep surface of the muscle. Intravascular injections can cause distant necrosis or the formation of temporal hematomas. (g) All layers of the temporal fossa are clearly visible. Note the number of vessels present within the muscular portion. It is therefore essential to always inject with the tip of the needle in close contact with the bone.

improved contours, elevation of descended brows, and an improved appearance of the eye area.

The deep fat compartment of the upper eyelid is called the ROOF (retro-orbicularis oculi fat) and it gives shape to the brow and upper eyelid above the supratarsal fold.

- Lies deep to the orbicularis oculi muscle and the inferior extension of the galea aponeurosis.
- Lies superficial to the pericranium.

Treatment goals of placing filler deep to the tail of the brow are [27]:

- Three-dimensional brow correction
- Vertical lifting
- Horizontal brow projection

PRACTICAL TIPS

- Baseline pretreatment photographs are mandatory.
- Pretreatment with neuromodulators may help to raise the brow above the orbital rim and facilitate synergistic effect with fillers.
- Be wary of placing fillers in the suprabrow hollow if the eyebrow position is below the orbital rim.
- Injection of HA at the supraorbital crest [19] will force the eyebrow up if the brow is above the promontory but force the eyebrow down if the brow is at or below the promontory.
- A lateral entry point at the tail of the brow and above the superior orbital rim is suggested.
- In the lower 2 cm of the forehead, arteries run deep on the bone.
- Product placement should be:
  - At or superior to the superior orbital plane.
  - Deep to the orbicularis oculi muscle.
  - In the subQ of the brow (just pre-periosteal).
  - Superior to the supraorbital arteries (not on the periosteum where the large vessels can be found).
  - Via anterograde and retrograde placement.
  - Tapered from medial to lateral, with slight accentuation at the predetermined peak of the brow.
- The non-injecting "smart hand" is essential for positioning the tissue while contouring the brows.
- Blending or molding after treatment with cool ultra- sound gel helps to achieve a smooth, graded result.

References

1. Liew S et al. *Aesthetic Plast Surg.* 2016;40(2): 193–201.
2. Kuonen F et al. *Dermatology.* 2017; 233(2–3):199–204.
3. Rohrich RJ & Pessa JE. *Plast Reconstr Surg.* 2012;129(5S):31–9.
4. Moss CJ et al. *Plast Reconstr Surg.* 2000;105(4):1491–4.
5. Wong C-H et al. *Plast Reconstr Surg.* 2012;129(6). Available from: https://journals.lww.com/plasreconsurg/Fulltext/2012/06000/The_Tear_Trough_Ligament___Anatomical_Basis_for.30.aspx
6. Stuzin JM et al. *Plast Reconstr Surg.* 1992 Mar;89(3):441–9; discussion 450–1. Available from: http://europepmc.org/abstract/MED/1741467
7. Stuzin JM et al. *Plast Reconstr Surg.* 1990 Jan;85(1):29–37. Available from: https:// doi.org/10.1097/00006534-199001000-00006
8. Wong C-H & Mendelson B. *Plast Reconstr Surg.* 2013;132(1). Available from: https://journals.lww.com/plasreconsurg/Fulltext/2013/07000/Facial_Soft_Tissue_Spaces_and_Retaining_Ligaments.9.aspx
9. Mitz V & Peyronie M. *Plast Reconstr Surg.* 1976 Jul;58(1):80–88. Available from: https://doi.org/10.1097/00006534-197607000-00013
10. Choi YJ et al. *Toxins (Basel).* 2016;8(9):1–10.
11. Kahn A et al. *J Oral Med Oral Surg.* 2018; 24(3):107–11.

12. Abul-Hassan HS et al. *Plast Reconstr Surg.* 1986 Jan;77(1):17–28. Available from: http://europepmc.org/abstract/MED/3941846
13. De la Plaza R et al. *Br J Plast Surg.* 1991;44(5):325–32. Available from: http://www.sciencedirect.com/science/article/pii/0007122691901438
14. Stuzin JM et al. *Plast Reconstr Surg.* 1989 Feb;83(2):265–271. Available from: https:// doi.org/10.1097/00006534-198902000-00011
15. Pitanguy IVO & Ramos AS. *Plast Reconstr Surg.* 1966;38(4). Available from: https://journals.lww.com/plasreconsurg/ Fulltext/1966/10000/The_Frontal_Branch_of_ the_Facial_NerveThe.10.aspx
16. Philipp-Dormston WG et al. *Dermatologic Surg.* 2018;44(1):0–0. Available from: https://journals.lww.com/dermatologicsurgery/Fulltext/2018/01000/Intracranial_Penetration_During_Temporal_Soft.13.aspx
17. Zayed OM et al. *Tanta Dent J.* 2015;12(3):156–62. Available from: http://dx.doi. org/10.1016/j.tdj.2015.03.001
18. Sunil Dutt C et al. *J Maxillofac Oral Surg.* 2015;14(2):171–5. Available from: http://dx.doi.org/10.1007/s12663-014-0641-9
19. Jones D & Swift A. *Injectable Fillers: Facial Shaping and Contouring.* Wiley-Blackwell, 2019.
20. Swift A. *Plast Reconstr Surg.* 2015;136:204S–18S.
21. Seckel B. *Facial Danger Zones*, 2nd ed. Thieme, 2010.
22. Carruthers JDA et al. *Plast Reconstr Surg.* 2014;134(6):1197–201.
23. Chatrath V et al. *Plast Reconstr Surg – Glob Open.* 2019;7(4). Available from: https://journals.lww.com/prsgo/fulltext/2019/04000/Soft_tissue_Filler_associated_Blindness__A.1.aspx
24. Lee W et al. *J Plast Reconstr Aesthetic Surg.* 2019 Feb 1;72(2):335–54. Available from: https://doi.org/10.1016/j.bjps.2018.10.008
25. Jiang X et al. *JAMA Facial Plast Surg.* 2014 May 1;16(3):227–9. Available from: https:// doi.org/10.1001/jamafacial.2013.2565
26. Juhász MLW & Marmur ES. *J Cosmet Dermatol.* 2015 Sep 1;14(3):254–9. Available from: https://doi.org/10.1111/jocd.12155
27. Sykes JM et al. Upper face: Clinical anatomy and regional approaches with injectable fillers. *Plast Reconstr Surg.* 2015;136(5S):204S–18S.

3 PERIORBITAL REGION AND TEAR TROUGH

Colin M. Morrison, Ruth Tevlin, Steven Liew, Vitaly Zholtikov, Haideh Hirmand, and Steven Fagien

The periorbital region is a confluent aesthetic unit consisting of anatomically distinct but visually interdependent units. These units comprise the lower eyelid and infrapalpebral area, which includes the tear trough and extends down onto the mid-cheek. The aesthetically attractive lower eyelid should display a relatively smooth transition between the preseptal and orbital portions of the orbicularis oculi muscle and continue into the upper malar region without a definable transition point [1]. Aesthetic improvement in this region is both challenging and rewarding and should be approached with conservativism and caution as even the most minor errors become evidently visible and can be unforgiving to treat.

BOUNDARIES

The periorbital is a confluent region which is surrounded by the eyebrows superiorly and temple laterally, which are linked at the lateral canthal region. Inferiorly it is bordered by the inferior palpebral groove and medially by the nasal sidewall (Figure 3.1).

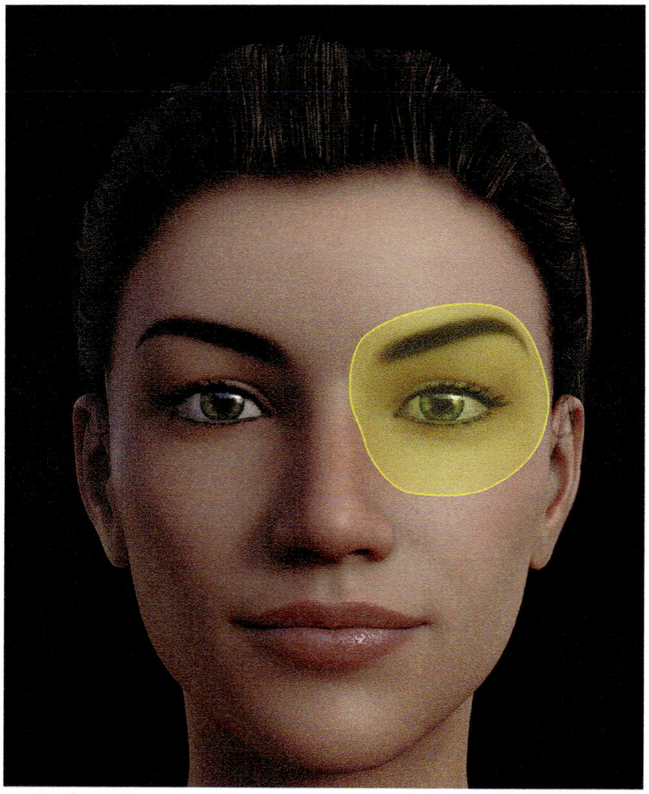

Figure 3.1 The periorbital area extending between the eyebrow (superiorly), inferior palpebral groove (inferiorly), nasal sidewall (medially) and lateral canthal region and temple (laterally).

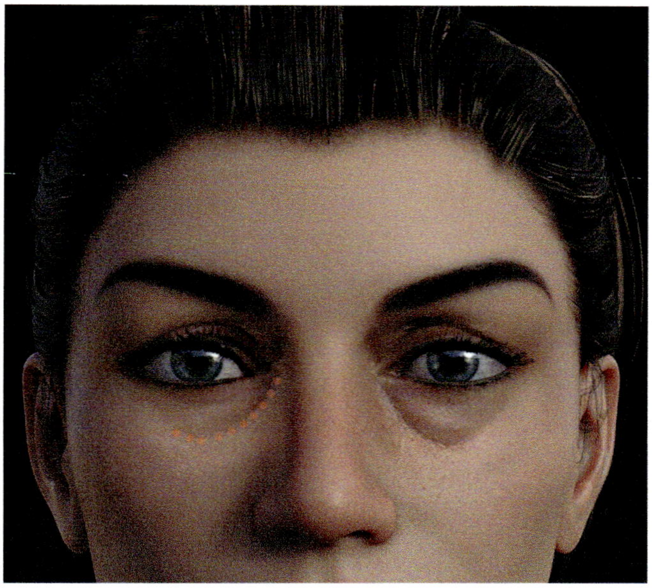

Figure 3.2 The tear trough (TT) deformity characterized by a sunken infraorbital appearance. Orange dots: lid-cheek junction (LCJ).

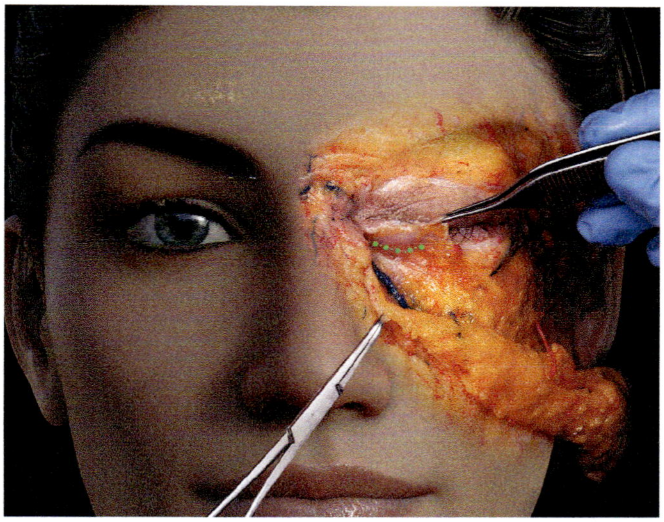

Figure 3.3 The TT is composed of thin skin adherent to orbicularis muscle attached to the orbital rim (green dots).

The tear trough (TT) is a distinct cutaneous groove extending inferolaterally from the medial canthus to approximately medial to the mid-pupillary line (Figure 3.2).

The medial border of the TT lies at the inferior orbital rim. This area has scant subcutaneous tissue, with skin adherent to muscle that is attached to bone.

The orbicularis oculi muscle has a direct osseous attachment extending from the anterior lacrimal crest to the medial limbus at the inferior orbital rim.

More laterally, the orbicularis oculi muscle attaches indirectly to bone via the orbicularis retaining ligament (ORL) (Figure 3.3).

At the level of the medial third of the orbital rim, the TT runs along fibers of orbicularis oculi [2], with the maximum distance from orbital rim to TT at the central aspect of the rim.

AGING

During aging, there is unequal evolution of the three infraorbital regions, characterized by:

- **Lower eyelid:** Herniation of the infraorbital fat
- **Infrapalpebral area and mid-cheek:** Volume loss in the superficial and deep fat compartments
- **Maxillary bone:** Resorption with subsequent loss of projection

The TT deformity first manifests as a depression at the medial aspect of the orbital rim, along the attachment of the orbicularis oculi muscle. It is a common characteristic of the lower orbital region and becomes progressively deeper and more visible with aging [2–5]. Over time, true indenta-tion develops which significantly impacts facial appearance and is regarded as a deformity when fully manifest [2,4,5]. The deep groove that commonly occurs near the junction of the eyelid and the cheek is the most consistently ignored major deformity of the orbital region. With a characteristic length of about 2 cm, it extends inferolaterally from the inner canthus of the eye, invariably giving the face an unhealthy, tired or even haggard appearance [1]. The TT is not

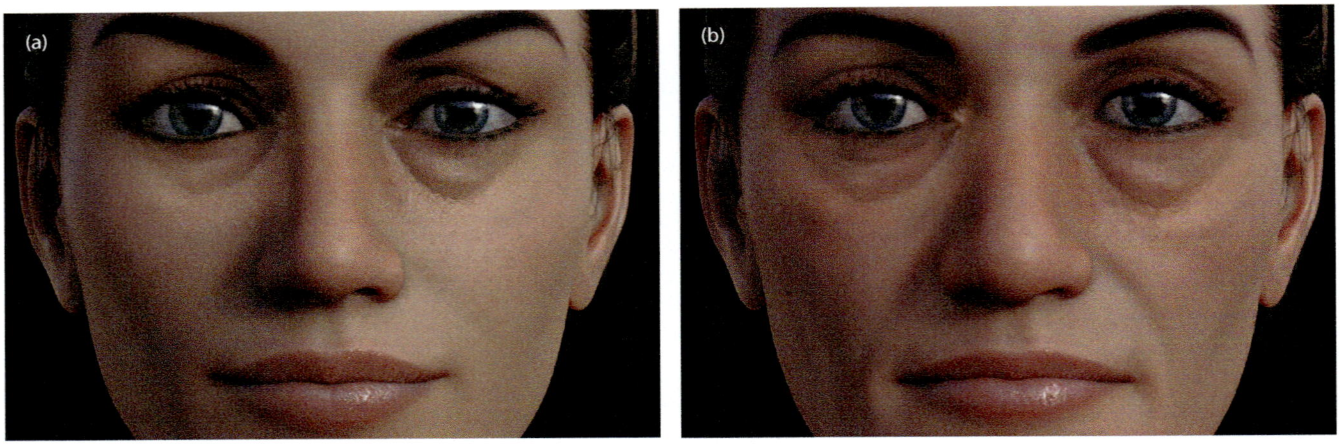

Figure 3.4 TT associated with thin skin in (a) the young and (b) the aged patient. Note progressive textural skin changes and sagginess.

exclusively age-related and may also be visible in youth when the orbicularis oculi muscle has thin overlying skin (Figure 3.4) [4]. The TT deformity represents an important aesthetic concern which is one of the most frequently discussed landmarks in facial aesthetic surgical and non-surgical treatments [1,4,6–33].

The cause is multifactorial and differentiating individual components may be challenging. Factors contributing to prominence include the contrasting quality and quantity of tissues both above and below the TT:

- **Above:** Thinner preseptal skin, absent subcutaneous fat, and noticeable hyperpigmentation [2,5].
- **Below:** Thicker skin and more abundant subcutaneous fat. Bulging orbital fat (above the ligament), maxillary retrusion, tissue descent, and atrophy account for the prominence of the TT deformity with aging [4].
- **Orbital fat herniation:** In advanced aging, there can be additional volume loss laterally or just below the orbital rim, where the retaining ligaments are thicker and less distensible. The concavity in the groove is often associated with orbital fat herniation in the lower lid fat compartment, thus accentuating the appearance of the TT. In addition, fat herniation in the lower lid distracts from the overall deficiency in the TT and periorbital volume loss.

SKIN

The skin varies in color, texture and thickness in the different facial regions (Figure 3.5). The development of dark undereye circles is one of the early signs of periorbital aging, causing a fatigued and aged appearance [2]. In the palpebral region, the skin is delicate, thin, and sometimes translucent. In fair-skinned Caucasians, the underlying orbicularis oculi muscle

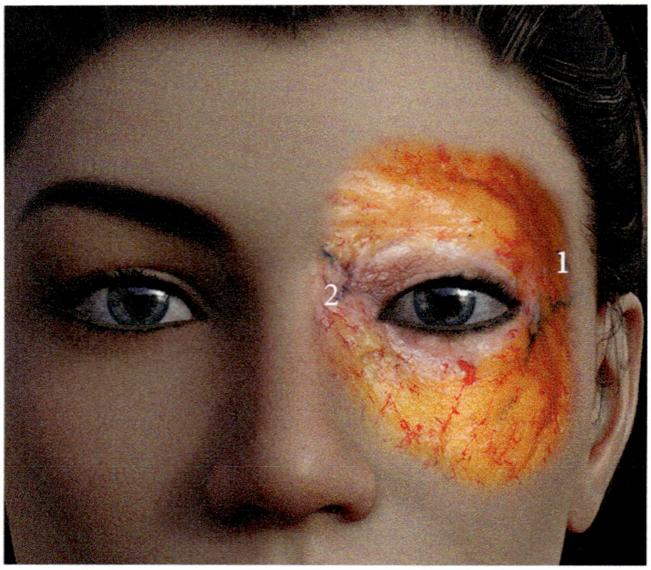

Figure 3.5 Superficial periorbital fat and vasculature. Note the sentinel vein (1) and angular vein (2).

may manifest as a reddish TT, while this area may be pigmented in darker-skinned individuals. In contrast, the skin of the cheek is generally lighter and thicker. With aging, the skin of the palpebral portion can become thin, atrophic, and hyperpigmented with subsequent accentuation of the lid-cheek junction. The thin upper eyelid skin is slightly thicker over the supratarsal crease where it folds in a predictable location.

FAT

The superficial fat compartments in the palpebral region (Figure 3.6) are usually very thin or absent between the skin and the preseptal orbicularis oculi muscle. Subcutaneous fat of the mobile upper eyelid is thin-ner and forms the transition point between the thick adipose tissue of the forehead and the thinner adi-pose tissue of the upper eyelid and corresponding crease. The subcutaneous fat in the lower eyelid is also thinner and becomes thicker in the cheek area. There is a distinct superficial boundary in the lower eyelid between eyelid and cheek, which is called the lid-cheek junction (LCJ) or lid-cheek crease (Figure 3.2).

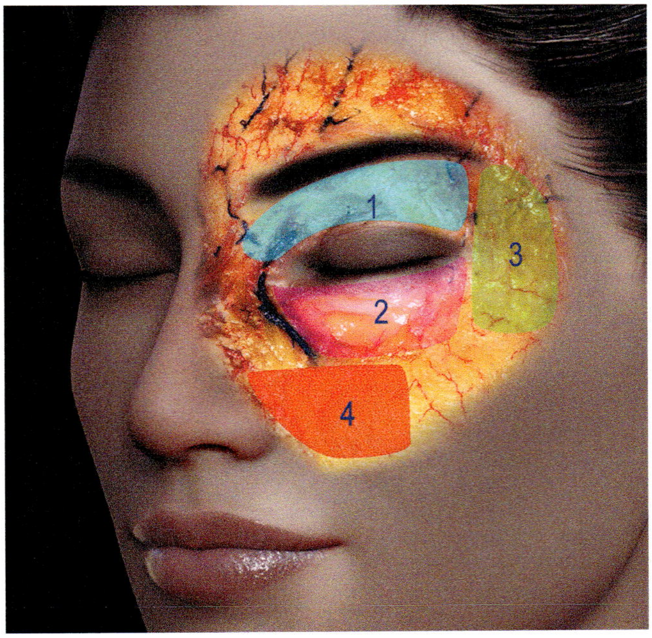

Figure 3.6 Skin and fat compartments of the periorbital area: (1) Superior palpebral superficial fat; (2) inferior palpebral superficial fat pads; (3) lateral palpebral superficial fat; (4) superficial medial cheek fat pad.

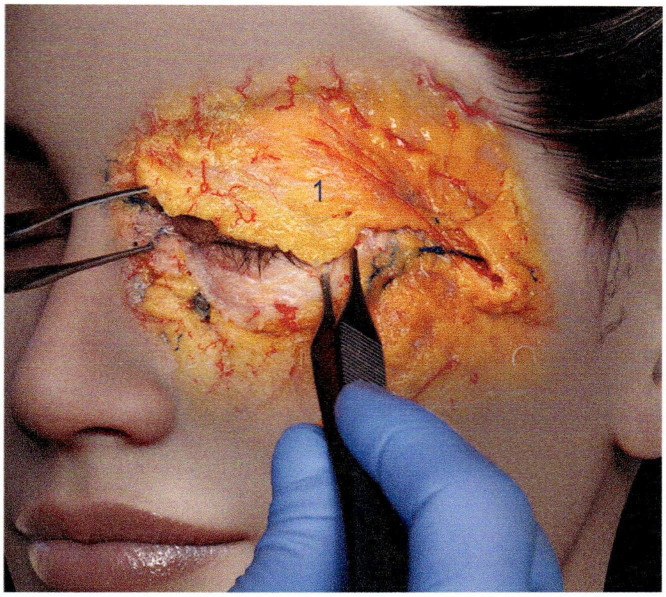

Figure 3.7 Deep supraorbital fat: (1) Retro-orbicularis oculi fat (ROOF).

In the cheek region, the cephalic margin of the nasolabial fat compartments covers the medial orbital portion of the orbicularis oculi muscle. Laterally, the superomedial angle of the infraorbital fat compartment covers the orbital portion of the orbicularis oculi muscle, which defines the lateral aspect of the TT deformity. The deep fat compartments comprise the ROOF (retro-orbicularis oculi fat pad) (Figure 3.7) the upper margin of the deep nasal-labial fat compartments (NLF) and the medial aspect of the medial suborbicularis oculi fat compartments (SOOF) (Figures 3.8 and 3.9).

MUSCLES

The orbicularis oculi muscle (OOM) is a circular sphincter that covers both the upper and lower eyelids (Figure 3.10).

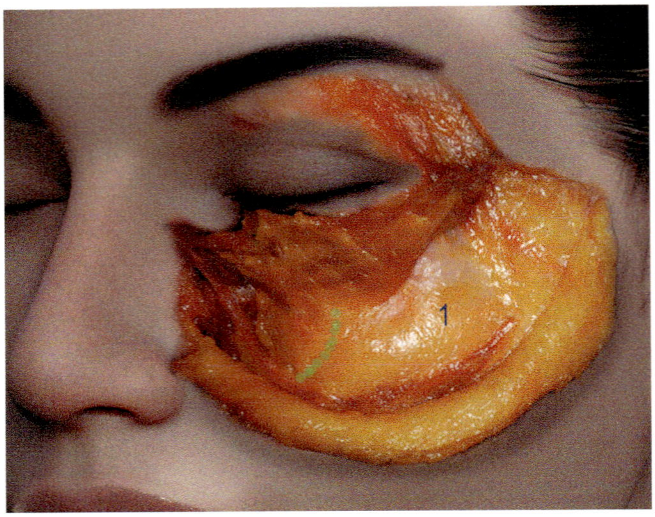

Figure 3.8 Deep fat compartments: (1) Suborbicularis oculi fat (SOOF). This compartment overlies the zygoma and is divided into medial and lateral SOOF at a vertical line (green) passing through the medial margin of the pupil.

The OOM lies in the same plane as the frontalis muscle. The ORL is the membrane created when the fascia beneath the OOM inserts into the periosteum 2–3 mm above the supraorbital rim. In the upper lid, it is also the deep boundary between the upper eyelid and the forehead, where it forms a fusion zone. In the lower eyelid, the ORL forms the deep boundary between the orbital rim and the cheek (Figure 3.11).

The OOM has a preseptal portion which is thinner and lighter in color and covers the medial septum and the intraorbital medial fat pad. The orbital portion of the OOM is thicker and darker and covers the frontal process of the maxillary bone, the upper part of the medial portion of the deep medial cheek fat compartments (DMCF), and the origin of the levator labii superioris alaeque nasi muscle (LLSAN). The superior origins of the levator labii superioris alaeque nasi muscle (medial)

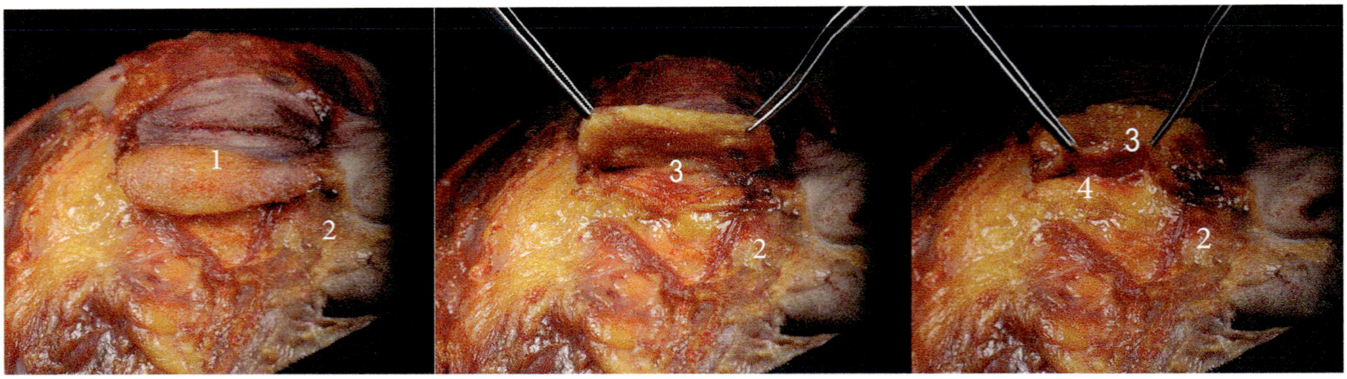

Figure 3.9 (1) Superficial infraorbital fat; (2) LLSAN; (3) OOM; (4) SOOF.

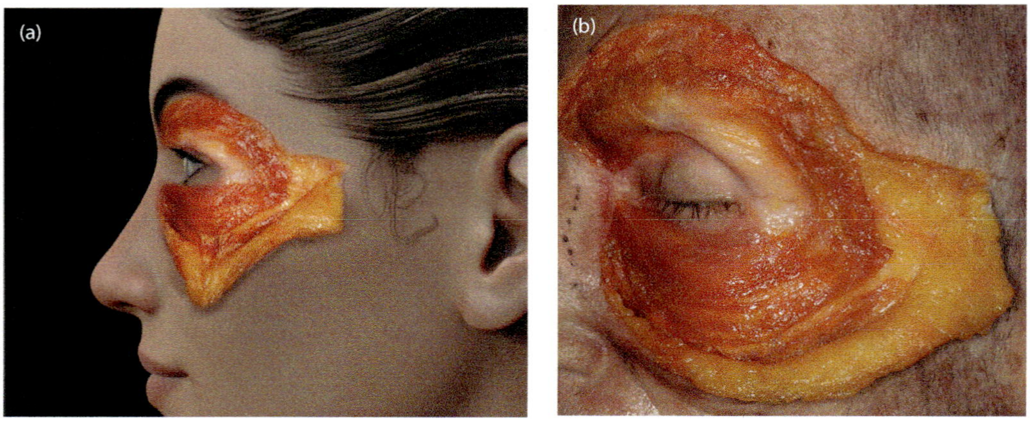

Figure 3.10 (a) The orbicularis oculi muscle (OOM) is a circular, sphincter muscle that covers both the upper and the lower eyelids. (b) The OOM is in the same plane as the frontalis muscle, separated from the forehead by the orbicularis retaining ligament (ORL).

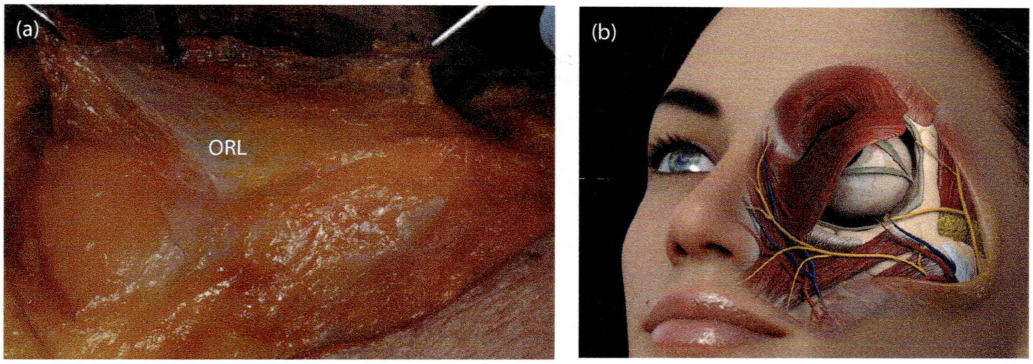

Figure 3.11 (a) The orbicularis retaining ligament (ORL) is the membrane created when the fascia beneath the OOM inserts into the periosteum of the supraorbital rim; (b) ORL in upper eyelid, is also the deep boundary between the upper eyelid and the forehead where it forms a fusion zone. ORL in lower eyelid forms the deep boundary between the orbital rim and the cheek.

and levator labii superior muscle (lateral) constitute the inferior margin of the TT deformity. They are fixed to the maxillary bone and covered by the upper margin of the medial aspect of the deep medial cheek fat compartment and by the inferior medial border of the orbital portion of the OOM.

VASCULARIZATION

The facial artery gives rise to the angular artery, which ascends medially to the TT adjacent to the nasal bone (Figures 3.12 and 3.13).

- Creases are usually defined by an underlying vascular arcade and regional differences in fat compartments.
- The nasojugal crease helps to mark the underlying infraorbital (IO) artery and accompanying nerve.
- The IO foramen lies at the junction of the nasojugal crease and lid-cheek junction.
- The lid-cheek junction marks the underlying infraorbital arcade to which the IO artery and branches of the transverse facial artery contribute.
- The inferior palpebral arcade runs just above the eyelid margin, while the superior palpebral arcade lies beneath the supratarsal crease.

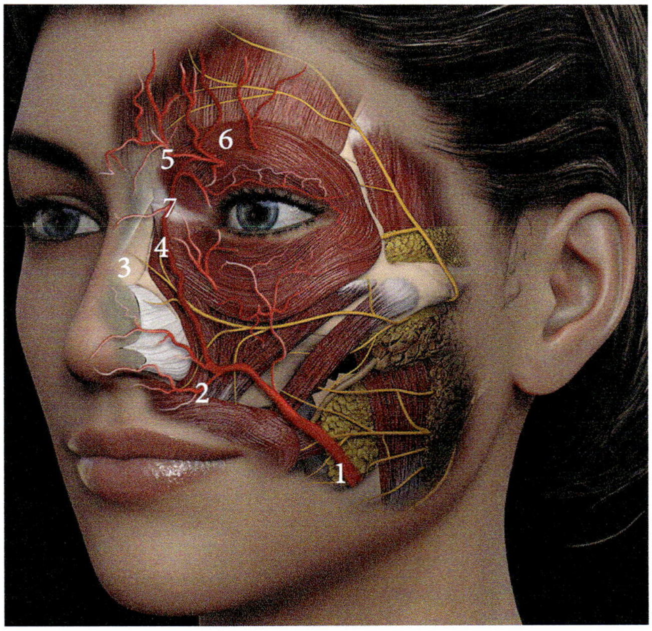

Figure 3.12 Periorbital vascularization: (1) Facial artery; (2) alar branch; (3) position of the dorsal nasal artery; (4) angular artery; (5) supratrochlear vessels; (6) supraorbital vessels; (7) lacrimal artery.

- The medial upper eyelid fat pad references an underlying vessel that communicates directly with the lacrimal, ophthalmic, and retinal arteries.
- The forehead-lid crease marks a more superior arcade defining the superficial boundary between the upper eyelid and forehead.

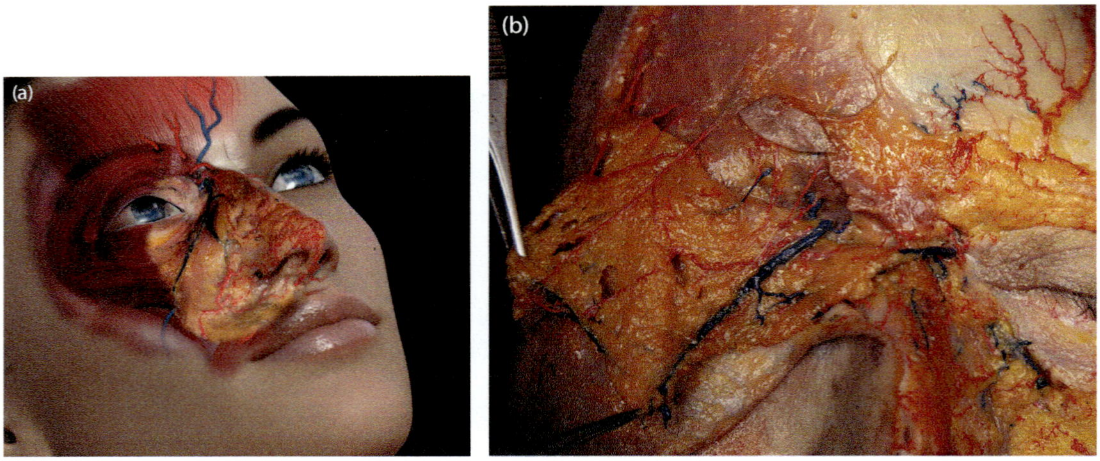

Figure 3.13 (a,b) Periorbital vascularization.

The blood supply of the eyelids is derived from the facial system, which arises from the external carotid artery, and the orbital system, which originates from the internal carotid artery along branches of the ophthalmic artery. The superficial and deep plexuses of arteries provide a vast blood supply to the upper and lower eyelids. The venous drainage of the eyelids can be divided into two portions: a superficial, or preseptal, and a deep system draining into the cavernous sinus.

Upper Eyelid

- Supplied by the lacrimal, supraorbital, and supratrochlear arteries that provide palpebral branches to the lateral, middle, and medial portions of the upper eyelid.

Lower Eyelid

- Supplied by the palpebral branch of the infraorbital artery and the lateral and medial palpebral branches from the lacrimal and supratrochlear arteries.
- The palpebral branch of the infraorbital artery emerges from the infraorbital foramen and courses superiorly and laterally to the orbital septum, piercing the septum close to the infraorbital rim.
- A small branch of the angular artery may also supply the medial lower eyelid.

Venous drainage of the eyelids can be divided into:

- Superficial/preseptal system that drains into the internal and external jugular veins
- Deep/post-tarsal system that flows into the cavernous sinus

The facial vein gives rise to the angular vein. The latter may sometimes be accompanied by the cephalic branch of the infraorbital artery, by a duplexed angular artery, or by a detoured facial artery, which all travel in the TT channel.

The ophthalmic artery (OA) is the artery of the orbit originating from the internal carotid artery within the middle cranial fossa. After traveling through the optic foramen, it divides into multiple arterial branches within the orbital cavity [34].

- The OA is considered a major arterial shunt between the internal and external carotid arteries.
- The OA provides anterior and posterior ethmoidal arteries that course through the anterior and posterior ethmoidal foramina, respectively.

- The anterior ethmoidal artery terminates as the external nasal artery which supplies the lateral nose.

INNERVATION

The upper eyelid: Sensory innervation is from the palpebral branches from the infratrochlear, supratrochlear, supraorbital, and lacrimal nerves, all originating from the ophthalmic nerve (Figure 3.14).

The lower eyelid: Sensory innervation is from the inferior palpebral branch of the infraorbital nerve (Figure 3.15). The inferior palpebral branch is often bifurcated, with one branch traveling laterally and the other medially, and sometimes the branch only innervates the medial or lateral part of the lower lid. If the lateral branch is absent, the zygomaticofacial branch of the zygomatic nerve may compensate; if the medial branch is missing, the external nasal branch may innervate the area. A palpebral branch of the infratrochlear nerve may also reach the medial aspect of the lower lid [35].

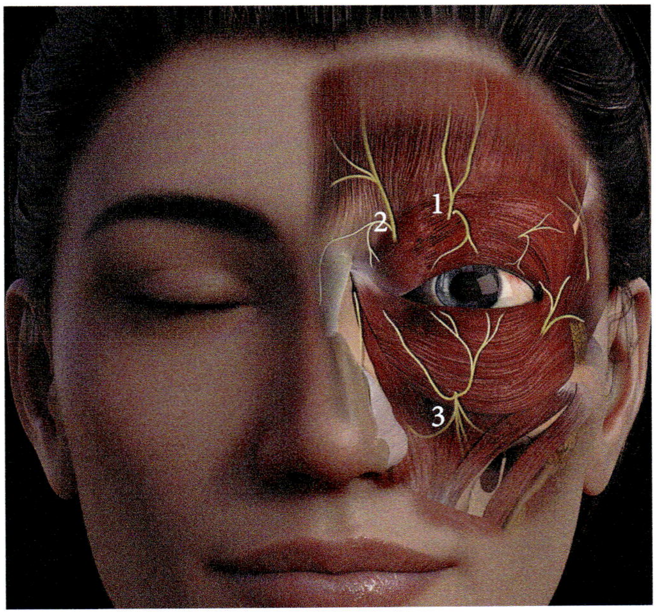

Figure 3.14 Periorbital innervation: Danger zone 5 at the superior orbital rim above the mid-pupil where the (1) supraorbital (CN V) and the more medial; (2) supratrochlear (CN V) neurovascular bundles are located; (3) infraorbital nerve.

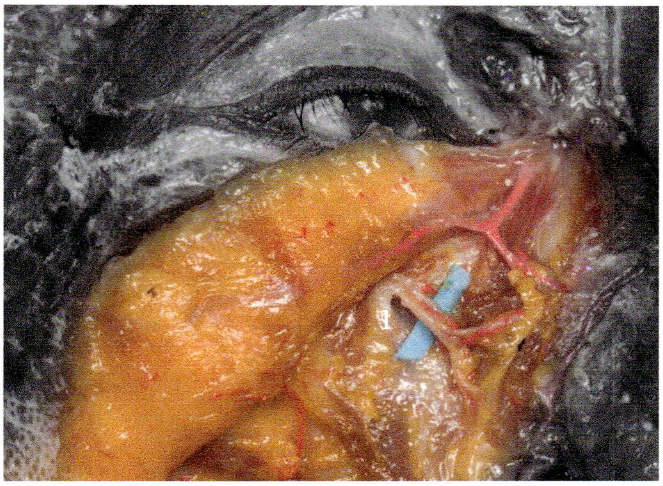

Figure 3.15 Periorbital innervation: Infraorbital nerve. It is 6–68 mm below the infraorbital bony margin and on the medial limbus line. (1) Infraorbital neurovascular bundel exiting foramen.

Orbicularis oculi has motor innervation from the zygomatic and temporal branches of the facial nerve (Figure 3.16).

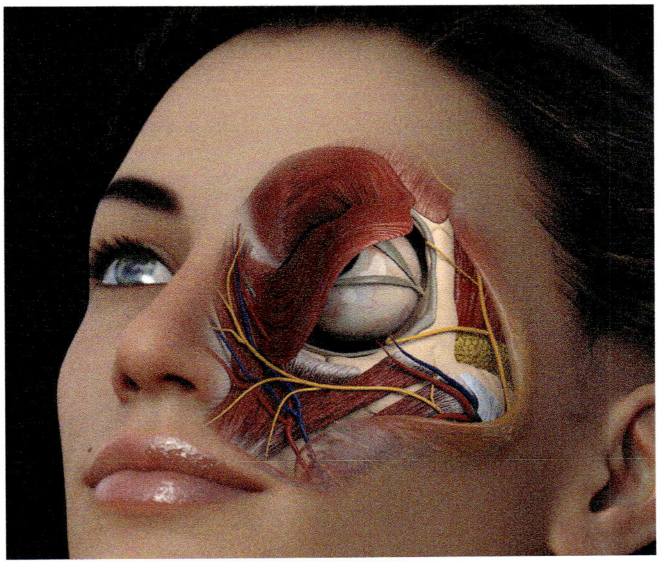

Figure 3.16 Periorbital innervation: The buccal branch of the facial nerve.

BONE

Bony structures undergo morphologic change with aging. This results in a widening of the orbital aperture that results in a change in the appearance of the overlying soft-tissue envelope. The overall widening of the orbital aperture results in a change in the relationship between the orbital contents and the surrounding bony framework. This may cause changes including the prominence of fat pads, deepening of sulci, or the enophthalmos and ptosis that may be seen with aging.

In the upper half of the orbit, the soft tissues may fall into the orbital aperture and thus cause the appearance of brow descent and lateral orbital hooding. In the lower half of the orbit, the tissues may fall over the recessed bony ledge, leading to lag of the lower lid, prominence of lower lid fat pockets, and deepening of the nasojugal groove. Since disproportionate tissue piles up, origin of the orbicularis is reshaped from its underlying bony attachment (Figure 3.17).

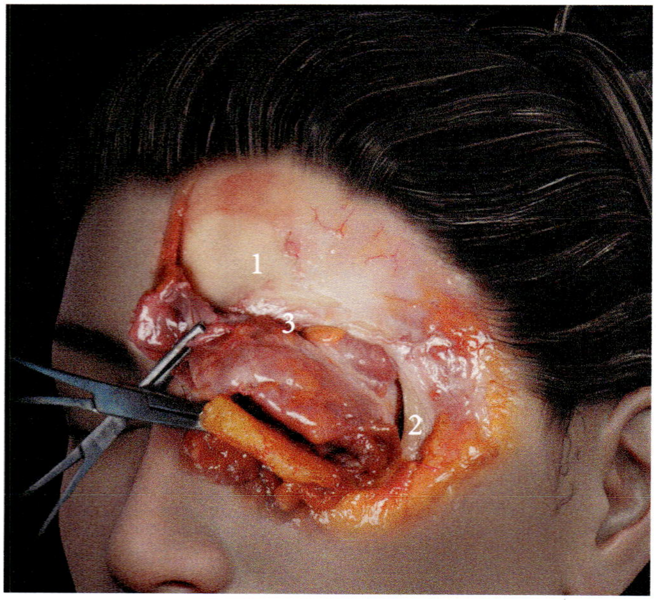

Figure 3.17 Periorbital bone. (1) Squamous portion of frontal bone; (2) lateral orbital rim; (3) superior orbital rim.

HOW I DO IT: BOTULINUM TOXIN

Botulinum toxin injections in the periorbital area involve the so-called crow's feet lines and the infraorbital pretarsal lines.

The glabella area was previously described in Chapter 1.

Crow's Feet Lines

We should distinguish between male and female injection in regard to the onabotulinum toxin A doses.

There are two patterns (A and B; Figure 3.18), both characterized by 4 U per injection point. Injections are done with a 32G 4 mm needle from medial to lateral, superficial to the orbicularis oculi muscle (Figure 3.19). There may be variations with regard to the lateral extension of the lines with larger OOM:

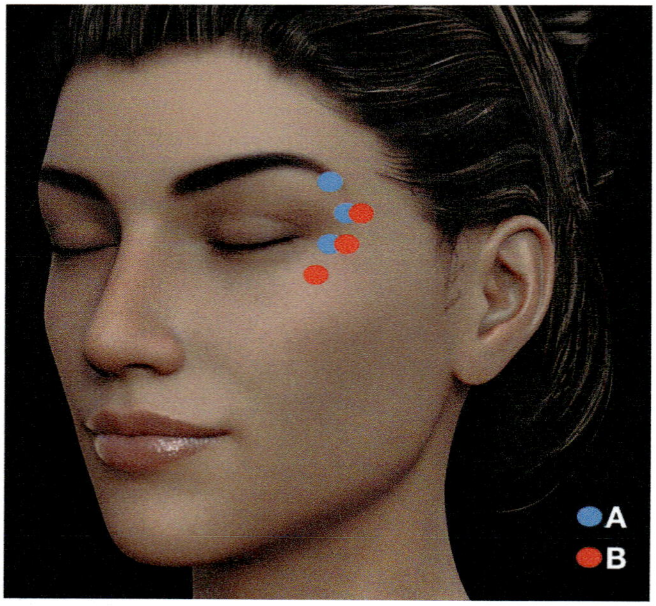

Figure 3.18 Periorbital injection points: The two patterns of crow's feet treatment with botulinum toxin injection. (A) Full fan pattern; (B) lower fan pattern.

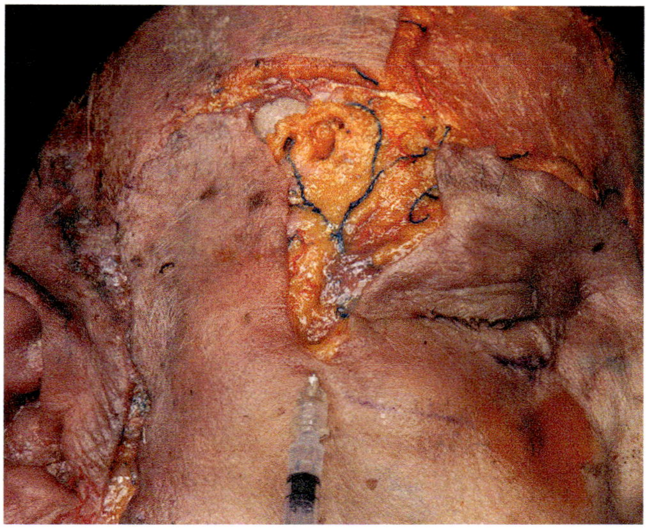

Figure 3.19 Periorbital toxin injection: Depth must be intradermal to avoid superficial vessels.

Male: Three more lateral points of 2 U per point
Female: Two or three more lateral points of 1 U per point (Figure 3.20)

Pretarsal Lines

0.05 U per point (Figure 3.21).

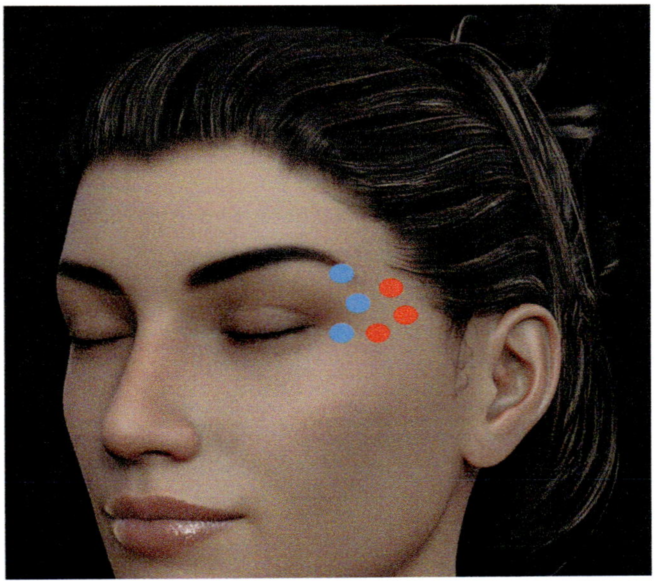

Figure 3.20 Periorbital lateral extension of botulinum toxin injection on orbicularis oris.

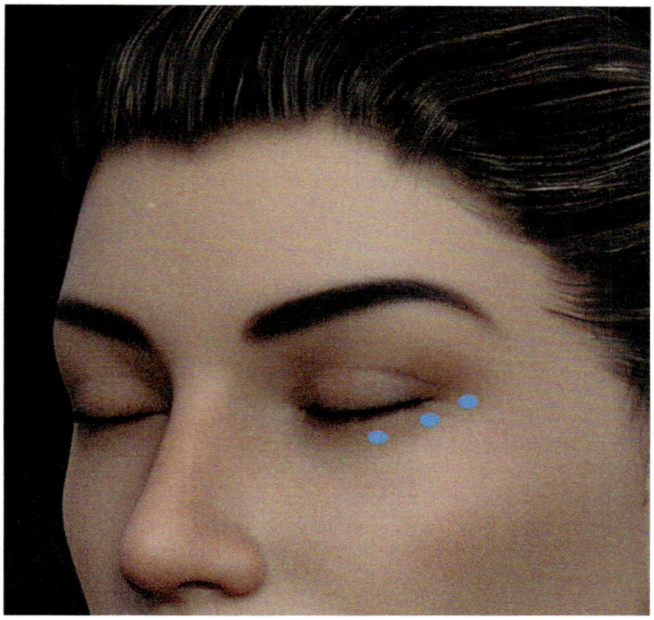

Figure 3.21 Periorbital lower-lid injection points.

HOW I DO IT: FILLER

Both non-surgical and surgical options exist to address the TT deformity. Patient selection is critical to obtaining good results. The best candidates for non-surgical correction are patients with good skin tone and minimal skin laxity, with mild to moderately deep TTs. Non-surgical treatment is ideal for patients seeking facial rejuvenation with minimal downtime. Poor nonsurgical candidates include those with excess orbital fat, thin skin, significant skin laxity, and deep TTs. Non-surgical techniques also have excellent utility in postsurgical patients who have uncorrected troughs or over-resected orbital fat [2]. Many surgical techniques have also been described. Most, however, do not fully correct the deformity, and some can accentuate it.

Non-Surgical Management

Correction of a TT trough deformity with non-surgical techniques presents unique challenges. Unlike other facial hollows (such as the nasolabial folds, which are easily camouflaged), the TT requires more technically demanding treatment due to the breadth of the hollow, skin quality changes (thinning), and the presence of adjacent orbital fat pads [1]. Lambros stressed that when a patient engages in non-surgical treatment for TT correction, it is essential to evaluate the following factors [36]:

- **Skin quality:** Patients with thick, smooth skin will have better results than those with thin, extremely wrinkled skin.
- **Definition of the hollow:** A more defined hollow is more amenable to filler.
- **The orbital fat pad:** Larger fat pads are more difficult to correct due to "puffiness" caused by the injection.
- **The color of the overlying skin:** Filler may improve shadowing but will not improve dark pigmentation.

Patients with very thin or transparent skin, those with significant skin laxity, and those with extremely deep TTs are poor candidates. These patients could still obtain improved appearance with the procedure; however, they need to be counseled as to the higher risk of visibility, irregularity and overall less than perfect results. Many of these patients still elect to proceed and rarely seek reversal even if the results are not perfect [2].

Patients who do best with non-surgical management of the TT deformity have thick, smooth skin, and a well-defined TT without overly large lower lid fat pads. Patients with extremely wrinkled skin and less of an actual indentation to fill do less well with injections. The larger the overhanging fat pads, the more the injection becomes a compromise procedure, as one tries to correct the shelving of the fat and the intrinsic indentation of the TT [5].

The presence of filler (e.g., hyaluronic acid) in the TT does not diminish the intrinsic color of the overlying skin, though it does diminish the shadow. Patients with deep pigmentation should be advised of this, although an indentation in the presence of dark pigmentation usually appears better corrected. In order to preserve harmony and aesthetic facial proportions, consider additional volume correction of the brow, sub-brow eyelid, or medial upper-lid A-frame deformity [2]. In addition, botulinum toxin can be used in the lateral orbicularis oculi or in the medial third along the orbital rim to prevent distortion and increase longevity of treatment.

Surgical Management

Patients who would benefit from surgery are those with orbital fat herniation and significant skin laxity. These patients are unlikely to obtain good results from injecting the TT alone and should be thus advised. It is helpful to simulate the effect of filling in the less-than-ideal candidate by pushing on the soft tissues just under the TT with the patient observing in the mirror while their reaction is assessed. This procedure is an effective adjunct to lower-lid blepharoplasty and can be recommended as part of the rejuvenation plan at the time of consultation.

Blepharoplasty has evolved from the old paradigm of pure fat and skin removal [37] to the modern practice of preserving orbital fat with limited resection to restore a youthful contour [38–40]. Rohrich proposed a "five-step lower blepharoplasty" that addresses both the TT and the lid-cheek junction [41]. This approach systematically treats both elements by evaluating and addressing the following:

- **Deep malar fat** augmentation
- **Orbicularis oculi muscle** preservation with conservative fat pad removal
- Selective release of the **orbicularis retaining ligament**
- Lateral **canthopexy**
- Conservative **skin excision**

Regardless of the particular technique utilized, it is important to evaluate each of these five steps to optimally treat the TT deformity.

TT deformities can also be accentuated by atrophy and/or descent of midfacial soft tissue, combined with infraorbital rim retrusion. Periorbital skeletal augmentation is thus another method of treating the TT deformity, as advocated by Yaremchuk [42], Flowers [43], and Terino [44].

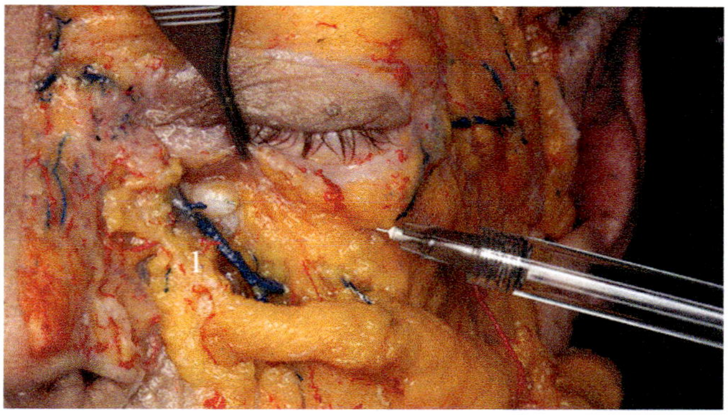

Figure 3.22 Periorbital HA injection: Blunt cannula (25G 38 mm length) is most commonly advised for injection in infraorbital area. (1) Angular vein.

Choice of Filler

Low G′ hyaluronic acid is the filler of choice for this region. Several companies have tried to address the challenge of adequate volumization without the sponge-like absorption of water, which can also compromise the delicate lymphatic tissue in this region. Sometimes the extremely thin soft-tissue coverage can show even the most minute irregularities. The following fillers are most prevalent on the market for this region: Allergan Volbella (VYC-15), Merz Belotero Balance, Teoxane Redensity-2 or RHA 2, and Galderma Restylane. It should be noted that Restylane may show a blue haze if injected superficially, which can be disturbing to the patient.

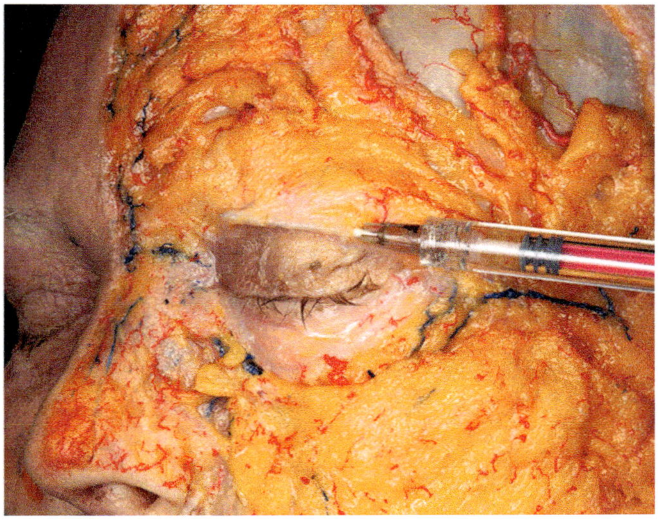

Figure 3.23 Periorbital HA injection: Upper lid injection with low G′ filler, using a cannula in a vascular danger zone.

Needle versus Cannula

Blunt cannulae (25G or 27G 38 mm length) are most commonly advised for injection, being introduced through a 23–25G needle hole for injection in the TT (Figures 3.22 and 3.23).

Blunt cannulae are recommended to reduce the chance of inadvertent intravascular injection but are not failsafe. Extreme care and experience are of vital importance in this region. Alternatively, a 30G or 32G needle can be used for small superficial aliquots in a subcutaneous level (Figures 3.24–3.26).

Technique

The TT area is treated only after thorough assessment and, where necessary, revolumization of the medial cheek fat compartment. This compartment is the founding layer for support and structure of the overlying TT. Small volumes are delivered in a retrograde fashion with each injection (0.01–0.05 mL). The injections are usually deep to the orbicularis muscle and just superficial to the periosteum of the orbital rim in the most medial aspect (Figure 3.27).

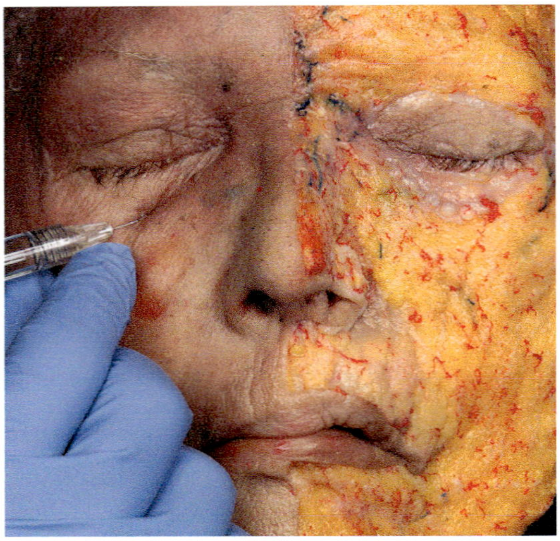

Figure 3.24 Periorbital HA injection: A 30 to 32G needle can be used for small superficial aliquots of HA.

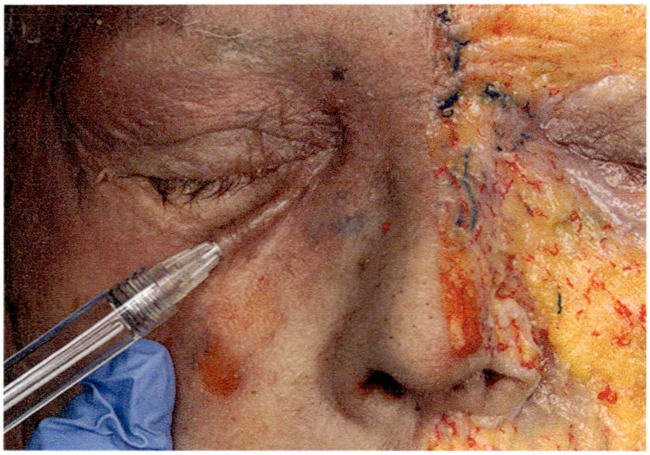

Figure 3.25 Periorbital HA injection: Subcutaneous injection of tear trough is considered an advanced technique.

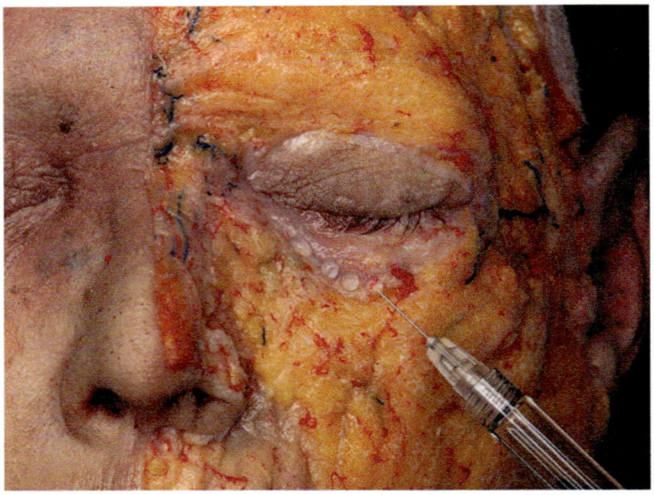

Figure 3.26 Periorbital HA injection: Micro aliquots of low G′ HA above the orbicularis oculi muscle.

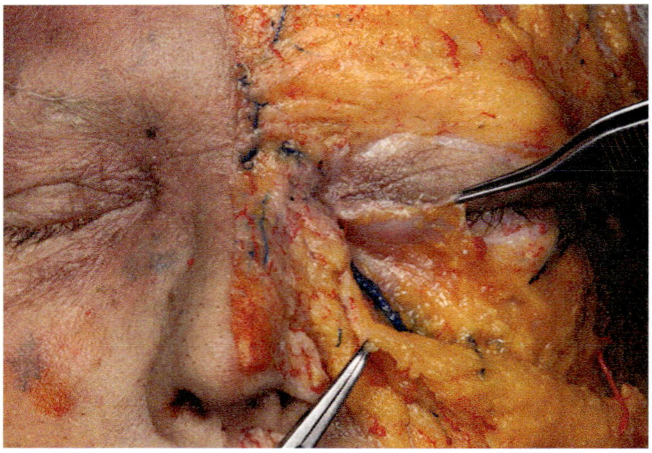

Figure 3.27 Periorbital HA injection: Injections are deep to the orbicularis muscle and superficial to the periosteum of the orbital rim in the most medial aspect.

Injection deep in the pre-periosteal plane reduces visibility of the product.

It is advised to inject discontinuously in the deformity from medial to lateral. It is important to avoid injecting a large continuous column of filler along the TT to prevent a resulting oval bulge or sausage appearance, which is accentuated on animation [2].

Alternatively, more entry sites can be made with depot injections to avoid long continuous retrograde injections. Typically, two to three injection sites are used medially and centrally, and one or two sites are used laterally. Gentle digital massage, or massage with a wet cotton-tipped swab, is performed to disperse and smooth out the filler in the intended location.

Note that the TT is at or below the infraorbital rim in all cases; thus, injections above the orbital rim are not necessary in the absence of volume deficiency within the confines of the orbit [2]. The key to aesthetic correction of the TT is to think beyond the TT. Depending on the depth and extent of volume loss, further injections are indicated to correct the central and lateral aspect around the orbital rim and all adjacent areas. Overcorrection of the TT deformity is not recommended. The most common total volume injected into the periorbital area is 0.2–0.5 mL on each side.

CAUTIONS

See Sharad [28] for detailed caution information.

- Vitamin E, alcohol, ginkgo biloba, and nonsteroidal anti-inflammatory drugs should be avoided at least five days before the treatment to prevent bruising. Similarly, antiplatelet agents should be avoided for 10 days before the procedure [2].
- Care should be taken in patients with a history of trauma, scarring, and/or lower eyelid blepharoplasty without lateral retinacular suspension.
- Patients that have a history of semi-permanent or permanent filler in the area should be avoided and referred to experts.
- Caution should be exercised while injecting around the orbital foramen to avoid injury to the neurovascular bundle.
- Careful and gentle molding of the filler is encouraged after injection for more homogenous distribution and even distribution in the lateral aspect of the hollow.

COMBINATION THERAPIES

Combination therapies include the use of ablative and non-ablative lasers and/or energy-based devices prior to the filler as thermal energy causes accelerated degradation of HA. Platelet rich plasma (PRP) and microneedling can be used prior to or after filler injection.

HOW I DO IT

- Mark TT with the patient sitting upright.
- Upward gaze accentuates deficit medially and centrally.
- Upward, outward gaze outlines deficit laterally on contralateral side.
- Mark surgical "roadmap" plan and review with patient.
- Cold packs are used before and after.
- Meticulous aseptic technique.
- Needle/cannula is inserted deep suborbicularly, supraperiosteal plane, in the medial aspect.
- Discontinuous deposition.
- Filler is massaged in place, and visual evaluation is performed.
- Multiple passes needed for full correction.
- It is important to evaluate the feature in *animation*
- to identify and correct bulging.
- "Less is more."

POST-TREATMENT REGIMEN

Regular makeup and skin care are discouraged for 24 hours post-procedure. Physicians often recommend a specific post-procedure regimen.

COMPLICATIONS

Ecchymosis (11%), edema (12%), and inflammation (11%) are the most common complications [6]. Ecchymosis usually occurs at injection sites and can take up to 10 days to resolve. Due to the hydrophilic nature of the filler, variable but subtle edema is not uncommon, and resolution can take 2–3 weeks [2,22].

Visible irregularity is a significant complication and more prevalent in patients with thin or lax skin. Irregularities can be effectively managed with massage over two weeks. Irregularities due to superficial placement are difficult to resolve and may persist well over two years. Thus, reversal with hyaluronidase is recommended after four weeks with persistent irregularities.

Visibility of product may occur [6]; deep injections reduce the risk, but in rare cases, underlying tissue characteristics may predispose to visibility regardless of technique [2]. Persistent and delayed edema may accentuate this complication. Visibility may be associated with a gray or blue color, a refractive phenomenon known as the "Tyndall effect." Patients who are photographed professionally may show skin surface deformities that are only visible temporarily during flash photography and should be forewarned. Sometimes this bluish hue cannot be avoided and should be discussed with patients prior to injection. In some cases, anterior migration of hyaluronic acid (HA) may ensue over time, causing more of a bluish hue. This problem may be addressed by dissolving the HA product with hyaluronidase.

Rare cases of blindness, stroke, and skin necrosis after inadvertent intravascular injections have been reported in many facial areas with both needles and cannula. The periorbital area is considered a high-risk area due to multiple communications between the internal and external carotid circulations. Retrograde and then anterograde movement of filler within vessels by means of the internal carotid artery and the ophthalmic artery can theoretically account for occlusion of the central retinal artery. To minimize the risk of intravascular injection, regardless of instrument, filler should only be injected under low pressure, in a discontinuous and retrograde manner.

Soft tissue ischemia is a recorded complication [45]. Signs of soft tissue ischemia include blanching on injection, pain, mottling, blister formation, bluish discoloration, and, later, pustules and tissue necrosis. Mottling in the area of a vascular distribution larger than the injected area is a clue that vascular ischemia is occurring. The mottled appearance can then change into a bluish discoloration, which may appear like a large bruise. Tissue necrosis or eschar formation appears even later. Once the deep dermal layers are affected, scarring will likely occur.

Various treatment protocols have been suggested in cases of soft tissue ischemia. Treatments such as aspirin to prevent platelet aggregation, warm compresses to improve circulation, nitroglycerin paste, other vasodilators, hyaluronidase and hyperbaric oxygen have been reported to have been used [45]. The only proven treatment for soft tissue ischemia is the use of early high-dose hyaluronidase. Reports suggest that for patients who present within 24 h and are treated with high-dose hyaluronidase until the resolution of ischemia (in the range of 400–1500 IU; can be repeated every 24h) in the entire area of the tissue, ischemia had no long-term scarring or sequelae [46]. Even if patients present after 24 h, it is still recommended to treat with high-dose hyaluronidase in order to reduce ischemia and scarring; however, the sooner the treatment is commenced, the better the outcome [47]. It is imperative to have hyaluronidase available whenever one is injecting hyaluronic acid [47].

It is critical that the periorbital pattern of volume loss is thoroughly evaluated and a comprehensive strategy for injection is planned. A corrected TT in the absence of repletion of volume loss at the lateral orbit or of the midface results in an overall unaesthetic appearance at rest and especially with animation. Further evaluation and treatment effectively correct this issue.

Poor candidates are unlikely to obtain the best results and may be dissatisfied. The goal is to identify those patients at the outset. If a patient who is a surgical candidate is injected with suboptimal results, reversal is indicated. Often injections can complement surgery in order to optimize outcomes.

"Less is more" applies well in this area, and softening of the hollow often suffices. This is easily corrected with additional application. Patients should be advised of this possibility before the procedure.

Acceptable correction may last for one to two years and the effect wears off slowly over time.

Reapplication or touch-ups are based on subjective parameters.

Botulinum toxin in the lateral orbicularis oculi or the medial third along the orbital rim is a useful adjunct for preventing distortion of the filler by muscular action and for increasing longevity.

Overall, the complication rates associated with injection of the TT with HA have been acceptable. The aesthetic results that can be achieved represent a significant improvement compared with traditional methods, creating a more effective rejuvenation of the lower lid and midface.

COMPLICATIONS

For general complications and the concept of "safety by depth," see Chapter G.

Seckel [48] divided the face into seven functional danger zones; the periorbital regions include danger zones 5 and 6.

The Periorbital Region

- The orbicularis retaining ligament (ORL) inserts 2–3 mm above the inferior edge of the supraorbital rim. This insertion is of extreme clinical importance as injections performed below the ORL may place material into the upper eyelid, causing injury to the underlying levator muscle. This is avoidable by palpating the supraorbital rim and ensuring placement at least 3 mm above the inferior border (above the insertion of the ORL) [2,34]. Inadvertent nerve injury may cause a painful neuroma.
- Intravascular injections adjacent to the nose and within the TT region may cause embolization into the angular artery. This vessel is a continuation of the facial artery which anastomoses with the ethmoidal arteries, which in turn anastomose with the internal carotid system and retinal artery. Embolization of filler may ultimately cause blindness (Figure 3.28).
- Danger zone 5 is located at the superior orbital rim above the mid-pupil where the supraorbital (Cranial Nerve V) and the more medial supratrochlear (CN V) neurovascular bundles are located. The supraorbital nerve lies deep to the corrugator supercilii muscle (CSM), and the supratrochlear nerve passes through the CSM. Nerve injury may cause numbness of scalp, forehead, upper eyelid, and nasal dorsum. This danger zone can be identified with a 1.5 cm circle with the supraorbital foramen at its center, which is easily palpated at the supraorbital rim at mid-pupil level (Figure 3.29).
- Danger zone 6 is located in the infraorbital region with the infraorbital (V2) neurovascular bundle exiting the infraorbital foramen. Nerve injury may

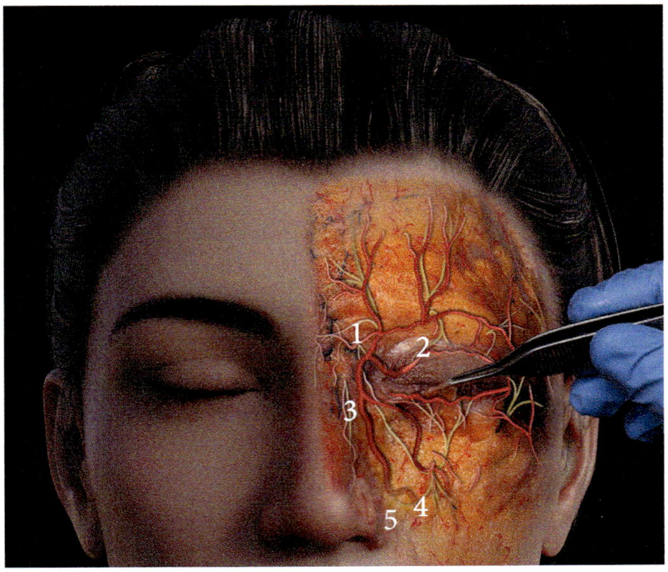

Figure 3.28 Periorbital danger area: Multiple areas of anastomosis between the internal and external carotid circulations, with risk of embolization to the ophthalmic circulation. (1) Supratrochlear; (2) supraorbital; (3) lacrimal; (4) infraorbital vessels; (5) facial artery becoming angular artery.

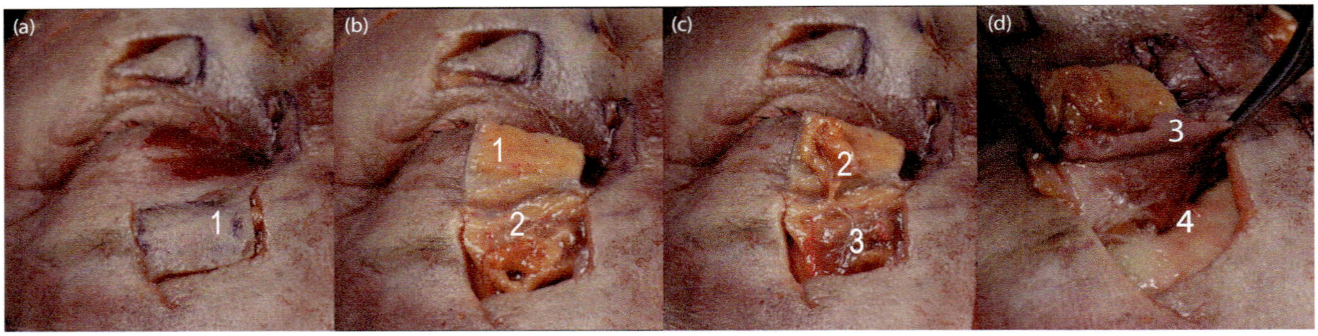

Figure 3.29 (a–d) Supraorbital danger area. (1) Skin; (2) superficial fat; (3) orbicularis muscle; (4) supraorbital nerve.

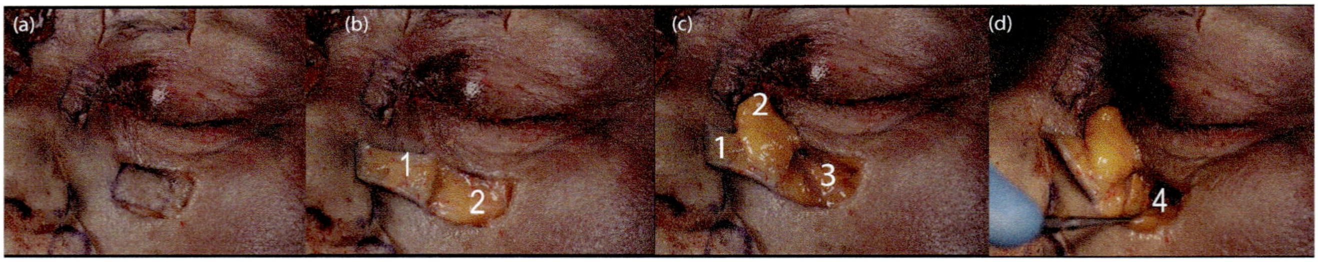

Figure 3.30 (a–d) Infraorbital danger area. (1) Skin; (2) superficial fat; (3) orbicularis muscle; (4) infraorbital nerve.

cause numbness of the lateral upper nose, cheek, upper lip, and lower eyelid. Zygomatic branches of the facial nerve also run in this zone to innervate the levator labii superioris muscle. This danger zone can be identified by drawing a 1.5 cm circle that centers around the infraorbital foramen located 1–1.5 cm below the infraorbital rim at mid-pupillary level (Figure 3.30).

References

1. Stutman RL & Codner MA. *Aesthet Surg J.* 2012;32:426–40.
2. Hirmand, H. *Plast Reconstr Surg.* 2010;125:699–708.
3. Flowers RS. *Clin Plast Surg.* 1993;20: 403–15.
4. Wong CH et al. *Plast Reconstr Surg.* 2012;129:1392–402.
5. Lambros VS. *Plast Reconstr Surg.* 2007;120:74s–80s.
6. Berguiga M & Galatoire O. *Orbit.* 2017;36(1):22–26.
7. Branham GH. *Facial Plast Surg Clin North Am.* 2016;24:129–38.
8. Brown M et al. *J Plast Reconstr Aesthet Surg.* 2014;67:e310–311.
9. Chiu CY et al. *Aesthet Plast Surg.* 2017;41: 73–80.
10. Davison SP et al. *Clin Plast Surg.* 2015;42: 51–6.
11. De Pasquale A et al. *Aesthet Plast Surg.* 2013;37:587–91.
12. Einan-Lifshitz A et al. *Ophthalmic Plast Reconstr Surg.* 2013;29:481–5.
13. Gierloff M et al. *J Plast Reconstr Aesthet Surg.* 2012;65:1292–7.
14. Hamman MS et al. *J Drugs Dermatol.* 2012;11:e80–84.

15. Hill RH 3rd et al. *Ophthalmic Plast Reconstr Surg.* 2015;31:306–9.
16. Huber-Vorlander J & Kurten M. *Plast Surgical Nursing.* 2015;35:171–6.
17. Huber-Vorlander J & Kurten M. *Clin Cosmet Investig Dermatol.* 2015;8:307–12.
18. Hwang K. *J Craniofac Surg.* 2016;27:1350–3.
19. Jiang J et al. *Postepy Dermatologii i Alergologii.* 2016;33:303–8.
20. Kashkouli MB et al. *Diplopia after hyaluronic acid gel injection for correction of facial tear trough deformity.* Orbit (Amsterdam, Netherlands). 2012;31:330–1.
21. Komuro Y et al. *Aesthet Plast Surg.* 2014;38:648–52.
22. Kridel RW & Sturm-O'Brien AK. *JAMA Facial Plast Surg.* 2013;15:232–4.
23. Liao SL & Wei YH. *Graefe's Archive Clini Experiment Ophthalmol.* 2011;249:1735–41.
24. Liapakis IE et al. *J Cranio-Maxillo-Facial Surg.* 2014;42:1497–502.
25. Lim HK et al. *J Cosmet Laser Ther.* 2014;16:32–36.
26. Mashiko T et al. *Plast Reconstr Surg Global Open.* 2013;1.
27. Pessa JE. *Plast Reconstr Surg.* 2012;129:1403–4.
28. Sharad J. *J Cutan Aesthet Surg.* 2012 ;5:229–38.
29. Smith CB & Waite PD. *Atlas Oral Maxillofac Surg Clin North Am.* 2016;24:135–45.
30. Viana GA et al. *Aesthet Surg J.* 2011;31:225–31.
31. Wang Y et al. *Aesthet Plast Surg.* 2015; 39:942–5.
32. Wattanakrai K et al. *J Plast Reconstr Aesthet Surg.* 2014;67:513–9.
33. Youn S et al. *Ann Plast Surg.* 2014;73:479–84.
34. Pessa J & Rohrich RJ. *Facial Topography: Clinical Anatomy of the Face.* Thieme; 2014.
35. Von Arx T et al. *Swiss Dent J.* 2017; 127(12):1066–75.
36. Lambros V. *Plast Reconstr Surg.* 2007;120:1367–76; discussion 1377.
37. Castanares S. *Plast Reconstr Surg (1946).* 1951;8:46–58.
38. Hamra ST. *Clin Plast Surg.* 1996;23:17–28.
39. Eder H. *Aesthet Plast Surg.* 1997;21:168–74.
40. Goldberg RA et al. *Semin Ophthalmol.* 1998;13:103–6.
41. Rohrich RJ et al. *Plast Reconstr Surg.* 2011;128:775–83.
42. Yaremchuk MJ & Kahn DM. *Plast Reconstr Surg.* 2009;124:2151–60.
43. Flowers RS & Nassif JM. Aesthetic periorbital surgery. In: Mathes SJ, ed. *Plastic Surgery,* Vol. 2. Philadelphia, PA: Saunders Elsevier; 2006, pp. 77–126.
44. Terino EO & Edwards MC. *Facial Plast Surg Clin North Am* 2008;16:33–67, v.
45. Cohen JL et al. *Aesthet Surg J.* 2015;35:844–9.
46. deLorenzi C. *Aesthet Surg J.* 2017;37(7):814–25.
47. Hwang CJ. *J Cutan Aesthet Surg.* 2016;9:73–9.
48. Seckel B. *Facial Danger Zones*, 2nd ed. Thieme; 2010.

Further Reading

Barton FE Jr et al. *Plast Reconstr Surg.* 2004;113:2115–21; discussion 2122–2113.

Born TM et al. Soft tissue fillers: Aesthetic surgery of the face. In: Neligan PC, ed. *Plastic Surgery.* 2013.

Carraway JH et al. *Aesthet Surg J.* 2001;21:337–43.

Coleman SR. *Aesthet Plast Surg.* 2008;32:415–7.

Mehryan P et al. *J Cosmet Dermatol.* 2014;13:72–8.

Rohrich RJ et al. *Plast Reconstr Surg.* 2003;112:1899–902.

Sadick NS et al. *J Cosmet Dermatol.* 2007;6:218–22.

Schierle CF & Casas LA. *Aesthet Surg J.* 2011;31:95–109.

Spector JA et al. *Aesthet Plast Surg.* 2008;32:411–4.

4 CHEEK AND ZYGOMATIC ARCH

Emanuele Bartoletti, Ekaterina Gutop, Chytra V. Anand, Giorgio Giampaoli, Sebastian Cotofana, and Ali Pirayesh

INTRODUCTION

Midface rejuvenation with fillers has marked a turning point in facial aesthetics. As such, the cheek and malar areas constitute aesthetically important regions which now form the foundation of modern aesthetic injectable practice. Both bone and soft tissues embody vitally important components of beauty which diminish with aging. As such, the targeted enhancement of midface fat compartments plays a pivotal role both in clinical facial aesthetics and in new research into facial layers.

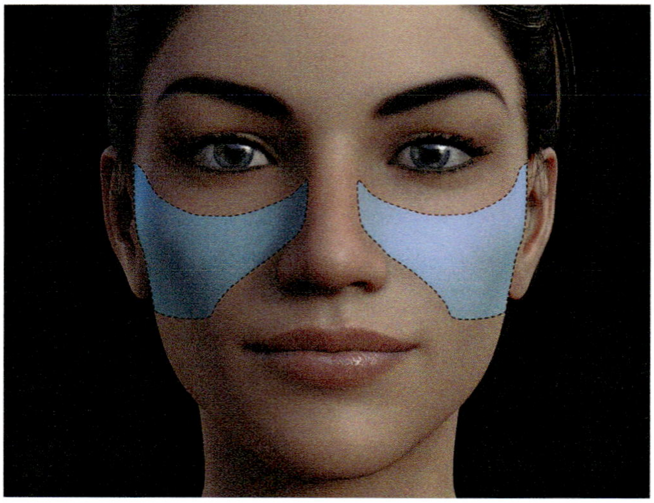

Figure 4.1 The malar region.

BOUNDARIES

The midface extends from the glabella to the subnasale, with the malar region overlying the zygoma and malar bone (Figure 4.1). The nasal-labial area is on the lower boundary and continues on the horizontal line that runs from anterior nasal spine to the earlobe insertion. The upper boundary runs from the glabella, following the infraorbital bony margin to the upper margin of the zygomatic arch.

AGING

Midface aging is a multifactorial process, with bone, soft tissue, retaining ligaments, fat compartments and the overlying skin envelope contributing in various ways to the characteristic stigmata. A fundamental understanding of salient tissue interactions is mandatory as the concept of compartment-specific volume augmentation has become integral to facial rejuvenation.

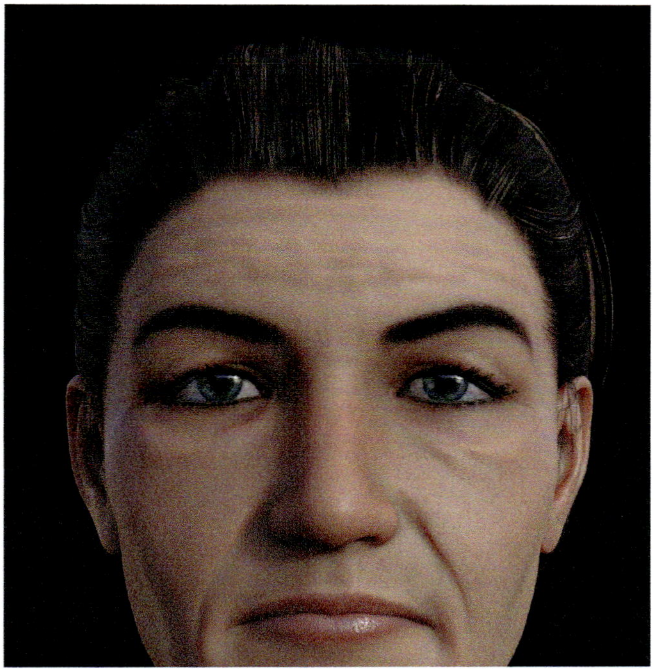

Figure 4.2 Midface aging: Note sagginess, heavy nasolabial folds and differential volume loss in various fat compartments.

There are two main theories of aging:

- A gravitational theory centered around changes in the ligamentous system of the cheek.
- A volumetric theory based on facial fat compartments deflation, particularly in the midface.

Midfacial aging most likely involves both gravitational ptosis and volume deflation (Figures 4.2 and 4.3) with pseudoherniation of the Bichat's fat pad probably also contributing. Insightful understanding of the degree of volume loss in both bone and facial fat is essential for effective planning and optimal outcomes.

SKIN

The midfacial skin envelope reflects the deflation and atrophic changes of underlying bone and soft-tissue compartments.

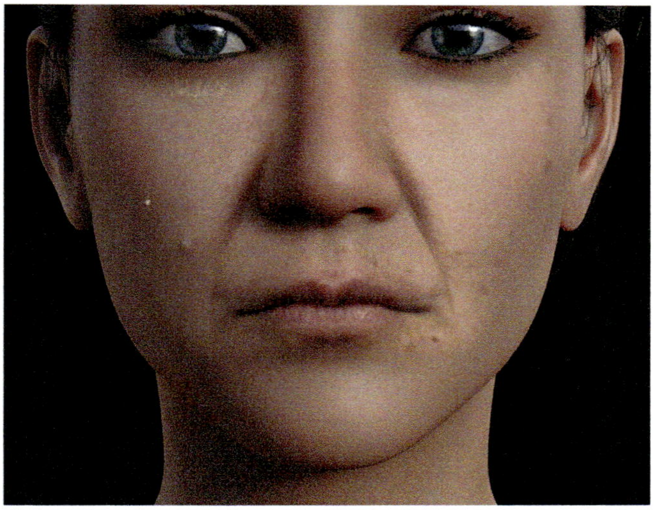

Figure 4.3 Severe ageing of midface.

Additionally, the skin undergoes intrinsic and extrinsic aging which is compounded by repetitive, dynamic facial muscle movements.

FAT

Since the first description of the superficial facial fat compartments (Figure 4.4) by Pessa and Rohrich (2007), understanding of the exact localization, anatomic boundaries, relevant clinical landmarks and

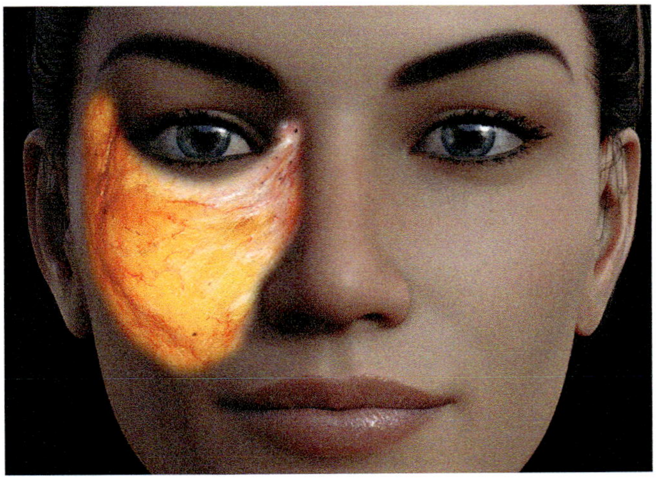

Figure 4.4 Exposed superficial fat compartments of the midface.

age-related changes of the facial fat pads has been constantly evolving. In addition to initial dissections, subsequent MRI and computed tomographical studies have facilitated accrual of new insights [16].

The facial fat compartments (Figures 4.5–4.10) may be categorized as either superficial or deep, and insightful understanding of their delicate functional anatomy enables clinicians to achieve optimal aesthetic outcomes. It is vitally important to understand that filling of certain compartments may exacerbate sagginess, whilst filling others is less prone to do so, probably due to more stable anatomic boundaries.

The superficial fat compartments have recently been described by Cotofana as comprising seven bilaterally distinct subcutaneous fat compartments

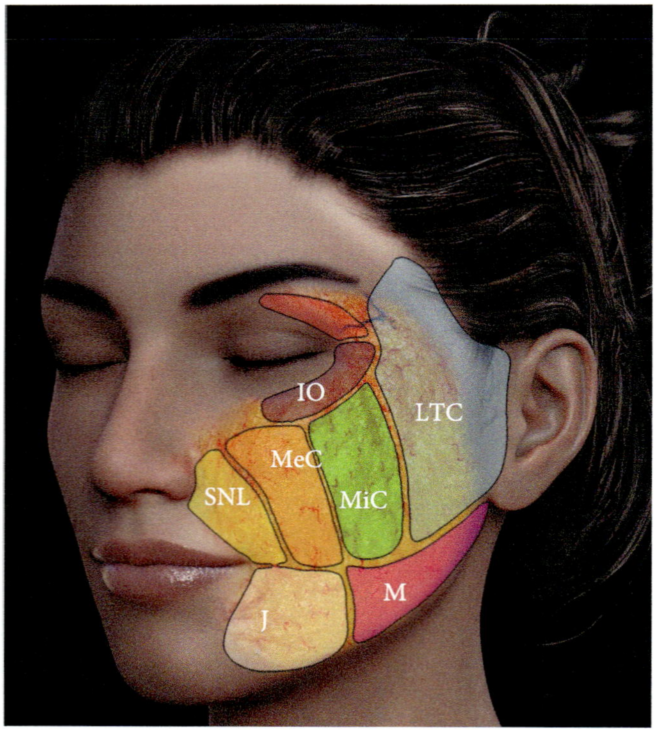

Figure 4.5 Illustration of fat compartments: IO, infraorbital fat; SNL, superficial nasolabial fat; MeC, medial cheek fat; MiC, middle cheek; J, jowl fat pad; LTC, lateral temporal cheek fat (now shown to be 2 separate compartments separated by zygoma).

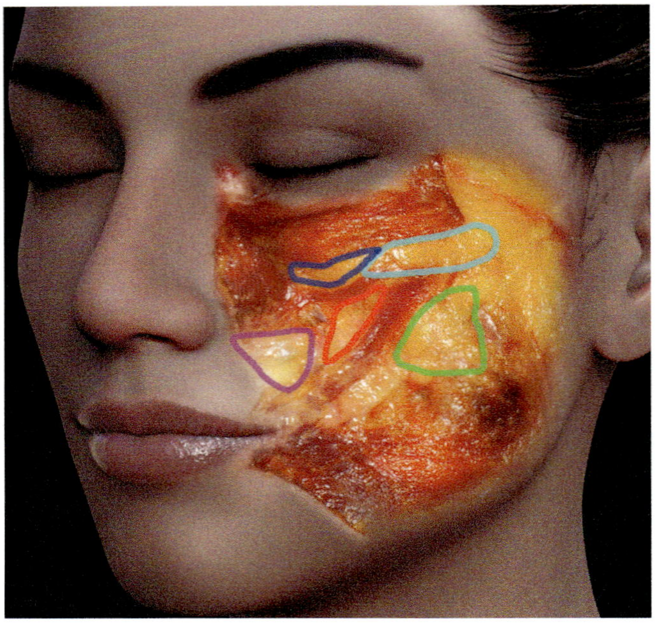

Figure 4.6 The deep fat compartments: SOOF: blue medial portion, light blue lateral portion; deep medial cheek fat: red medial portion, green lateral portion; Purple: deep nasolabial fat.

(excluding the superficial forehead compartment) which are separated by delicate fibrous septae. These superficial fat compartments do not cover the tear trough, lateral orbital thickening or zygomatic arch. Superior and Inferior superficial Jowl fat pads lie below the superficial medial and middle cheek fat pads. It is clinically important to realize that the various superficial (subcutaneous) fat compartments behave differently on filling: whilst the inferior aspect of the nasolabial, middle cheek, and jowl compartments descend on filling, this is not observed for the medial or lateral cheek compartments.

The superficial fat compartments [13] comprise the

1. Superficial nasolabial
2. Superficial medial cheek
3. Superficial middle cheek
4. Superficial lateral cheek
5. Superior temporal
6. Inferior temporal
7. Jowl fat compartment

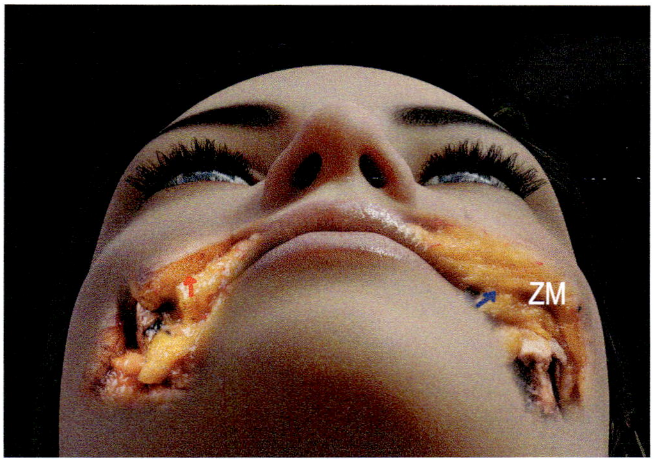

Figure 4.7 Deep fat compartments: The middle cheek fat compartment lies between medial cheek and lateral temporal cheek fat. The superior border is defined by the superior cheek septum (SCS). A zone of fixation (red arrow) is noted where this compartment adjoins the middle compartment and inferior orbital compartment. (Right) The cross-sectional anatomy illustrates the anatomic principle that fusion planes exist between adjacent fat compartments. A dense fascial system (blue arrow) exists where the medial and middle fat compartments meet. The zygomaticus major (ZM) muscle is noted deep to this fusion plane.

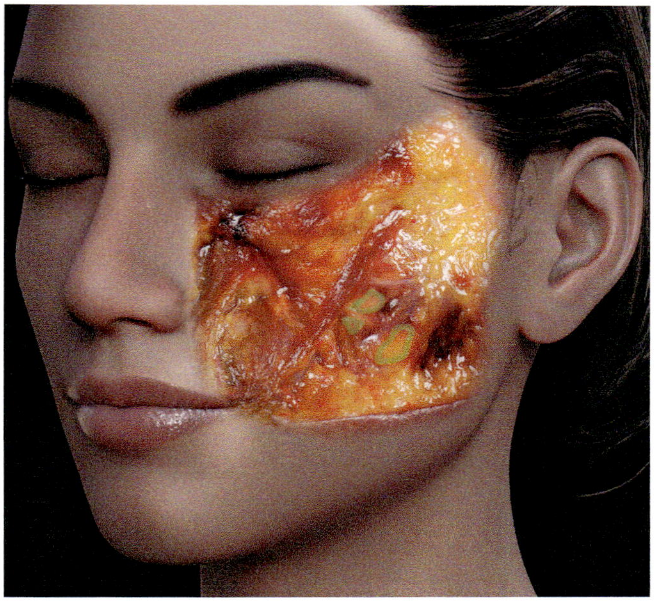

Figure 4.9 Green: buccal fat compartment; the buccal fat pad has a buccal, pterygoid and temporal extension and paler yellow colour.

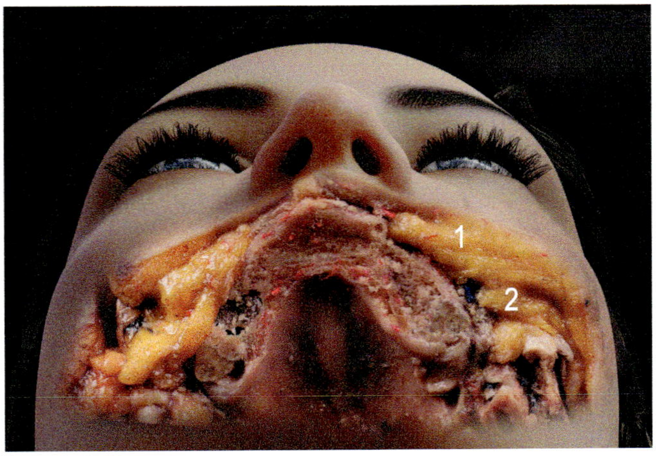

Figure 4.8 (1) Deep medial cheek fat compartment; (2) deep middle fat pad compartment.

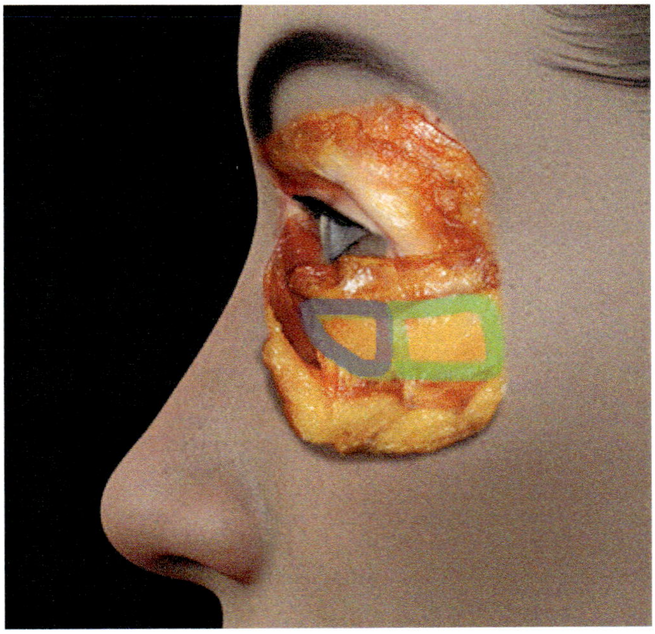

Figure 4.10 Green: suborbicularis oculi fat compartment (SOOF); this compartment is divided into a medial (blue) and lateral (green) SOOF; a vertical line through the medial margin of the pupil forms the boundary. The upper border is formed bye ORL and the lower border by the zygomaticocutaneous ligaments.

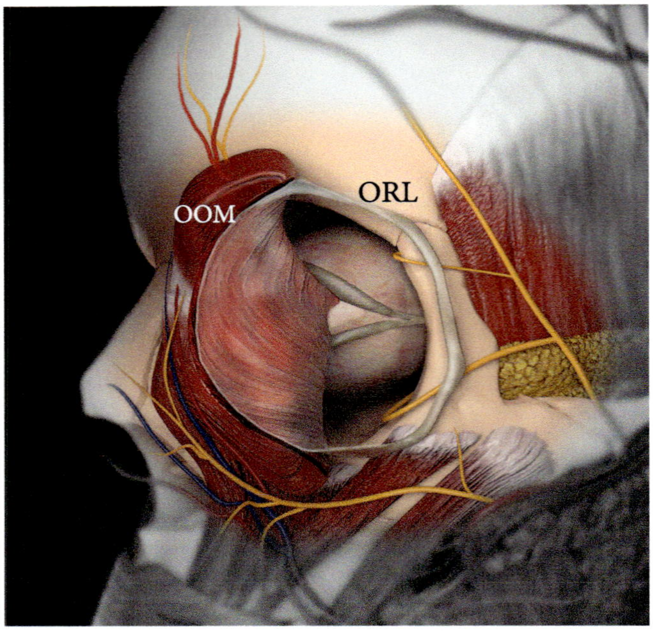

Figure 4.11 ORL: the orbicularis retaining ligament inserts 2–3 mm from the orbital margin and inserts into the dermis, stabilizing the orbicularis oris muscle (OOM).

Superficial Fat Compartments

Infraorbital Fat

Description of this fat compartment has been included here for comprehensiveness. The superior margins of the infraorbital fat compartment correspond to the skin surface of the tear trough and palpebral malar groove. DMCF is divided into: Deep medial cheek fat medial part and deep medial cheek fat lateral part. The superior boundary is formed by the orbicularis retaining ligament (ORL) (Figure 4.11) which originates from the orbital bone 2–3 mm inferior to the margin of the orbit and passes through the orbicularis oculi muscle to insert in the dermis [1,2]. The ORL contributes to the formation of the tear trough and palpebromalar groove. The palpebral part of the orbicularis oculi muscle (OOM) is found cranially to the ORL, immediately subcutaneous to eyelid skin; caudally, the orbital OOM is covered by infraorbital fat which is bordered by the zygomatic cutaneous ligament [3] (Figure 4.12a and b). Mendelson described

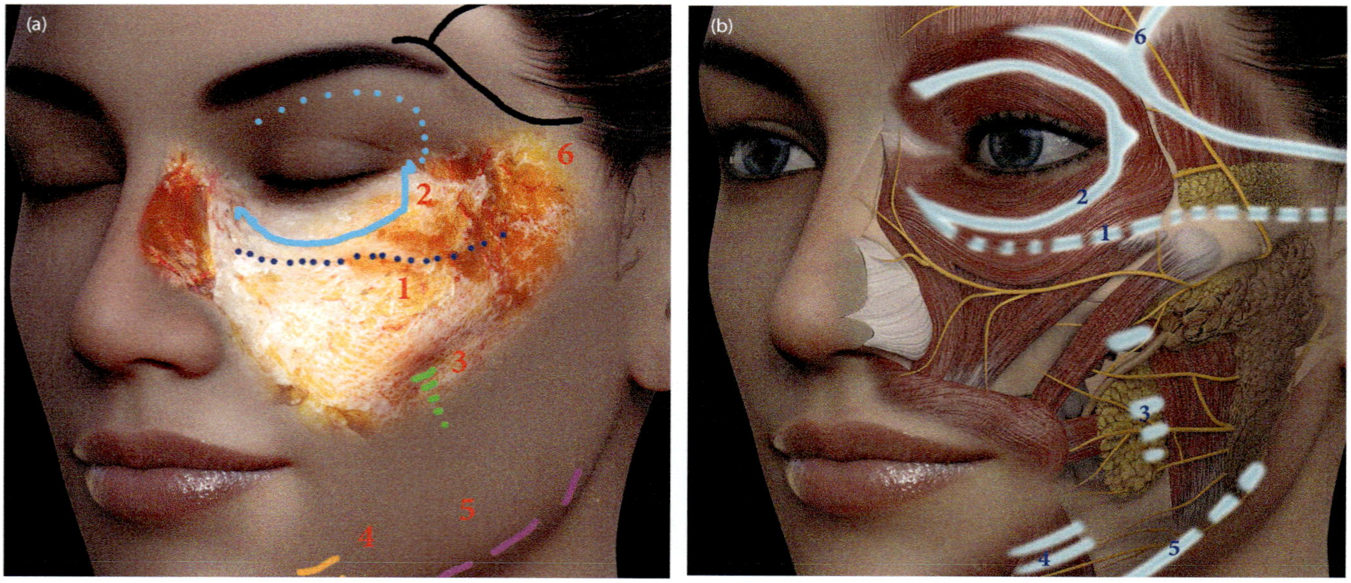

Figure 4.12 (a and b): 1 = Zygomatic cutaneous ligament; 2 = ORL; 3 = anterior masseteric ligaments; 4 = mandibular ligaments; 5 = mandibular ligaments; 6 = temporal fusion line.

the zygomatic ligaments medial to the junction of the arch and body of zygoma, located at the origins of the muscles of facial expression (zygomaticus major, zygomaticus minor, and levator labii superioris [4]). At the junction of the arch and body of the zygoma, just lateral to the origin of the zygomaticus major muscle, this ligament becomes thicker and stronger and denoted as McGregor's patch [5].

The infraorbital fat has a high tendency for water retention and is prone to persistent edema [6,7].

Superficial Medial Cheek Fat

Forms an inverted triangle with its upper horizontal border at the level of the inferior orbital rim. The superior boundary is closely related to the orbicularis retaining ligament whilst the inferior boundary is related to the zygomaticus major muscle.

Superficial Nasolabial Fat

This compartment has an oblique longitudinal axis extending from the lateral nose to the angle of the mouth. The orbicularis retaining ligament represents the superior border of this compartment. It borders superolaterally with the medial cheek fat, inferomedially with the nasolabial fold and overlaps inferiorly with the jowl fat (Figure 4.13).

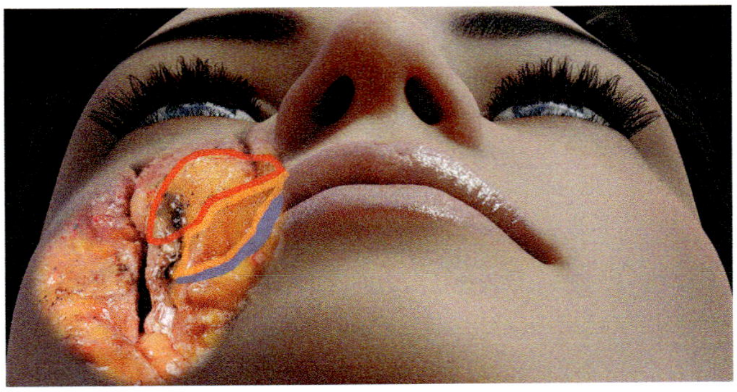

Figure 4.13 Nasolabial fat compartment: Red: superficial; Orange: deep; Blue: lip fat compartment.

Superficial Middle Cheek Fat

This rectangular compartment is located between the zygomatic arch and the mandible and lies lateral to the lateral canthus.

Superficial Lateral Cheek Fat

This rectangular compartment which was previously considered part of the lateral temporal cheek fat pad, extends from a discrete border at the zygomatic arch to the mandible. It lies between the superficial middle fat compartment and the auricle. Its stability may be due to its position on the midfacial SMAS which is strongly adherent to the underlying parotideomasseteric fascia, thus limiting inferior displacement upon filling.

Jowl Fat

This compartment lies inferior to the medial cheek fat, lateral to the superficial nasolabial fat compartment, medial to the superficial middle cheek fat and superior to the mandible. It is situated superficial to the SMAS and separated from the buccal space.

Deep Fat Compartments

The muscles of facial expression contribute to formation of the boundaries of the deep midfacial fat compartments in the premaxillary space (1) deep pyriform, (2) deep medial cheek, (3) deep lateral cheek, and (4) deep nasolabial), and the (5) medial and lateral suborbicularis oculi fat (SOOF). These muscles have a stable location and course during the aging process.

Suborbicularis Oculi Fat (SOOF)

The SOOF is divided into distinct medial and lateral compartments, with the bilaminar ORL forming the superior boundary. The inferior boundary is formed by the zygomaticocutaneous ligament and/or the zygomaticus minor muscle. A vertical line passing through the medial margin of the pupil forms the medial boundary. The angular vein is embedded in this boundary and courses toward the medial canthus inferior to the tear trough area, which is not connected to the SOOF. The lateral boundary has recently been visualized to be open and connected to the inferior temporal compartment via the temporal tunnel. The lateral orbital thickening forms the superior margin and McGregor's patch the inferior margin of this tunnel. McGregor's patch also constitutes the starting point of the zygomaticocutaneous ligament. The SOOF lies on a thin sheet of fibrous connective tissue extending from the superficial lamina of the deep temporal fascia. It is thus separated from the prezygomatic space, which lies deep to this fat compartment, between the fascia and periosteum. Neither the position (superior versus inferior boundary) nor extent (vertical versus horizontal) changes with increasing age.

Deep Nasolabial Fat

The triangular deep nasolabial fat lies within the premaxillary space, superficial to the levator labii superioris alaeque nasi (LLSAN) and deep to the orbital part of the orbicularis oculi muscle in its upper part, adjacent to the the midcheek SMAS in its lower part. The medial wall is formed by the lateral nasal wall and lateral nasal vein, whereas the lateral boundary is formed by a thin sheet of fibrous connective tissue covering the angular vein. The cranial boundary is formed by the angular vein and its fascia, inferior to the tear trough, whilst the inferior boundary is formed by the fascial fusion of the midcheek SMAS and the LLSAN. With aging there is no significant relationship to any change in position or extent of their compartment.

Deep Pyriform Fat

This deep fat compartment is located between the levator anguli oris and LLSAN. It is bounded superomedially by the lateral nasal wall and inferiorly by the depressor septi nasi. The lateral wall is formed by the fascial sheet surrounding the infraorbital neurovascular bundle emerging from its foramen, thus separating this fat compartment from the deep medial cheek fat. The inferior boundary is formed by the fusion of LLSAN and the levator anguli oris muscle at the level of the nasolabial sulcus, whereas the superior boundary is formed by the oblique (medial superior to lateral inferior attachment of the LLSAN to the maxilla.

Deep Lateral Cheek Fat (DLCF)

This inverted triangle overlies the area around the zygomatico-maxillary suture and is in direct contact with the bone. The superior boundary is formed by the zygomaticocutaneous ligament and/or the zygomaticus minor muscle and the medial boundary by a thin layer of connective tissue enveloping the angular vein. The lateral and inferior boundary is formed by the zygomaticus major muscle and the transverse facial septum. The orbital part of the orbicularis oculi muscle and the midcheek SMAS form the anterior boundary. This compartment has no connections to the buccal fat pad.

Deep Medial Cheek Fat

The deep medial cheek fat lies between the LAO and the LLSAN in the same plane as the deep pyriform fat compartment. The medial boundary is formed by the fascial sheet surrounding the infraorbital neurovascular bundle emerging from its foramen, whereas the lateral boundary is formed by a thin sheet of connective tissue enclosing the angular vein. The superior boundary is formed by the bony attachment of the LLSAN and the inferior boundary by the fusion of the levator anguli oris and the LLSAN medially and the zygomaticus major and the transverse facial septum laterally [16].

Aging of the Fat Compartments

Although widely accepted that the facial skeleton undergoes significant changes during aging, it is currently unknown how these effects ultimately influence the overall functional anatomy of the deep midfacial fat compartments.

Individual facial fat compartments appear to age differently, most probably depending on their location. Whilst some may change position, others remain stable because of their ligamentous connections to underlying bone. Aging significantly influences inferior displacement of the superficial nasolabial and jowl compartments, thus substantialy influencing the appearance of the aging face. It is important to understand that whereas the inferior nasolabial, middle cheek, and jowl compartments descend on filling, the medial and lateral cheek and superficial temporal compartments do not.

Injection procedures should be consciously targeted in terms of fat compartments and fascial planes as each have unique tissue responses to injected soft-tissue fillers. In a recent study by Cotofana et al. the SOOF revealed the highest surface-volume coefficient after filling, whilst the deep medial cheek fat compartment demonstrated the lowest tissue response.

Buccal Fat

The buccal fat extension appears to undergo hypotrophic aging, with several authors reporting decreasing volume of buccal extension in older patients [8,9]. Deflation leads to lack of medial and middle cheek support, thus aggravating descent of these compartments. Antero-inferior protrusion of buccal fat may also increase cheek convexity and jowl ptosis [10,11].

MUSCLES

Clinically relevant, albeit less commonly described cheek muscles, include the **malaris** and **buccinator muscles**.

Malaris is a bilaminar muscle with mesial and lateral heads of which the mesial head corresponds to the tear trough. This muscle forms the medial and lateral non-sphincteric aspects of the orbicularis oculi muscle, enveloping the medial and lateral sphincteric orbicularis oculi. It does not insert into the malar bone, whereas the zygomaticus major and zygomaticus minor originate from the zygomatic bone and insert respectively into the modiolus and upper lip. The malaris muscle may interdigitate with the upper lip levators before inserting superficially into the upper lip adjacent to the zygomaticus minor [12].

Buccinator is a thin, quadrilateral muscle lying between the maxilla and mandible with fibers con-verging toward the modiolus. It inserts into the deep layer of perioral muscles and often connects with orbicularis oris, depressor anguli oris (DAO), levator anguli oris (LAO), platysma, and deep slip of zygomaticus major. In many cases, a slip inserts into the mentalis.

In the temporal-malar region the fascial layer demonstrates a trilaminar structure:

- **Superficial layer**, or **SMAS,** enveloping the muscles around the periorbital and perioral apertures
- **Middle** layer beneath facial nerves, connecting with the parotid fascia
- **Deep** layer identical to the temporal fascia

The **SMAS** is a midlevel fibromuscular layer separating the superficial and deep facial fat.

The fasciae enveloping individual facial muscles are interconnected, thus forming **myofascial continuity**. This continuity, explained as the "anatomical trains", is of clinical relevance as it helps to explain the indirect effects of fillers effected via SMAS expansion (see Chapter D on Myomodulation). The layered periorbital and perioral muscles, with their enveloping SMAS layers, are capable of intricate facial movements and expressions.

Pessa described several variations in midface musculature [6]. From medial to lateral, these muscles are (Figures 4.14 and 4.15)

1. **Levator labii superioris alae que nasi (LLSAN)**
2. **Levator labii superioris (LLS)**
3. **Zygomaticus minor (Zyg min)**
4. **Zygomaticus major (Zyg maj):** the morphology may be either single or bifid
5. **Risorius (Ris)**

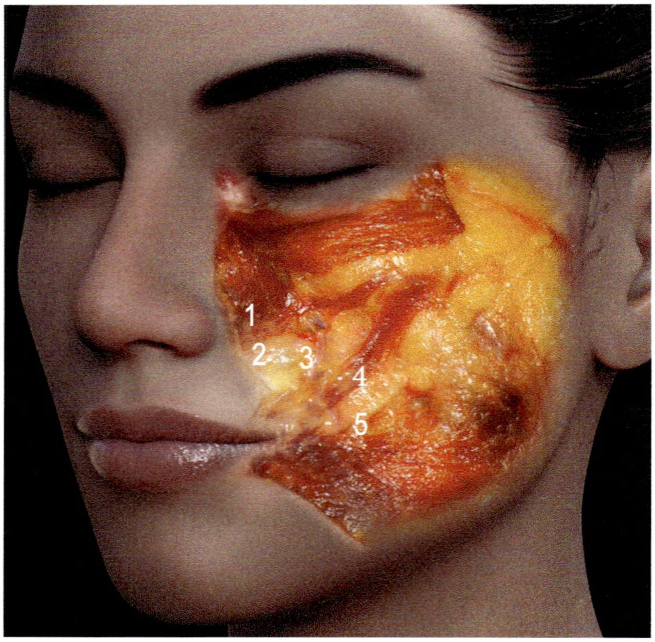

Figure 4.14 Muscle origins and insertions: Levator labii superioris alae que nasi (LLSAN), levator labii superioris (LLS), zygomaticus minor (Zyg min), zygomaticus major (Zyg maj), risorius (Ris).

1. Levator labi superioris alae que nasi (LLSAN)

Origin	Upper frontal process of maxilla, medial infraorbital margin
Insertion	Skin of lateral nostril and upper lip
Innervation	
Motor	VII (zygomatic branch)
Vascularization	Facial artery and maxillary artery
Action	Dilates nostril; elevates and inverts upper lip "Elvis muscle"

2. Levator labii superioris (LLS)

Origin	Broad sheet, medial infraorbital margin; extending from side of nose to zygomatic bone
Insertion	Skin and muscle of upper lip
Innervation	
Motor	VII (buccal branch)
Vascularization	Facial artery
Action	Elevates upper lip

3. Zygomaticus minor (Zyg min)

Origin	Lateral part of zygomatic bone medial to zygomaticus major
Insertion	Skin of lateral upper lip; extends to nasolabial sulcus
Innervation	
Motor	VII (buccal branch)
Vascularization	Superior labial branch of the facial artery
Action	Pulls the upper lip backward, upward, and outward Aids in deepening and elevating the nasolabial sulcus

4. Zygomaticus major (Zyg maj)

Origin	Temporal process, anterior zygomatic bone
Insertion	Modiolus
Innervation	
Motor	VII (zygomatic and buccal branch)
Vascularization	Superior labial branch of the facial artery
Action	Elevates and draws angle of mouth laterally

5. Risorius (Ris)

Origin	Pre-parotid fascia
Insertion	Modiolus
Innervation	
Motor	VII (buccal branch)
Vascularization	Facial artery
Action	Draws back corner of mouth

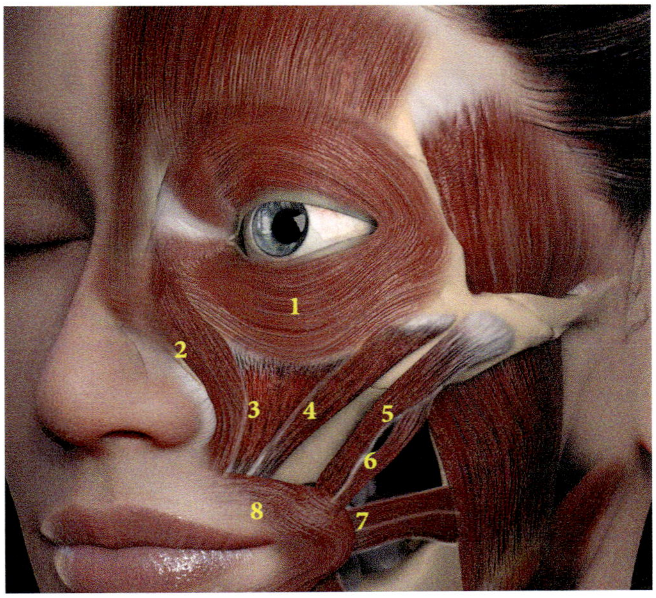

Figure 4.15 Muscle origins and insertions of mimetic muscles. (1) Orbicularis oculi; (2) LLSAN; (3) levator labii superioris; (4) zygomaticus minor; (5) zygomaticus major; (6) levator anguli oris; (7) risorius; (8) orbicularis oris.

VASCULARIZATION

- The main facial blood supply is provided by the facial, transverse facial, and infraorbital (IOA) arteries, which are in hemodynamic balance (Figure 4.16).
- The facial arteries originate either
  - Directly from the external carotid artery (facial artery, superficial temporal artery), or
  - From branches of the external carotid artery (transverse facial artery from superficial temporal artery, infraorbital artery from maxillary artery)

The **superficial temporal artery (STA)** is a terminal branch of the external carotid and arises within the parotid gland at the level of the maxillary artery bifurcation from the external carotid artery. The STA ascends over the posterior root of the zygomatic arch approximately 1 cm anterior to the ear.

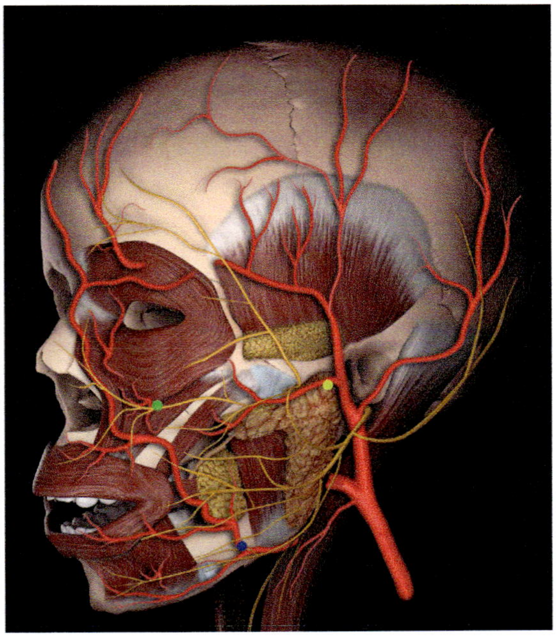

Figure 4.16 Facial blood supply to the cheek is provided by the facial (blue), transverse facial (yellow), and infraorbital (IOA) (green) arteries.

The **transverse facial artery (TFA)** (Figure 4.17) originates from the STA within the parotid gland and courses anteriorly and sometimes slightly downward, to the cheek.

- The transverse facial artery may anastomose with the facial artery.
- The main blood supply to the cheeks is from arterial perforators originating from the
    - **Transverse facial artery**: Posterosuperior parts of the cheek (zygomatic and parotid-masseteric regions).
    - **Facial artery**: Lower anterior cheek (buccal region).
    - The **buccal artery** (originating from the maxillary artery) perfuses the lower anterior portion of the cheek (buccal region).

The zygomatic area of the cheek further receives arterial supply from the **zygomaticofacial branch of the lacrimal artery** (see Figure 4.17b).

- The zygomaticomalar branch (ZMB) of the infraorbital artery (IOA) becomes superficial ~17 mm medial to the edge of the zygomatic arch and runs through the malar fat pad before ending at the skin of the cheek.
- Cutaneous perforators of the ZMB of the IOA were present in 77% of cases in a recent cadaver study.
- This study found that the mean calibers of the IOA branches were 0.5 mm for the nasal branch (NB), 0.6 mm for the ZMB, and 0.7 mm for the vestibular branch, which makes them too small to be injured using a cannula.
- The lateral third of the zygomatic bone constitutes a danger zone for more superficial injections and should preferably be injected in the supraperiosteal plane.

INNERVATION

Sensory

The skin of the zygomatic prominence is innervated by the zygomaticofacial branch of the zygomatic nerve, which originates from the maxillary nerve within the pterygopalatine fossa (Figures 4.18 and 4.19).

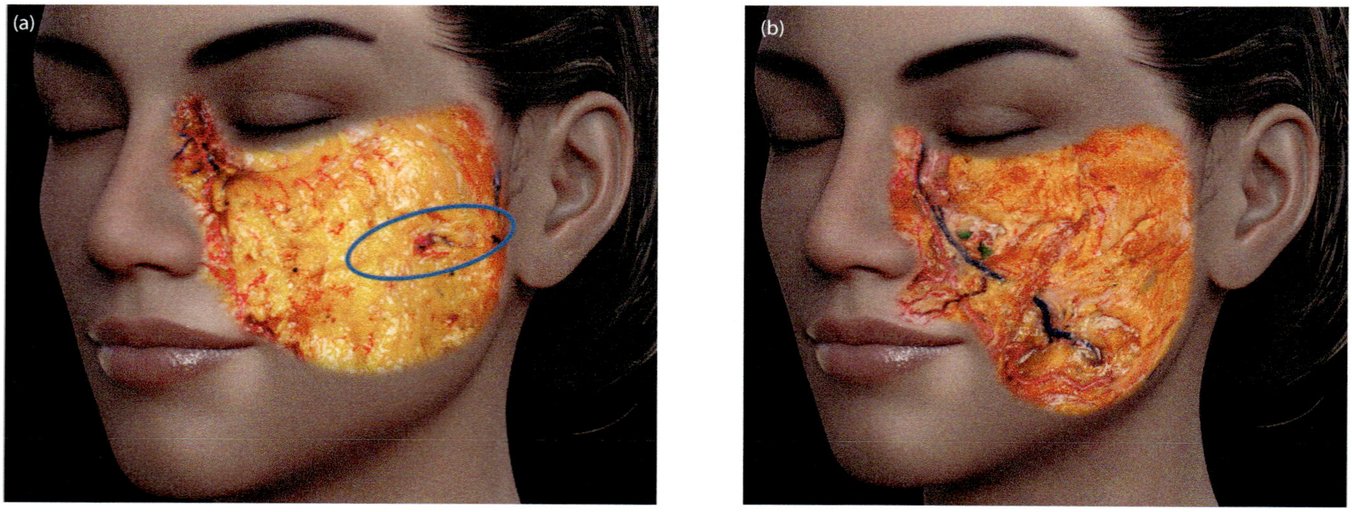

Figure 4.17 (a) The transverse facial artery (TFA) originates from the superficial temporal artery within the parotid gland and courses anteriorly and sometimes slightly downward to the cheek. (b) Zygomaticofacial branch of the lacrimal artery.

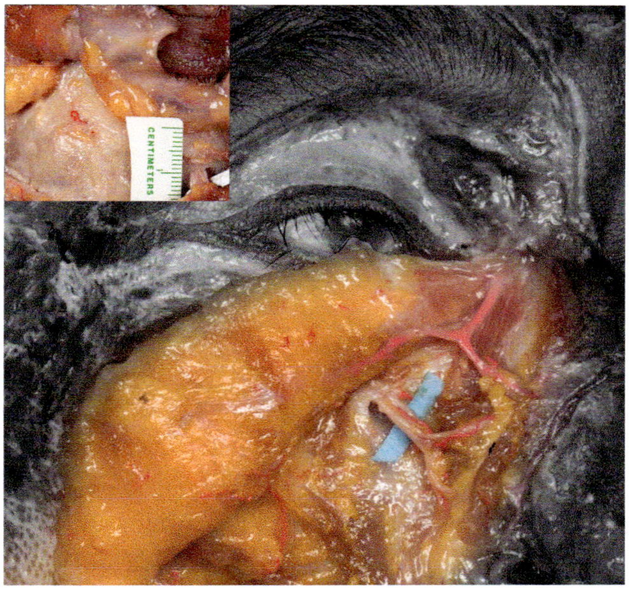

Figure 4.18 Infraorbital neurovascular bundle exits infraorbital foramen.

The skin of the infraorbital region is innervated by branches from the infraorbital nerve (ION), mainly by twigs from the superior labial branch, but also the other ION branches.

The skin of the upper anterior part of the cheek is supplied by lateral rami of the large superior labial branch from the ION.

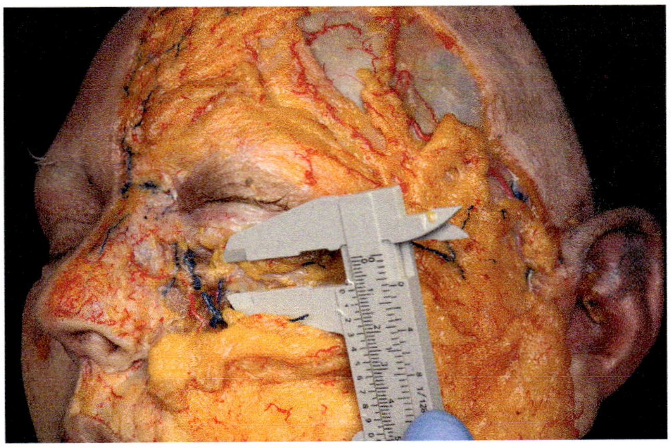

Figure 4.19 ION: position is usually low (0.8–1 cm below infraorbital rim) and on a vertical line that passes through the mid-limbus.

Motor

The facial muscles are supplied by the facial nerve (cranial nerve VII), with each nerve serving one side of the face (Figure 4.20). It courses through the facial canal in the temporal bone and exits through the stylomastoid foramen, after which it divides into five terminal branches at the anterior edge of the parotid gland. The facial nerve provides motor innervation to the muscles of the face and parasympathetic innervation to the glands of the oral cavity and lacrimal gland. It also supplies sensory innervation to the anterior two-thirds of the tongue, the external auditory meatus and the pinna of the ear.

Five branches can be identified:

- The **temporal** branch, innervating the frontalis and orbicularis oculi muscles and the muscles in the upper part of the face
- The **zygomatic** branch, innervating the middle part of the face

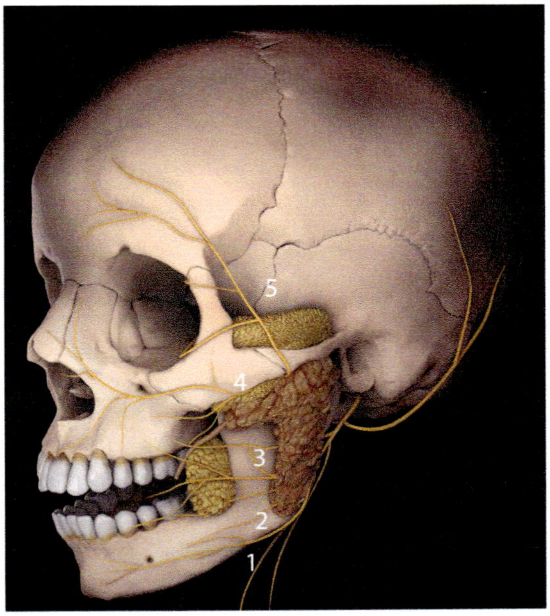

Figure 4.20 The five branches of facial nerve VII; of these, the frontal, marginal mandibular, and cervical branches could be in danger from aesthetic treatments.

- The **buccal** branch, innervating the cheek muscles, including the buccinator muscle and orbicularis oris
- The **marginal mandibular** branch, innervating muscles of the lower part of the face
- The **cervical** branch, innervating the muscles below the chin and, among others, the platysma muscle

The skin of the cheek prominence is innervated by the zygomaticofacial branch of the zygomatic nerve, which originates from the maxillary nerve within the pterygopalatine fossa. The skin of the infraorbital region of the cheek is innervated by branches from the ION.

BONE

The zygomatic bone (cheekbone/malar bone) is a paired irregular bone which articulates with the maxilla, temporal bone, sphenoid bone, and the frontal bone (Figure 4.21). It is situated at the upper lateral part of the face and forms:

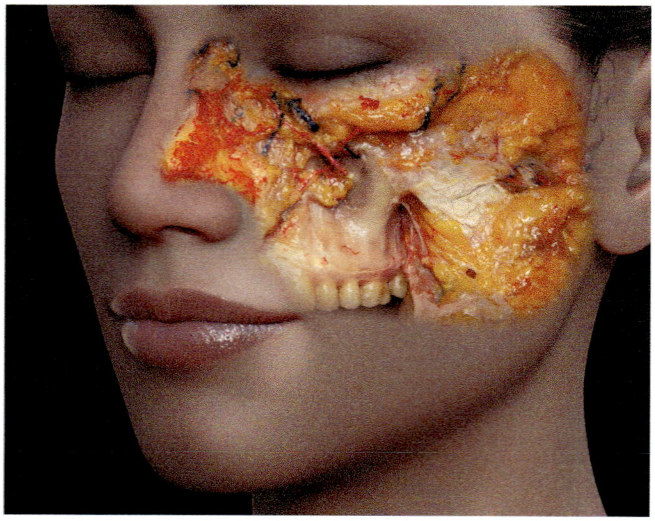

Figure 4.21 The midface skeleton, particularly the maxilla, pyriform region, and superomedial and inferolateral orbital rims, is prone to resorption.

- The cheek prominence
- Part of the lateral wall and floor of the orbit
- Parts of the temporal fossa
- The infratemporal fossa

It presents

- A malar and a temporal surface
- Four processes (the frontosphenoidal, orbital, maxillary, and temporal)
- Four borders

The orbital surface of the frontal process of the zygomatic bone forms the anterior lateral orbital wall. Usually, a small paired foramen, the zygomaticofacial foramen, opens on its lateral surface.

The temporal process of the zygomatic bone forms the zygomatic arch along with the zygomatic process of the temporal bone. These two processes join at a clinically important palpable suture.

Paired zygomaticotemporal foramens open on the medial deep surface of the bone.

The orbital surface of the maxillary process of the zygomatic bone forms a part of the infraorbital rim and a small part of the anterior part of the lateral orbital wall.

Bone aging and resorption occur in a specific and predictable manner, and correction of the skeletal framework is increasingly viewed as a new frontier in facial rejuvenation. The midface skeleton, particularly the maxilla, pyriform region, and superomedial and inferolateral orbital rims, is prone to resorption.

HOW I DO IT: BOTULINUM TOXIN

- Avoid placing lateral canthal toxins inferior to the superior zygomatic arch as this risks spread into

the zygomaticus major and minor muscles with subsequent ipsilateral facial paralysis or lip ptosis.
- Over-treatment of the lateral canthal area decreases the function of orbicularis oculi as the only elevator of the cheek and may increase palpebral oedema in predisposed individuals.
- Avoid inadvertent treatment of risorius, with subsequent asymmetric smile, by remaining in the safe zone 1 cm post to the anterior border of masseter when treating the masseter with botulinum toxin.

HOW I DO IT: FILLERS

Assessment

- Evaluate patient in anterior, oblique, and lateral views.
- Lateral assessment is vital in evaluating negative vectors in the midface.
- Deficient malar and midfacial projection leave the soft tissues poorly supported, resulting in premature lower lid and cheek descent, eye bags, scleral show, and a more aged appearance. These deficiencies should be accurately assessed and insightfully addressed.
- Assess the face both at rest and in animation. Upgrading in animation is usually predictive of a favorable outcome after correct volumization.
- Carefully assess the function and synergy of the upper-lip levators in order to plan optimal depth of placement, especially in the central cheek area (see Chapter D on Myomodulation).

Technique

Lateral Zygoma (Cheek Point 1)

- Mark the lid-cheek junction (LCJ) with the patient in the upright, "chin down, eyes up" position. This position accentuates the LCJ (Figure 4.22).

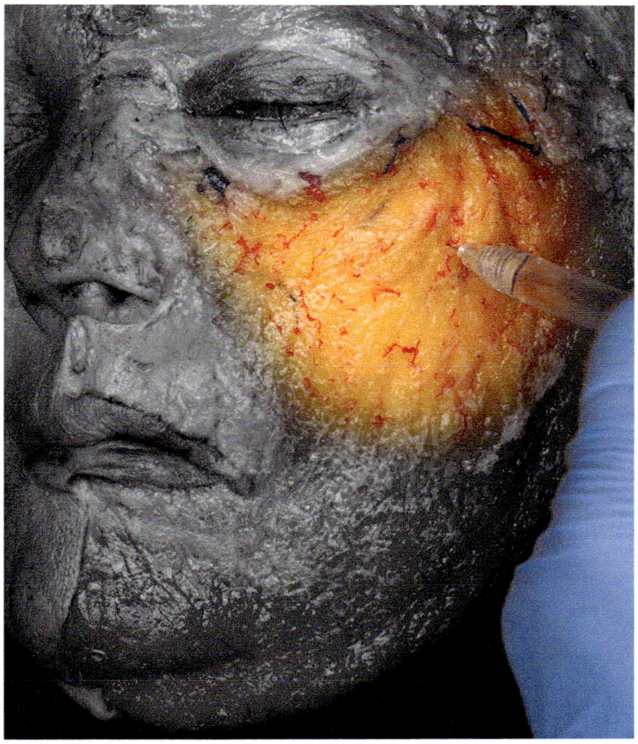

Figure 4.22 Malar Eminence injection (Cheek Point 2).

- Palpate the zygomatic bone (with second and third fingers) and mark the superior and inferior borders meticulously. These are vital landmarks as the middle temporal vein and transverse facial artery run parallel with the zygoma at a distance of 1 cm superior and inferior, respectively, to the bone. Inaccurate needle angulation carries the risk of vascular compromise.
- Palpate and mark the suture between the zygomatic and frontal bones.
- Mark two additional points 1 cm anterior and posterior to the suture if additional lifting/support is desired.
- Cleanse meticulously.
- Retract the skin (while palpating the zygoma). Aspirate for 4–6 seconds while stabilizing the needle tip. It is important to realize that this manoeuver cannot completely exclude intravascular placement. Thus, concomitant vigilant injection technique with slow injection speed and low extrusion force is mandatory.

- Inject a bolus anterior to the marking in the supraperiosteal plane, with the needle perpendicular to the bone.
- Always have an awareness of watershed circulation regions such as the glabella and nasal tip.
- When clinically indicated, place an additional bolus anterior and then posterior to the first point.

Malar Eminence (Cheek Point 2)

- Palpate and mark the malar eminence (Figure 4.23).
- Inject a supraperiosteal bolus.
- Injection technique is as for the lateral malar point.

Mid-Cheek (Cheek Point 3, Which is More an Area Than a Point)

This area may be volumized at different three levels, depending on clinical needs (Figure 4.24):

- On the bone
- In the deep medial cheek fat pad (DMCF)
- In the medial SOOF

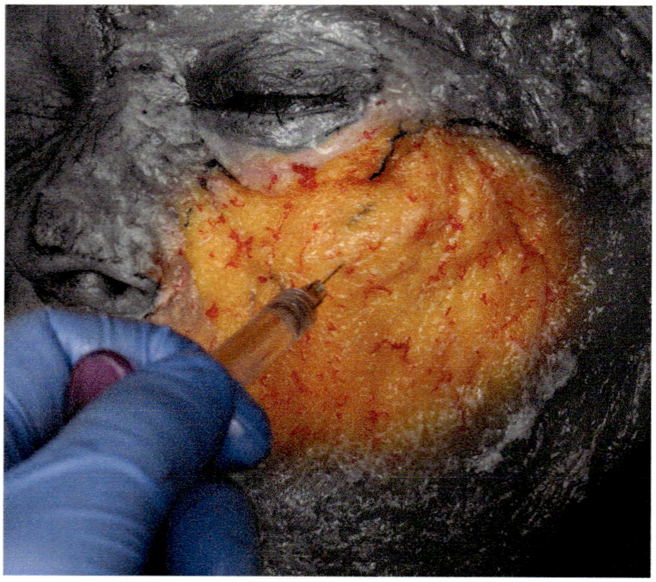

Figure 4.23 Supraperiosteal injection at the malar emnence. This injection is also in the lateral SOOF.

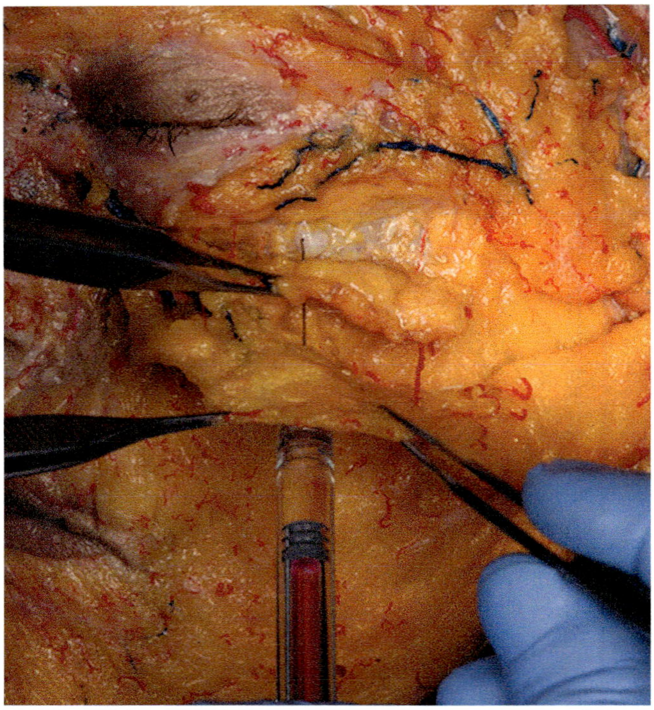

Figure 4.24 Deep medial cheek fat pad (using a cannula).

Accurate clinical assessment is vital as product placement above the upper-lip levators may lengthen the upper lip, whereas placement below the levators may strengthen their action. These principles are discussed in Chapter D on Myomodulation.

Injecting Deep on the Bone to Address Bone Deficiency (Using a Needle)

- Mark the infraorbital foramen:
  - Draw a vertical line medial to the mid-pupillary line.
  - Mark the foramen at a point just medial to the line and ~6–8 mm inferior to the inferior orbital rim.
- Mark the area of volume deficiency after evaluation in upright, lateral and supine positions.
- Intravascular injury of the main IOA trunk may be minimized by injecting from lateral to medial in a plane perpendicular to the axis of the IOA. The

bony "hood" over the foramen gives added protection to the IO foramen when using this lateral approach.
- Aspirate (as previously mentioned).
- Inject a bolus deep on the bone while maintaining vigilant aseptic technique and constant awareness of the signs of possible vascular compromise (watershed areas, blanching, mottling, pain).
- Massage gently.

Deep Medial Cheek Fat Pad (Using a Cannula)

- Mark the volume deficiency (as previously mentioned).
- Mark the cannula entry point, using a medial approach.
- Cleanse meticulously and maintain stringent aseptic technique.
- Pinch the skin and make needle puncture (one gauge larger than the cannula, e.g., 23G needle for 25G blunt-tipped cannula). Make the entry point in the same direction as the proposed cannula tract.
- Introduce the cannula at an angle of approximately 60° to the skin. This should guide placement below the upper-lip levators and in the correct plane.
- Using a fanning technique, gently place product in the marked area.
- Depending on product choice, 0.5 mL may be an initial practical volume.
- Massage.
- Evaluate in all angles, both at rest and in animation.

Injecting the Medial SOOF

- Mark the deficiency (as previously mentioned).
- Mark cannula entry, using a lateral approach (as previously mentioned).
- Cleanse and maintain stringent aseptic technique.
- Puncture skin with a sharp needle (as previously mentioned).
- Introduce cannula, using an angle of approximately 30° to the skin. This should guide more superficial placement above the upper-lip levators and into the medial SOOF.
- Gently place product, using a fanning technique.
- Massage.
- Evaluate in all angles, both at rest and in animation.
- Less is more!

Wide Malar Enhancement ("Top model look")

This is a method of accentuating the zygomatic arch (Figures 4.25 and 4.26).

- Cleanse meticulously.
- Mark upper and lower border of the zygomatic bone.
- Mark entry point at the malar eminence (cheek point 2).
- Pinch skin and puncture with a sharp needle.
- Introduce a 25G cannula and advance along the zygoma.
- Inject using retrograde linear technique, molding product between fingers.
- Average volume required is $\sim$0.5 mL.

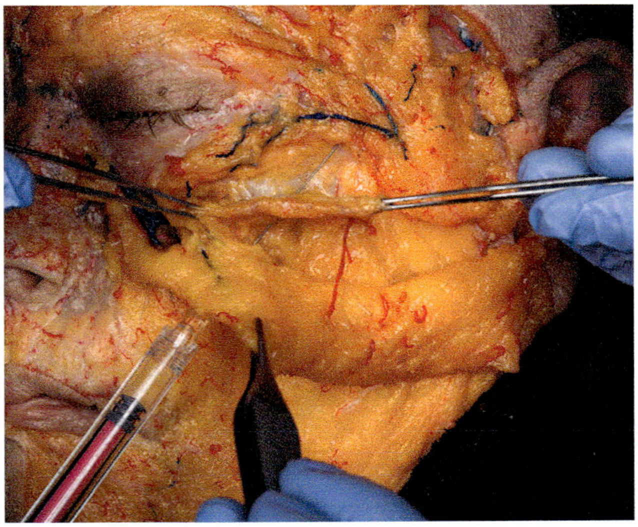

Figure 4.25 Wide malar enhancement.

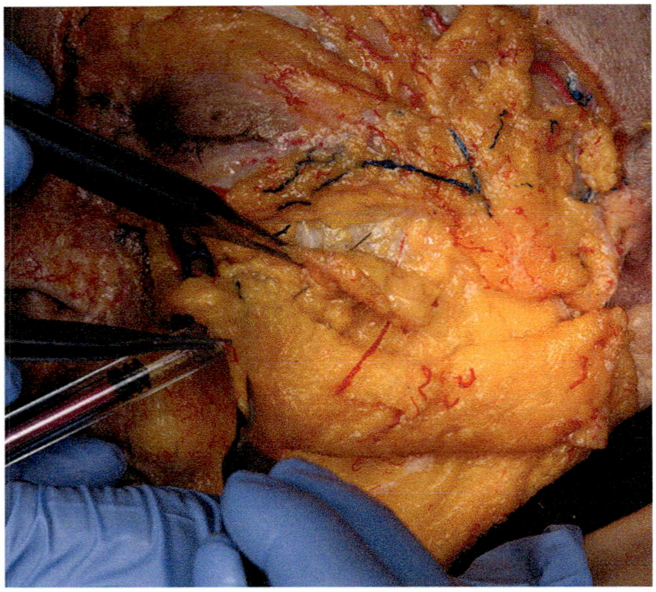

Figure 4.26 Wide malar enhancement.

Lower Malar Enhancement

- Cleanse meticulously (Figure 4.27).
- Mark upper and lower border of the zygomatic bone.
- Mark entry point below the malar eminence (lower cheek point).
- Pinch skin and puncture with a sharp needle.
- Introduce a 50 mm 25G cannula and advance below the zygoma.

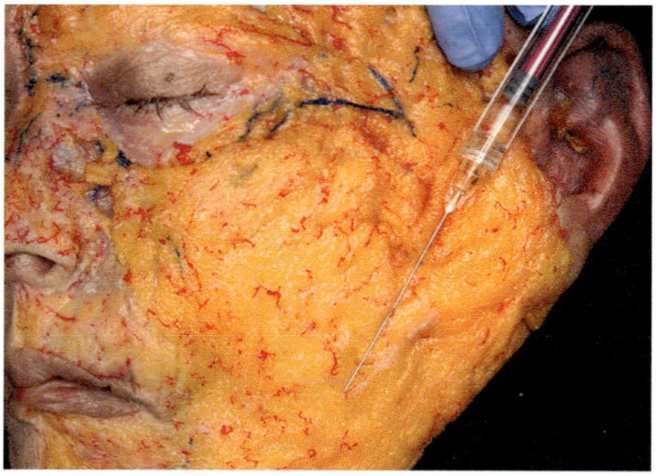

Figure 4.27 Lower malar enhancement.

- Inject using retrograde linear technique, molding product between fingers.
- Average volume required is ~1 mL.

"BEAUTIPHICATION" of the Cheek

This is a method of cheek augmentation based on the phi proportion (as described by Dr. Arthur Swift [15]):

- Draw a line from the lateral oral commissure to the lateral canthus of the ipsilateral eye. This line establishes the anterior extent of the malar prominence (Hinderer's line).
- Draw a second line from the lateral commissure to the inferior tragus of the ipsilateral ear, denoting the lateral and inferior boundary of the malar prominence (base of the triangle).
- Mark the highpoint of the cheek by drawing a horizontal line at the level of the limbus of the lower eyelid.
- Draw the cheek oval within these boundaries and tangential to the lines drawn.
- Feathering of the edges of the oval with subcutaneous filler product is done as necessary to create a smooth, egg-shaped mound.
- Lastly, draw a line from the lateral canthus down to the base of the triangle, perpendicular to the latter (the height of the triangle).
- The cheek apex lies phi (about one-third of the way) from the lateral canthus along this line. This defined point is in an eccentric position within the cheek oval.
- This same apex injection point can be obtained by the intersection of a line drawn from the nasal alar groove to the upper tragus and a line drawn down vertically from the midpoint of the lateral orbital rim.
- The final injection (0.25–0.5 mL of product placed on periosteum by vertical puncture) is performed at this precise point to create a beauti"phi"ed apex.

Lateral Zygoma

Inject a bolus anterior to the marking in the supraperiosteal plane, with the needle perpendicular to the bone.

Malar Eminence

- Inject a supraperiosteal bolus.
- Injection technique is as for the lateral malar point.

Mid-Cheek

Volumize at three different levels, depending on clinical needs:

- On the bone
- In the deep medial cheek fat pad (DMFP)
- In the medial SOOF

Wide Malar Enhancement

- Introduce a 25G cannula and advance along the zygoma.

Lower Malar Enhancement

- Inject using retrograde linear technique, molding product between finger.

COMPLICATIONS

For general complications and the concept of "safety by depth," see Chapter G.

Seckel [14] divided the face into seven functional danger zones; the malar region includes danger zone 4.

The most important complication to be aware of is embolization of the ophthalmic artery, which can lead to blindness. Should this embolization occur, the clinician has the possibility of retro-bulbar injection of hyaluronidase with a 25G cannula within a timeline of 90 minutes. Options can be injecting hyaluronidase through a cannula either 8 mm below the inferior tarsal strip, following the orbital floor with a downward curved direction at a depth of 3 cm from the bony orbital rim, or with entry 1 cm above the medial canthus directed 30° medially following the medial orbital wall. The dose of hyaluronidase differs among reports; however, we suggest 300–1500 IU of hyaluronidase repeated at frequent intervals (every 2–4 hours). Urgently refer patient to an Ophthalmologist.

Toxin Safety Considerations

- Lateral canthal botulinum toxin is a useful adjunct in preventing filler distortion due to muscular action.

Filler Safety Considerations

- The complication rates associated with HA injections in the malar area are generally deemed acceptable.
- It is of vital importance to mark both the upper and lower borders of the zygomatic arch before malar injections. The middle temporal vein runs parallel to the superior border, and the transverse facial artery parallels to the lower zygomatic border. Inappropriate needle angulation poses a risk for intravascular injection.
- Visible irregularity may be a significant problem in patients with thin or lax skin but can be effectively managed with massage over several weeks. Irregularities due to superficial placement of HA are more difficult to resolve and may persist well over two years, thus necessitating reversal with hyaluronidase.
- The infraorbital foramen constitutes an important danger area in the medial midface and should be

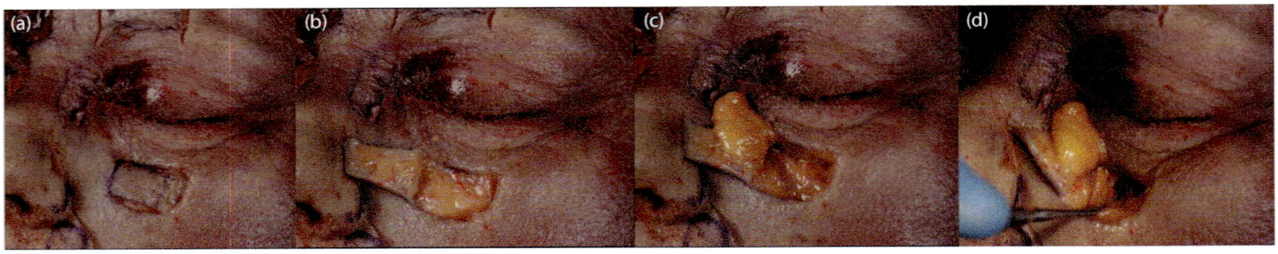

Figure 4.28 Lateral approach to the medial midface.

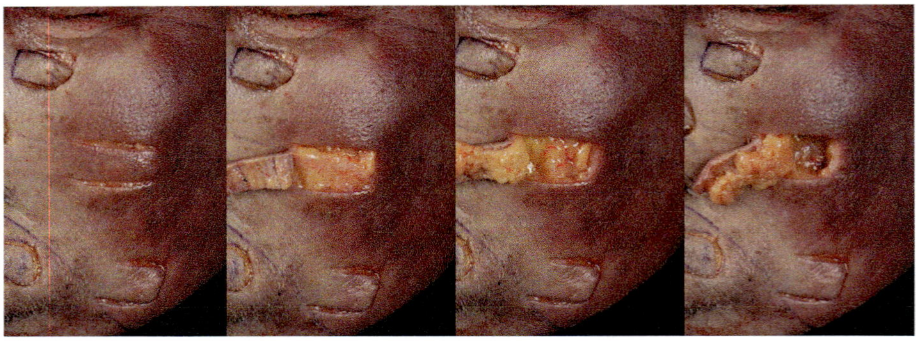

Figure 4.29 The buccal branch of the facial nerve.

carefully localized and marked before treatment. A lateral approach is advised when injecting with a needle in the deep plane as the bony hood over the foramen may add protection when using a lateral approach (Figure 4.28).

- The buccal branch of the facial nerve is deep to the superficial fat pad and must be avoided during lateral cheek injections (Figure 4.29).

References

1. Kikkawa DO et al. *Ophth Plast Reconstr Surg.* 1996;12:77.
2. Wong CH et al. *Plast Reconstr Surg.* 2012;129:1392–402.
3. Defatta RJ & Williams EF. *Arch Facial Plast Surg.* 2009;11:6–12.
4. Mendelson BC et al. *Plast Reconstr Surg.* 2002;110:885–911.
5. McGregor M. *Face lift techniques.* Presented to the Annual Meeting of the California Society of Plastic Surgeons. Yosemite, California, 1959.
6. Pessa JE & Rohrich RJ. *Facial Topography. Clinical Anatomy of the Face.* QMP; 2012.
7. Pessa JE & Garza JR. The anatomic basis of malar mounds and malar edema. *Aesth Surg J.* 1997;17:11–7.
8. Gierloff M et al. *Plast Reconstr Surg.* 2012;129:264.
9. Loukas M et al. *Surg Radiol Anat.* 2006;28:254–60.
10. Stuzin JM et al. *Plast Reconstr Surg.* 1990;85:29–37.
11. Li WT et al. *Chin J Clin Anat.* 1993;11:165–70.
12. Park JT et al. *J Craniofac Surg.* 2011 Mar;22(2):659–62.
13. Schenk et al. *Plast Reconstr Surg.* 2018;141(6):1353–9.
14. Seckel B. *Facial Danger Zones,* 2nd ed. Thieme; 2010.

15. Swift A & Remington K. *Clin Plas Surg.* 2011;38(3):347–77.
16. Cotofana et al. *Plast Reconstr Surg.* 2019:53–63.

Bibliography

Ghassemi A et al. *Aesth Plast Surg.* 2003; 27:258–64.

Har-Shai Y et al. *Plast Reconstr Surg.* 1996; 98:59–70.

Mitz V & Peyronie M. *Plast Reconstr Surg.* 1976; 58:80–8.

Muzaffar AR et al. *Plast Reconstr Surg.* 2002; 110:873.

Owsley JQ & Roberts CL. *Plast Reconstr Surg.* 2008;121:258.

Pessa JE & Rorich RJ. *Plast Reconstr Surg.* 2012;129:274.

Pontius AT & Williams EF. *Facial Plast Surg Clin N Am.* 2005;13:411–9.

Rohrich RJ et al. *Plast Reconstr Surg.* 2008;121:2107–12.

Rorhich RJ et al. *Plast Reconstr Surg.* 2009;124:946.

Rorich RJ & Pessa JE. *Plast Reconstr Surg.* 2007;119:2219.

Rorich RJ & Pessa JE. *Plast Reconstr Surg.* 2008;121:1804.

Tower JI et al. *Aesthet Surg J.* 2019. doi: 10.1093/asj/sjz185.

Further Reading

Cohen JL et al. *Aesthet Surg J.* 2015;35:844–9.

Coleman SR. *Aesthet Plast Surg.* 2008;32:415–7.

Hwang CJ. *J Cutan Aesthet Surg.* 2016;9:73–9.

Park JT et al. *J Craniofac Surg.* 2011 Mar;22(2):659–62.

Rees EM et al. *Plast Reconstr Surg.* 2008;121:1414–20.

Rohrich RJ et al. *Plast Reconstr Surg.* 2003;112:1899–902.

Schierle CF & Casas LA. *Aesthet Surg J.* 2011;31:95–109.

Spector JA et al. *Aesthet Plast Surg.* 2008;32:411–4.

5 NOSE

Dario Bertossi, Fazıl Apaydın, Paul van der Eerden, Enrico Robotti, Riccardo Nocini, and Paul S. Nassif

INTRODUCTION

Whilst the nose has primarily a breathing function, it also represents an aesthetically defining facial feature. The term non-surgical rhinoplasty is preferentially used for non-surgical aesthetic improvement with injectable fillers and toxins, whereas the term rhinoplasty is reserved for surgical nasal reshaping. Due to their reversibility, high G′ HA fillers are considered the safest material for non-surgical rhinoplasty. It is advisable that non-surgical rhinoplasty is performed only by highly experienced injectors with an intimate knowledge of injection anatomy and appropriate technique. Patient and product selection, accurate clinical assessment and correct injection techniques are of critical importance as the rich vascular network of the nose renders it a high risk area for severe complications.

NASAL BOUNDARIES

The nose is centrofacially situated, surrounded by important anatomical structures and has a profound impact on facial appearance. Even minimal shadowing or asymmetry may lead to obvious aesthetic dysharmony.

The glabella forms the upper nasal boundary, whilst the inferior border is formed by the nasal base and inferior nostril border. The lateral border is defined by an imaginary line between the ascending process of the upper maxilla and the nasal alar attachment (Figure 5.1a). The lateral end of the aesthetic brow forms the tip of a line running from the nasal ala and past the lateral canthus (Figure 5.1b).

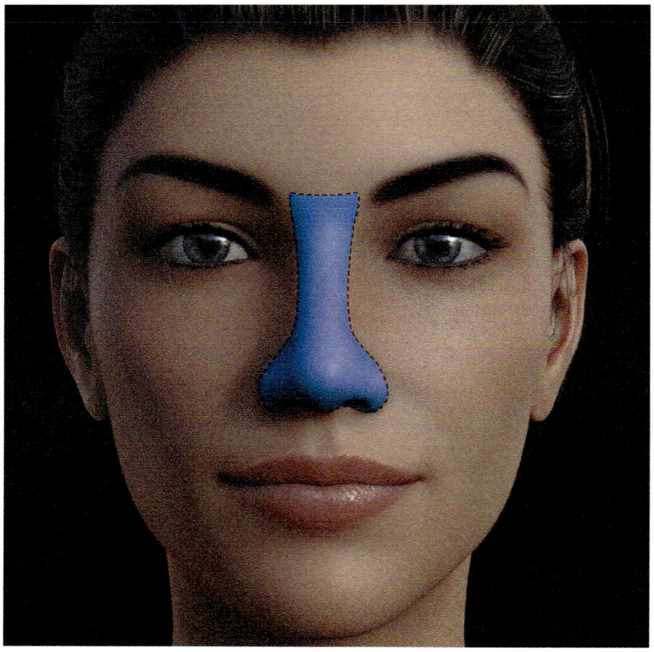

Figure 5.1a Nasal boundaries: The nose lies between the two medial canthi. The glabella forms the upper limit and a horizontal line through the inferior nasal spine the lower limit.

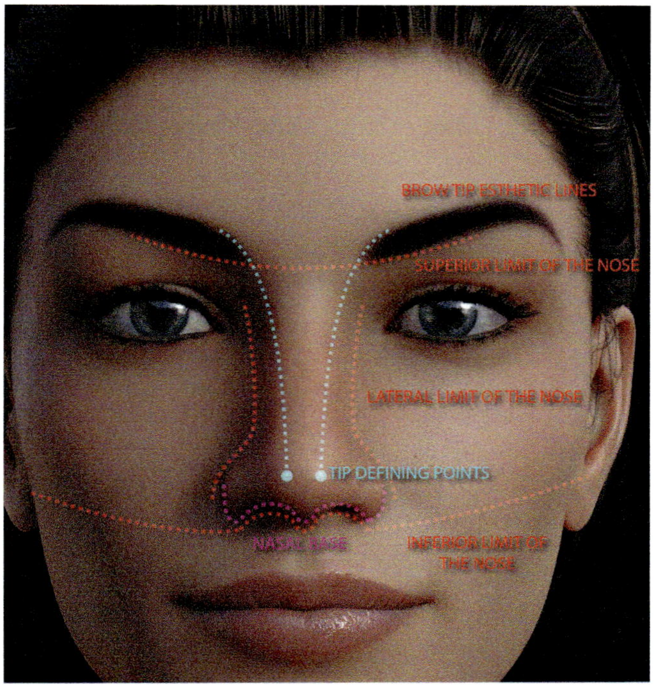

Figure 5.1b Brow tip defining lines and tip defining points.

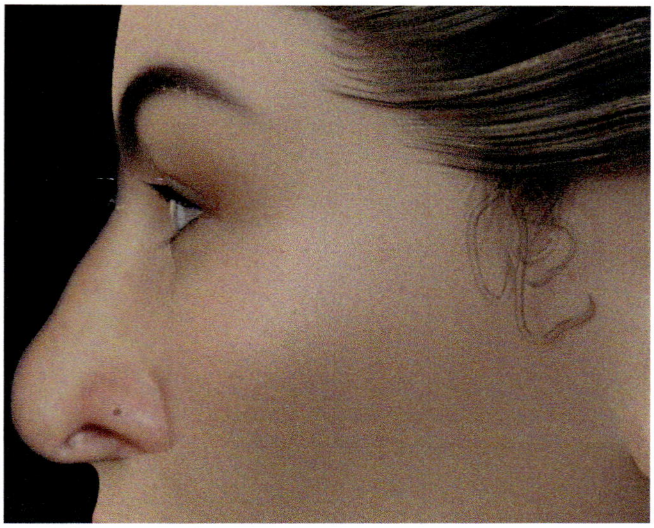

Figure 5.2 With aging, there is soft tissue deflation and less upper maxillary support, with resultant loss of nasal tip projection.

AGING

Craniofacial growth continues after the age of 16–18 years, with continual nasal reshaping occurring thereafter. Changes in soft-tissue, muscle, skin and cartilage result in continual evolution as the underlying nasal structure (unlike bone and cartilage) continues to evolve over time. Insightful and detailed observation of specific, age-related changes provides the necessary clinical information for optimal non-surgical correction techniques.

Nasal measurements have proven to be significantly affected by age, with an increase documented in volume, area, and linear distance. In the majority of study groups, elderly subjects tend to have larger noses than younger members of the same gender and ethnicity. The nasolabial angle—the angle between the lower border of the nose and the subnasal line that connects to the upper lip border—has consistently been found to decrease, implying that the nose tends to droop with age (Figure 5.2).

The nasal pyramid is the most influential aesthetic aspect of the middle third of the face. Although the aesthetic impact of the nose in profile view has been widely documented [1–14], the analysis of nasal proportions during the growth phase is less well documented than in mature populations, making assessment of the younger patient more complex.

Nasal soft tissue growth is greater, and occurs earlier, in adolescent girls than in age-matched boys. Nasal height increases the most, doubling from birth to the age of 20. Overall, males have larger noses than females, but noses seem to grow more quickly in girls when measurements are compared over a lifetime. In 3–4 year old females, the volume of the average nose is approximately 42% of early adult size (at 18–30 years of age); for males, the average volume has been found to be approximately 36%.

By the age of 30, nasal growth slows down considerably. Between 50 and 60 years of age, nasal volume will typically increase by a further 29% in men and 18% in women.

SKIN

Bone and cartilage form the supporting framework of the nose. From the glabella to the bridge, to the tip, the nasal skin is anatomically considered in vertical thirds (Figure 5.3).

- In the upper third, the skin is thick and relatively distensible (flexible and mobile). It then tapers, becoming tightly adherent to the osseocartilaginous framework, thinning towards the dorsal nasal bridge.
- The middle third overlying the nasal bridge (mid-dorsal section) has the thinnest, most adherent and least distensible, skin.
- The skin of the lower third is of equal thickness to the upper nose, due to more sebaceous glands, especially at the nasal tip.

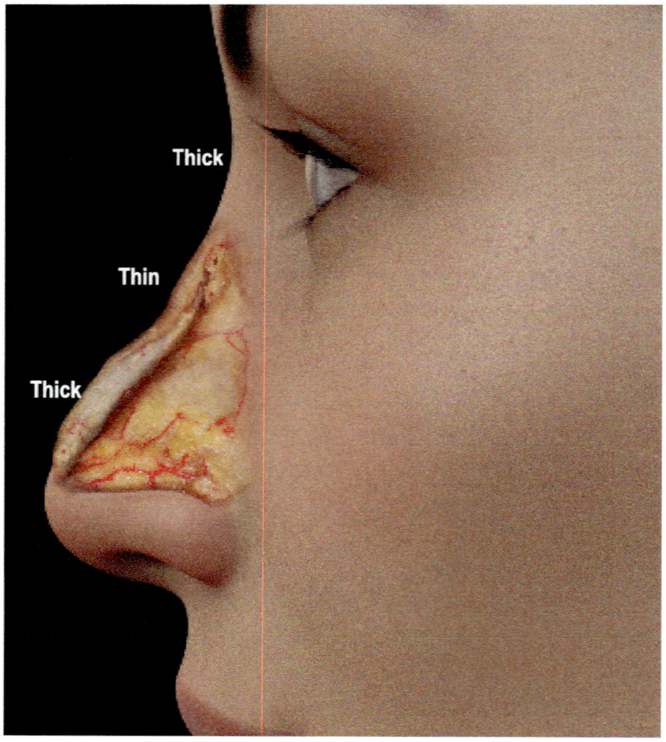

Figure 5.3 Skin on the nose is shown in elevation. The dorsal nasal skin is thinner, making every mistake visible.

FAT

The nose consists of a framework of skin, cartilage, and bone, with six distinguishable layers: skin, superficial fatty layer, fibromuscular layer (the superficial muscolar aponeurotic system, SMAS), deep fatty layer, periosteum-perichondrium, and bone-cartilage (Figure 5.4). Nasal subcutaneous tissue exists in discrete compartments that are determined by the underlying perforator blood supply [15].

- The skin is thicker in the radix area, becomes extremely thin in the mid-vault region, and thickens in the supra-tip area (see Figure 5.4).
- Immediately beneath the skin, there is a superficial fatty layer comprising predominantly adipose tissue containing vertical fibers and septae extending from the skin to the underlying SMAS.
- The distinct nasal SMAS is in continuation with the facial SMAS.
- Subcutaneous fat is concentrated in the glabella, lateral nasal wall, tip, and supra-tip areas (see Figure 5.5).

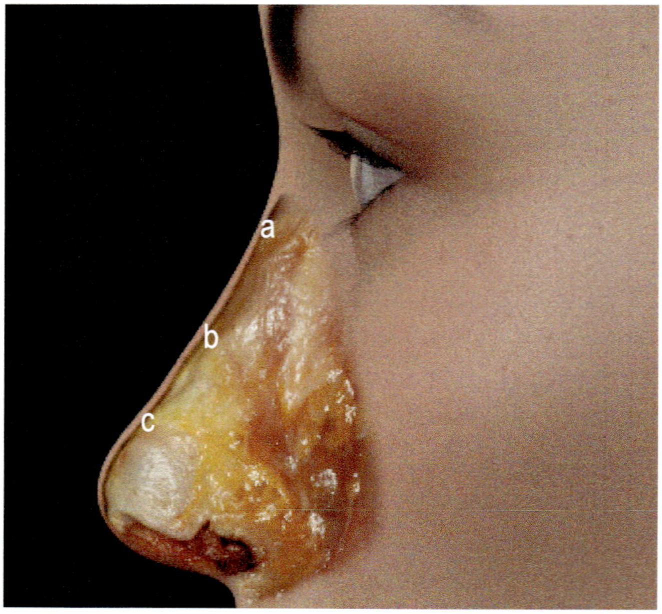

Figure 5.4 Deep nasal fat is related to the nasal SMAS deep layer: (a) Radix; (b) mid-vault; (c) supra-tip.

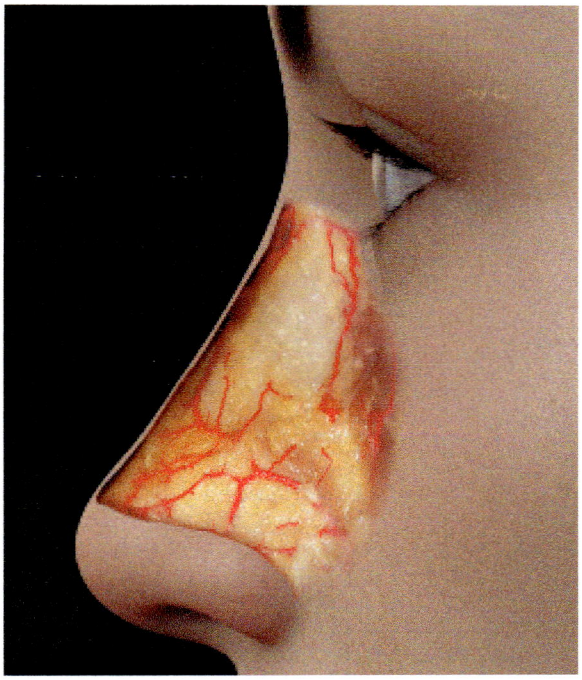

Figure 5.5 Nasal fat is very thin. Note the superficial vessels in the lateral aspect.

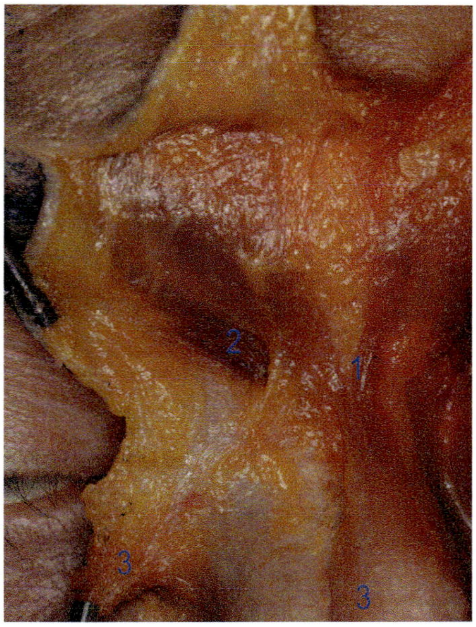

Figure 5.6 (1) Procerus muscle; (2) depressor supercilii; (3) transverse nasalis.

- Distribution of the sub-SMAS fat is similar to that of the superficial facial fat, with an additional layer of fat beneath the transverse nasalis muscle and an interdomal fat pad confirmed in cadaver studies (see Figure 5.4).

MUSCLES

The nasal SMAS is a continuation of the facial SMAS; this layer ensheathes the muscles and is highly vascular. All the nasal muscles are innervated by cranial nerve VII.

Procerus

The procerus is the most cephalic muscle of the nose. It arises from the glabellar area, extends caudally in a vertical fashion, and joins with the wing-shaped transverse nasalis muscle covering the caudal portion of the nasal bones. The main function of the procerus is depression of the eyebrows, which can create horizontal wrinkles over the cephalic portion of the nose in aging patients (Figure 5.6).

Nasalis

The nasalis muscle has two components: The transverse nasalis or compressor nasi and the pars alaris (Figure 5.7A and B).

The transverse part of the muscle spans the dorsum of the nose, covering the upper lateral cartilages. This muscle, also called pars transversa, arises from the lateral cephalic portion of the subpyriform crescent. The pars transversa joins with the procerus muscle and the opposite muscle in the midline to form the nasalis–procerus aponeurosis which compresses and elongates the nose, contracts the nostrils, and narrows the vestibules.

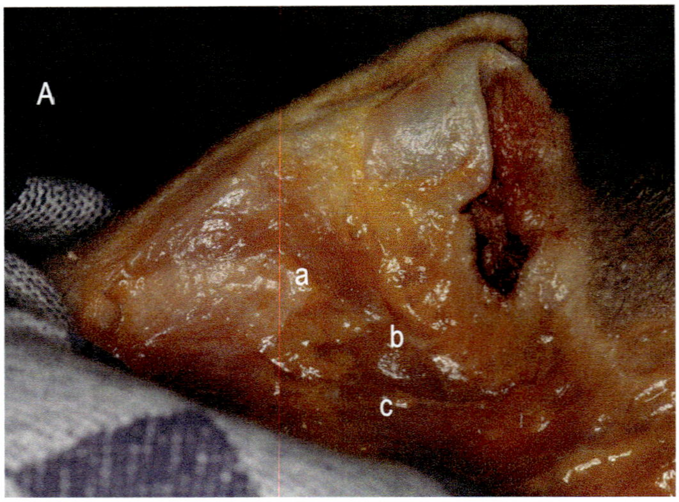

Figure 5.7A (a) Transverse nasalis; (b) compressor nasalis; (c) LLSAN muscles.

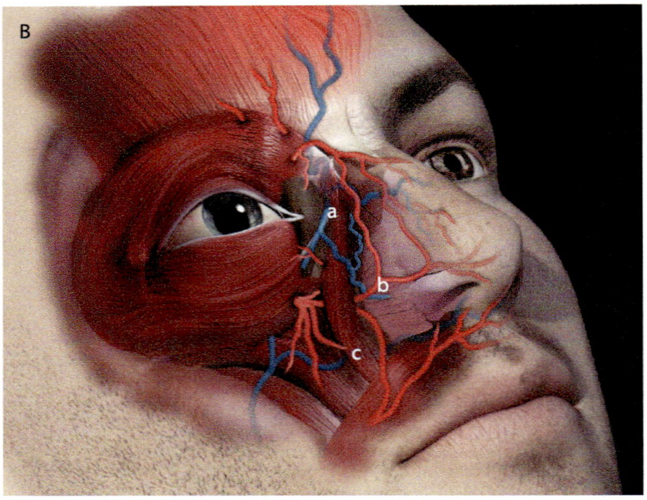

Figure 5.7B (a) Transverse nasalis; (b) compressor nasalis; (c) LLSAN muscles.

The second component of the nasalis muscle, the pars alaris (alar nasalis), arises from the crescent origin of the maxilla and is more lateral and slightly caudal to the bony origin of the depressor septi nasi muscle. The alar portion partially covers the lateral crus of the lower lateral cartilages and assists in dilatation of the nares. Damage to this muscle may result in collapse of the external nasal valve. In ethnic noses, the pars alaris is stronger and far more developed.

Depressor Alae or Myrtiforme

The depressor alae muscle originates from the border of the pyriform crest and then rises vertically, in a fan-like pattern, to the ala, acting as a depressor and constrictor of the nostrils.

Levator Labii Superior Alaeque Nasi (LLSAN)

LLSAN plays an important functional role. It extends lateral to the nose in a cephalocaudal direction and has fibers that are attached to the nostril, thus contributing to dilatation of the nares. Paralysis of these muscles will contribute to collapse of the external valve.

Depressor Septi Nasi

Depressor septi nasi arises from the maxilla just below the nasal spine, sometimes fuses with fibers of the orbicularis oris muscle, extends along the columellar base, and attaches to the foot-plate. Occasionally, fibers of this muscle extend to the middle genu. Some authors believe that these muscle fibers extend to the membranous septum. The depressor septi nasi depresses the nasal tip on animation and alters air turbulence. Additionally, it is of aesthetic importance as its contraction narrows the labio-columellar angle. Release of this muscle not only eliminates the depressor effect on the tip but may also cause slight ptosis of the upper lip, which may or may not be beneficial, depending on the visibility of the patient's incisor teeth.

VASCULARIZATION

The arterial blood-vessel supply to the nose is two-fold: There is internal vascularization through

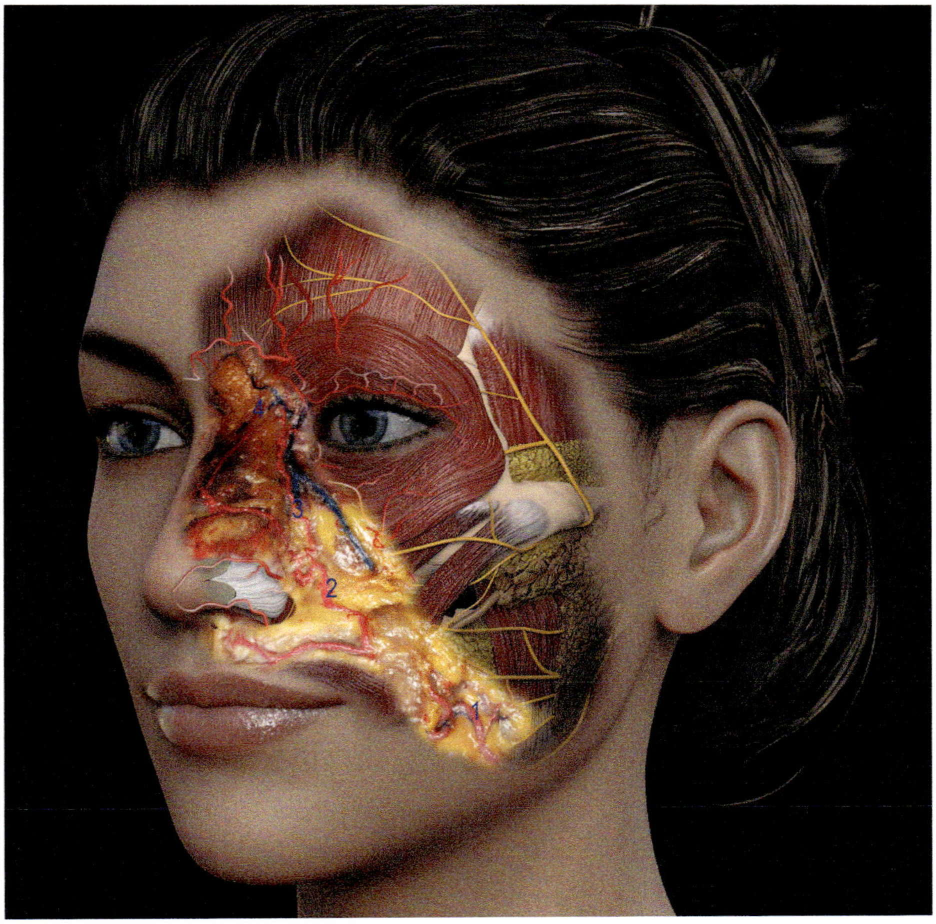

Figure 5.8 (1) Facial artery; (2) angular artery; (3) lateral nasal artery; (4) anastomosis with the ophthalmic artery (internal carotid system).

branches of the internal carotid artery - a branch of the anterior ethmoidal artery, and a branch of the posterior ethmoid artery, which derive from the ophthalmic artery; and branches of the external carotid artery - the sphenopalatine artery, and the greater palatine artery coming from the internal maxillary artery, the superior labial artery, and the angular artery coming from the facial artery. The latter becomes the angular artery in the proximity of the nasal ala and then courses over the superomedial aspect of the nose go become the lateral nasal artery (Figures 5.8 and 5.9). The dorsal nose is supplied by branches of the internal maxillary artery (infraorbital) and the ophthalmic arteries, deriving from the internal carotid artery. This anastomotic area between the internal and external carotid circulations is very important as it may lead to intravascular embolization of injected fillers (Figure 5.10).

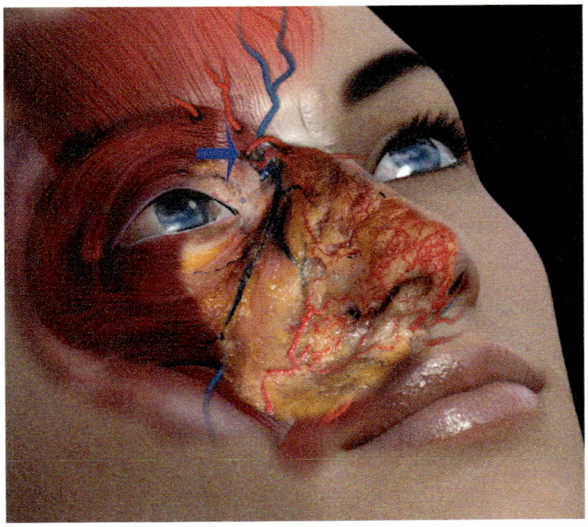

Figure 5.9 Blue arrow: Danger area where the lateral nasal artery (external carotid system) anastomoses with the ophthalmic artery (internal carotid system).

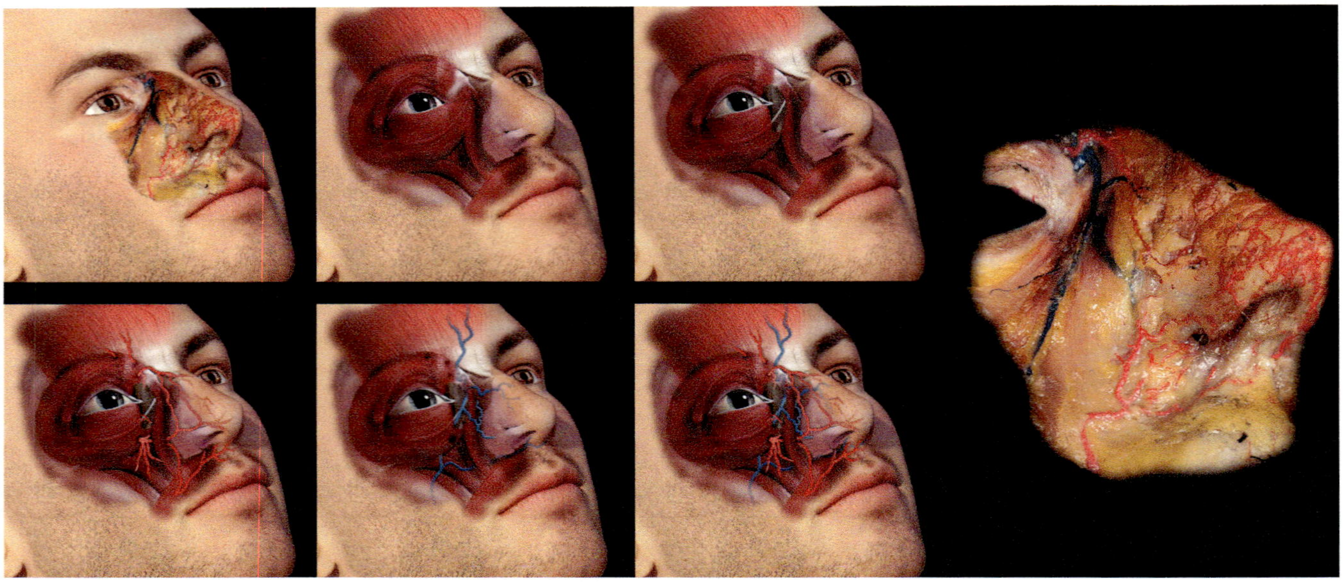

Figure 5.10 Danger areas: Anastomoses of the internal and external carotid systems.

The superior labial and the angular artery are the main branches that respectively form the columellar branches and the lateral nasal branches (Figure 5.11). The lateral nasal vessels are 2–3 mm above the alar groove and, together with the columellar artery, arise deep at the nasal base to end at the tip in the subdermal plexus [16]; both supply the tip of the nose. Internally, the lateral nasal wall is supplied by the sphenopalatine artery (from behind and below) and by the anterior and posterior ethmoid arteries (from above and behind). The nasal septum also is supplied by the sphenopalatine, anterior and posterior ethmoid arteries, with additional contribution by the superior labial and greater palatine arteries. These three vascular supplies to the internal nose converge in the Kiesselbach plexus (Little's area), a region in the antero-inferior third of the nasal septum. Furthermore, the venous supply of the nose generally follows the arterial pattern of nasal vascularization. The nasal veins are biologically significant because they have no valves, and communicate directly with the cavernous sinus. This may potentially cause intracranial spread of bacterial infections originating from the nasal region. Intra-arterial injections in this area may lead to skin necrosis and even blindness. Danger zones exist particularly in the areas where the internal and external carotid systems communicate (angular artery and columellar artery). Due to great anatomic variability, the midline position as a safe reference may sometimes be unsafe for injection. Therefore, we emphasize the principle of "staying deep," just above periosteum and perichondrium (Figure 5.12).

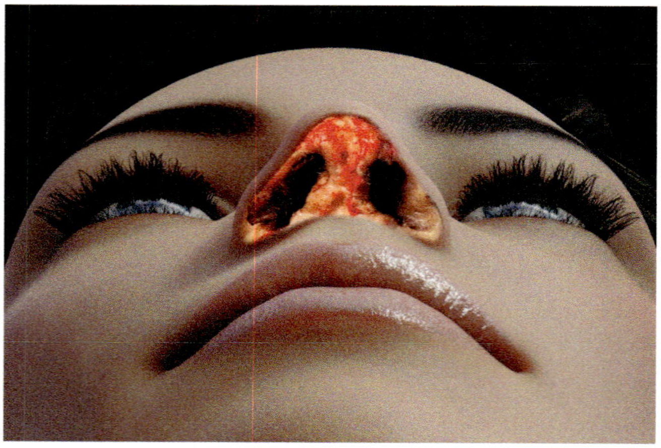

Figure 5.11 Skin removal showing vascularization of the nasal base; note the columellar arteries.

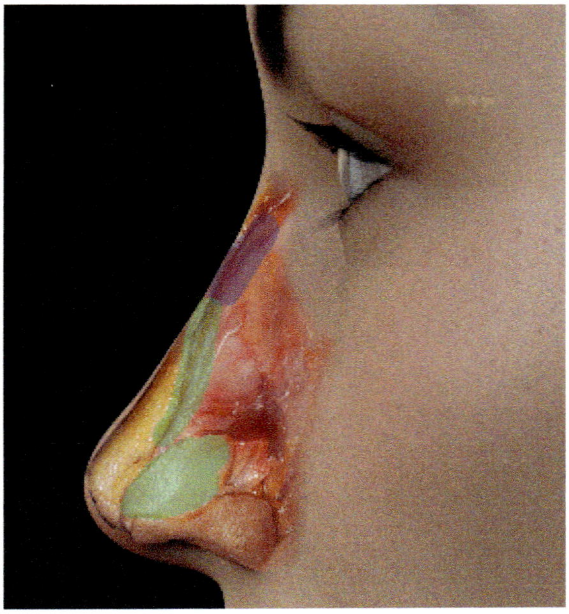

Figure 5.12 Suprapericondral (green) and supraperiosteal (blue) planes.

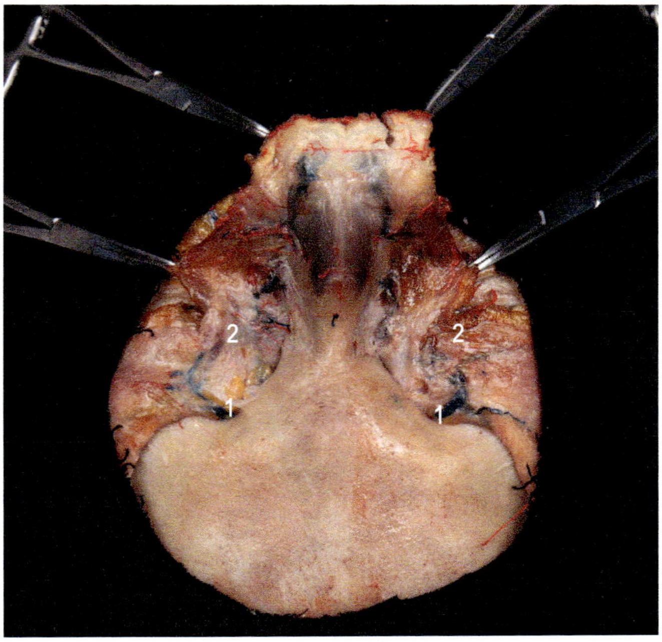

Figure 5.13 Innervation of the nose, seen from above: (1) Supraorbital nerve; (2) infraorbital nerve.

INNERVATION

Nasal sensory innervation is derived from the supraorbital and infraorbital nerves; motor innervation is via the buccal branch of the facial nerve (Figure 5.13).

BONE

The skeletal component of the nose consists of bone and cartilage. The paired nasal bones and the frontal process of the maxilla form the lateral aspect whilst the lateral surfaces of the upper two-thirds join in the midline at the nasal dorsum. Supero-laterally the paired nasal bones connect to the lacrimal bones, and infero-laterally they attach to the ascending processes of the maxilla. Postero-superiorly, the bony nasal septum is composed of the perpendicular plate of the ethmoidal bone. The vomer lies postero-inferiorly and partially forms the choanal opening into the nasopharynx.

The nasal floor is formed by the pre-maxillary and the palatine bones, which also form the roof of the mouth.

The bony nasal vault comprises the paired nasal bones and the ascending frontal process of the maxilla. This part of the nose is pyramidal in shape, the narrowest portion being at the intercanthal line. The average length of the nasal bone is 25 mm; although there may be both individual and significant ethnic variation (African American noses often have short nasal bones). Laterally the nasal bones join with the frontal process of the maxilla.

The circle created with the nasal spine, the thin portion of the frontal process of the maxilla, and the thin caudal border of the nasal bones is called the pyriform aperture. The nasal bones fuse with the superior edge of the perpendicular plate of the ethmoid bone cephalad to the intercanthal line. The confluence of cartilaginous nasal septum, ethmoid bone, and nasal bone is called the keystone area (Figure 5.14).

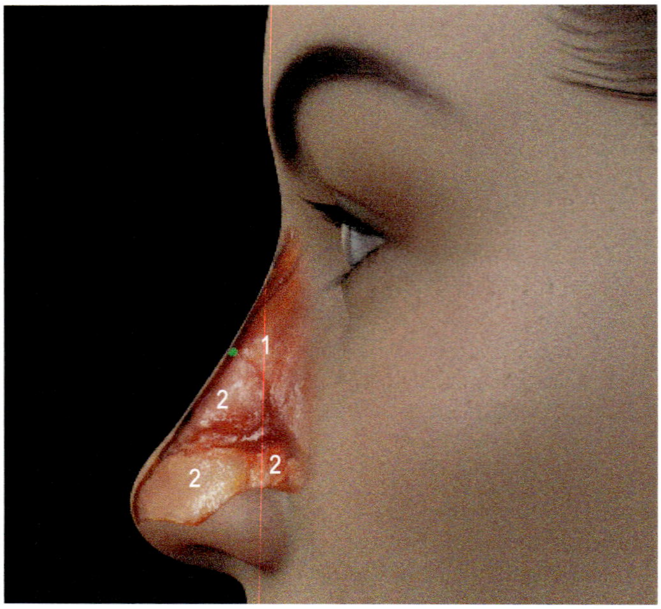

Figure 5.14 Nasal bone (1) and cartilages (2) are visible. Green dot: the keystone area.

CARTILAGE

The cartilaginous nasal frame consists of a pair of upper and lower lateral cartilages and the nasal septum (Figure 5.15).

The **upper lateral cartilages** are paired rectangular cartilages that support the lateral nasal walls. These cartilages join the septum in the midline, although the fusion between the upper lateral cartilages and the septum occurs in a manner which almost creates a single unit cephalically. The lateral border of the upper lateral cartilages frequently terminates at the level of the lateral nasal bone suture line. This leaves a space between the bone and upper lateral cartilage, which is termed the external lateral triangle. It is surrounded by the caudal border of the upper lateral cartilages cephalically, the frontal process of the maxilla laterally, and the cephalic border of the lower lateral cartilage caudally. The cephalic portion of the upper lateral cartilage is overlapped by the nasal bone. The amount of overlap is highly variable and can range from 2 to 11 mm.

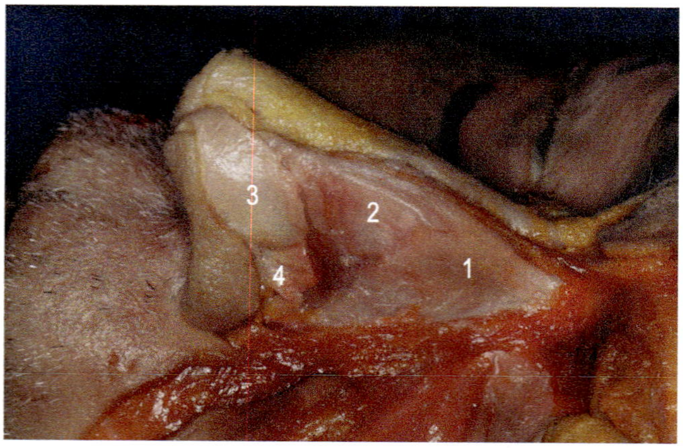

Figure 5.15 Figure illustrating the Nasal bone (1) and triangular cartilages (2), lateral crura cartilages (3), sesamoid cartilages (4).

The **lower lateral cartilages** have four components: the medial crus, middle crus, dome, and lateral crus.

Medial Crus: The medial crus has two distinct segments: the footplate and the columella. The footplate varies in size and in the degree of lateral angulation. This angulation of the footplate governs the width of the base of the columella. The columellar segment of the medial crus varies in length and width; the longer the columellar portion, the longer the nostril and thus the potential for a more projected nasal tip. Cephalad to this portion of the medial crura is the membranous septum, which is composed of two layers of soft tissues encasing some ibrous bands named septocolumellar ligaments.

Middle Crus: This part of the lower lateral cartilage extends between the medial crus and the domes and its length and width largely control the configuration of the infratip lobule.

Dome: The domal segment is the narrowest and thinnest portion of the lower lateral cartilage; yet, it is the most important in relation to the tip shape. There is tremendous variation in its shape; on rare occasions, it has a convolution that, when present, invariably results in bulbosity of the tip. The area posterior and caudal to the domes, between the medial and lateral segments, contains two segments of soft tissue, with no cartilage, is externally covered with skin and internally with the vestibular lining, and is called the soft triangle.

The medial and middle crura are tightly bound together by fibrous bands. The most anterior one is called the interdomal ligament. Additionally, there are fibrous bands more anteriorly binding the domes to each other and the overlying dermis; these are called the Pitanguy ligament. There are additional fibrous bands at the level of the footplates and between the upper and lower lateral cartilages.

Lateral Crus: This portion of the nasal lobule is the largest component. It is narrow anteriorly but becomes wider in the mid-portion and narrows again laterally. The lateral crus of the lower lateral cartilage (LLC) is usually in contact with the first chain of the accessory cartilages that abut the pyriform aperture. Medially, the lateral crus is continuous with the domal segment. The anterior portion of this cartilage can curve in a variety of directions and controls the convexity of the ala. It also provides support to the anterior half of the alar rim. However, posteriorly, it diverges and does not have much contribution to the ala, yet does contribute to the function of the external valve. Generally, this cartilage is oriented at a 45° angle to the vertical facial plane. The curled junction of the cephalic edge of the lateral crus and the caudal edge of the upper lateral cartilage is referred to as the scroll area. The magnitude of curling can vary from patient to patient and is sometimes significant enough to cause external visibility and fullness in this area. The lower lateral cartilage is commonly short and weak in non-Caucasian noses.

The **accessory cartilages** are a series of small cartilages situated on the nasal ala close to the tail of the alar cartilages.

The **nasal septum** is situated on the central part of the nose and its connected with its inferior surface with the upper maxillary crest, the posterior and the anterior nasal spine, and is connected to the nasal bones in the key area where the two upper lateral cartilages are also connected to it, forming the internal nasal valve.

HOW I DO IT: BOTULINUM TOXINS

Bunny Lines

Bunny lines are generated by the transverse portion of the nasalis muscle in synergy with the levator labii superioris alaeque nasi muscle. The dose per injection site is 2 U per side in both men and women (Figure 5.16).

The injection is performed at a 45° angle to the skin with a low-to-high direction. A single injection is performed on each side of the nose, in the center of the affected area. Needle penetration is limited to the tip only, as the muscle lies immediately under the skin. Care should be taken not to inject too laterally in order to avoid functional interference with the levator labii superioris alaeque nasi muscle, which would produce an undesirable elongation of the upper lip.

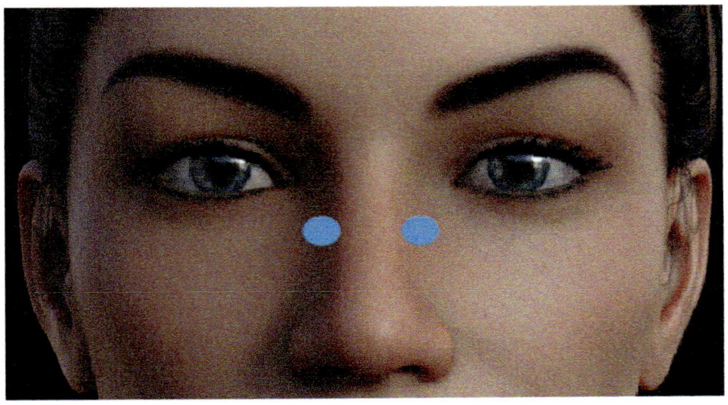

Figure 5.16 Nasal botulinum toxin injections for bunny lines.

Often, when treating the bunny lines, procerus treatment is performed concomitantly to manage the horizontal lines at the nasal root.

Sagging Nasal Tip

The target muscle for treatment of a sagging nasal tip is the depressor septi nasi. When hypertonic, the depressor septi nasi lowers the tip of the nose, which is usually more visible upon smiling. To treat a sagging nasal tip, a single injection with a 2–4 U dose is recommended in both men and women (Figure 5.17).

Treatment is performed by inserting one-quarter of a 30G × 1/2″ needle, at the base of the columella, pointing toward the nasal spine. The treatment produces upward rotation of the nasal tip. However, clinical assessment is crucial for correct patient selection as treatment of the sagging nasal tip should be avoided in patients with a long upper lip. A long caudal septum is also a contraindication to toxin treatment as it prevents the desired tip rotation.

HOW I DO IT: FILLERS

Patient selection is of utmost importance for nose reshaping with fillers. Both patients with thin and thick skin are suitable candidates for filler rhinomodulation.

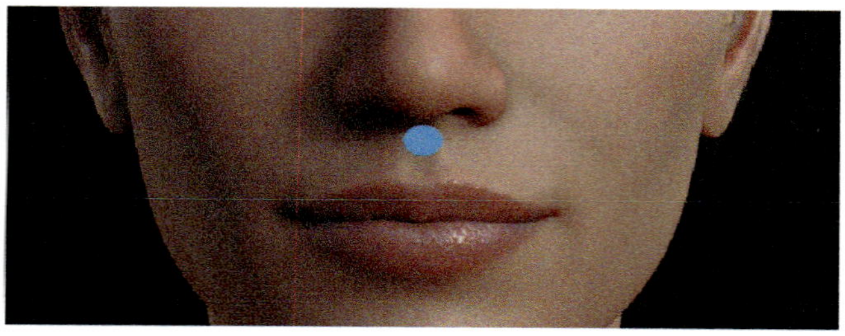

Figure 5.17 Nasal botulinum toxin injections for sagging nasal tip.

Patients with thinner skin usually require less product. In these patients in particular, however, any mistake (too much material either absolutely or relatively) can be visible during and after treatment. Biodegradable substances, although temporary, are thus the best to start with. Thicker skins do not expand as easily as the thinner ones and usually require more product or larger molecules.

As a general rule, HA should be injected in small quantities for every treated area with constant checkup of the patient during injections and after 3 and 10 days. Injection volume and skin color should be assessed regularly to avoid any compromise of vascular perfusion. It is best to conduct a nasal grid analysis immediately before filler injection and during treatment (see Figure 5.18a). The nasal grid is traced with standard make-up pencils and analysis allows identification of primary defects: deep glabella, nasal hump, pseudohump, double dome or defective nasal projection, nasolabial angle and hidden columella, crooked nose, saddle nose, and nasal base asymmetry.

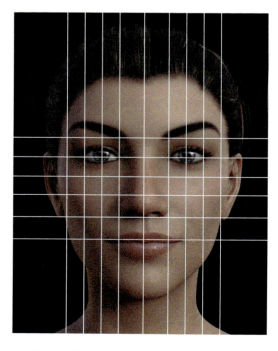

Figure 5.18a The nasal grid.

Injection Plan and Procedure

Skin is disinfected with a 75% alcohol solution. The nasal grid analysis is traced and the treatment performed by sole injector following the injecting protocol. Select a HA gel with a high G′, 20 or 25 mg/mL with 0.3% lidocaine, characterized by intrinsic viscosity and cohesivity. The main injection guidelines include the following:

1. To avoid vascular complications, it is prudent to **stay in the midline** [9,10], as the "major" vessels (angular arteries, columellar arteries, and dorsal arteries) normally lie laterally. In some patients, dorsal nasal vessels cross the midline, as apparent in some anatomic dissections, usually at the middle third of the nose [17]. Variations in the anatomy could put some patients at higher risk for intravascular injection. Always aspirate for a 5–7 seconds before injection.
2. **A 27G 13 mm needle** should be used (or a 38 mm 25G cannula).
3. Two distinct planes of injection are strictly adhered to, in order to minimize vascular accidents:
   - **Supraperiosteal injection** in the glabella/nasal dorsum/anterior nasal spine/columella [3].
   - **Deep dermal injection** in the nasal ala/tip (and also permitted in the glabella in addition to the supraperiosteal injections).
4. **Slow injection with small volumes** is recommended, with constant patient monitoring mandatory for signs of vascular compromise.
5. **Pinching soft tissue in midline**: The treatment area is constantly pinched up and compressed during injection to avoid lateral HA displacement.
6. **Lateral defects**, where there is increased risk of intravascular injection, can be most safely corrected by midline injection followed by molding and purposeful lateral displacement of the body of HA. This technique is useful where there are lateral defects for correction and allows for avoidance of an increased risk of intravascular injection by leaving midline.
7. **Smoothing massage** at the end of every injection, with wet gloves, help to avoid "bumps."

Treatment Plan Design

A sequence of injections is used in order to achieve the following aims:

- **Tip support and rotation (Sn)** (Figures 5.18b and 5.19), where there are two columellar arteries following the medial cartilaginous crus.
- **Nasal base support (Rnb, Lnb)** (Figures 5.20 and 5.21), where the lateral nasal artery creates a subdermal plexus (Figure 5.22).
- **Nasal tip projection (Nt)** (Figures 5.23 and 5.24), where columellar arteries and lateral nasal arteries create arcades.

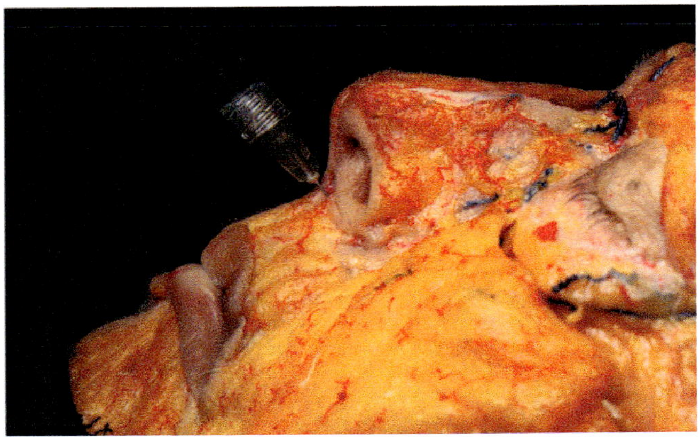

Figure 5.18b Anterior nasal spine injection.

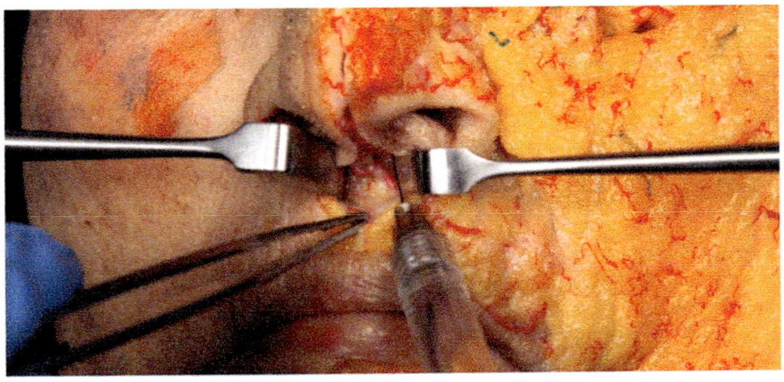

Figure 5.19 Depth of anterior nasal spine injection.

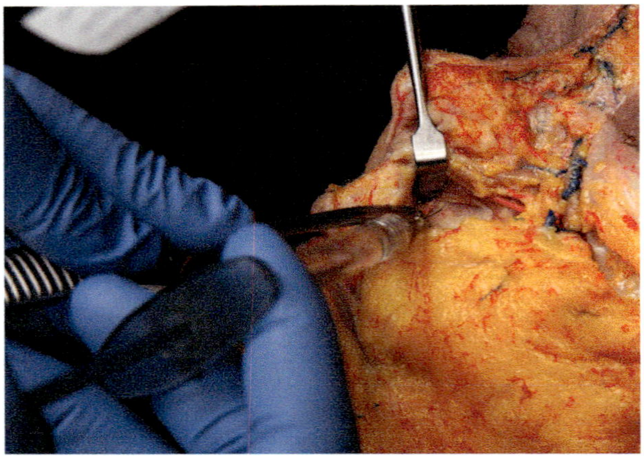

Figure 5.20 Depth of nasal base deep injection.

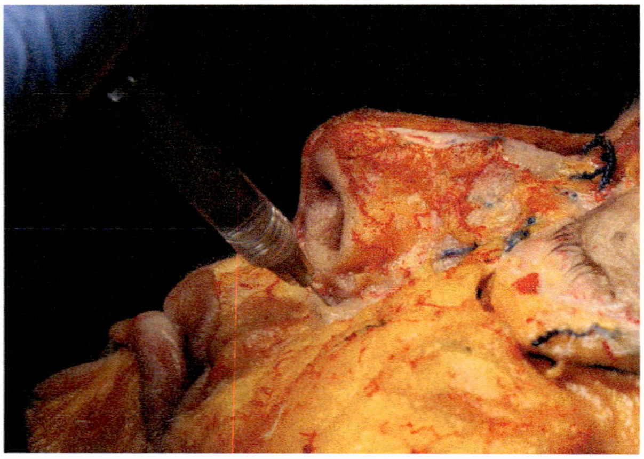

Figure 5.21 Depth of nasal base superficial injection.

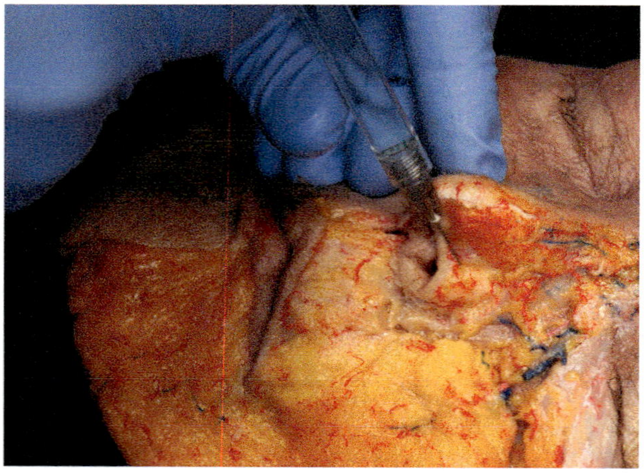

Figure 5.22 Depth of nasal ala superficial injection.

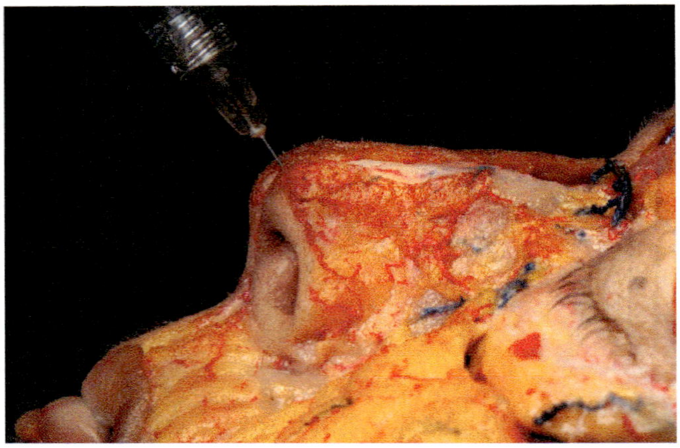

Figure 5.23 Depth of nasal intradomal deep injection.

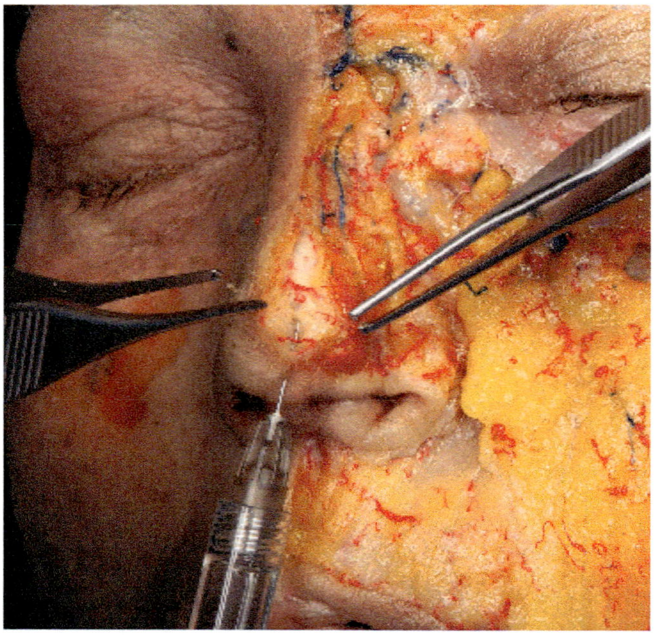

Figure 5.24 Depth of interdomal tip deep injection.

- **Glabella** is the next step (Figures 5.25 and 5.26).
- Then, inject in the midline on **nasal dorsum (nasion = Na and nasal dorsum = Nd)** (Figure 5.27), where nasal dorsal arteries provide vascularization from the angular and the ophthalmic arteries [16].
- The nasal dorsum can also be treated with the cannula (Figures 5.28–5.30).

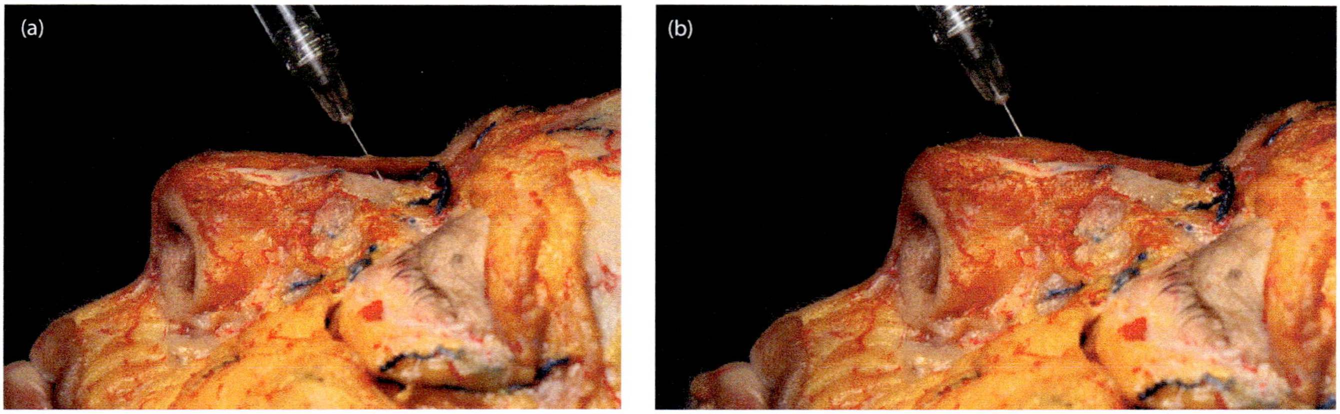

Figure 5.25 (a) Depth of nasal glabella deep injection. (b) Depth of nasal dorsum deep injection.

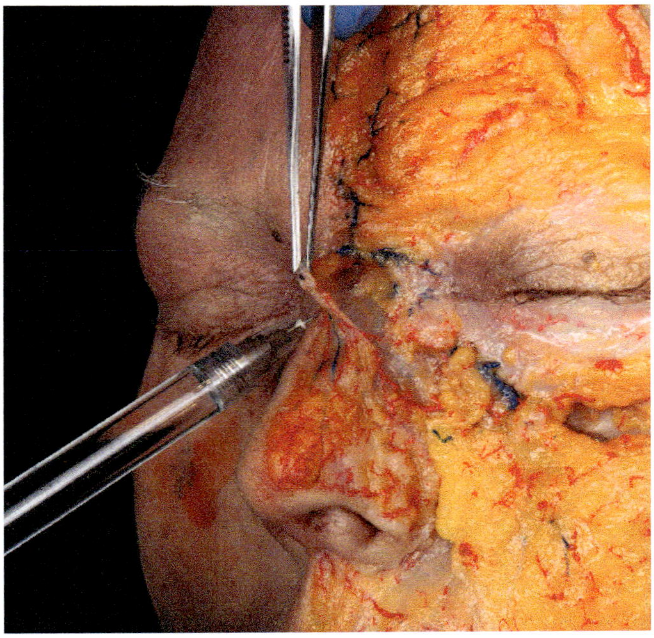

Figure 5.26 Depth of nasal glabella deep injection.

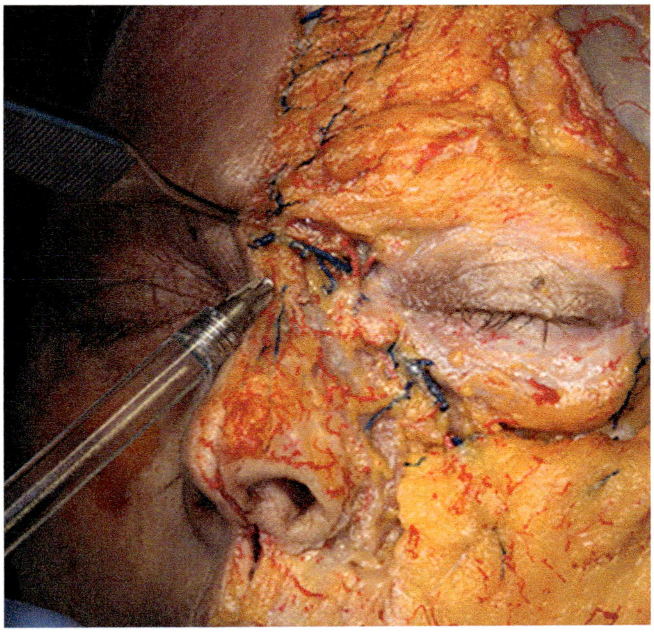

Figure 5.27 Depth of nasal glabella deep injection with danger area.

Following the nasal grid points, associated defects of the nasal structure should be treated with this sequence: Sn, Rnb and Lnb, Nt, Na and Nd. Remaining points through the grid are right and left nasal ala and right and left nasal base (Rna, Lna and Rnb, Lnb) for each side.

Columellar refinements are also possible in superficial fat or deep between the domes (Figures 5.31 and 5.32).

Isolated Defects

Deep glabella: Start with glabella and proceed caudally with few drops on the nasal dorsum and proceed with molding.

Nasal Hump: Treat first by injecting above the hump, extending and defining the nasofrontal angle. Overfilling of this area and the resulting straight-line

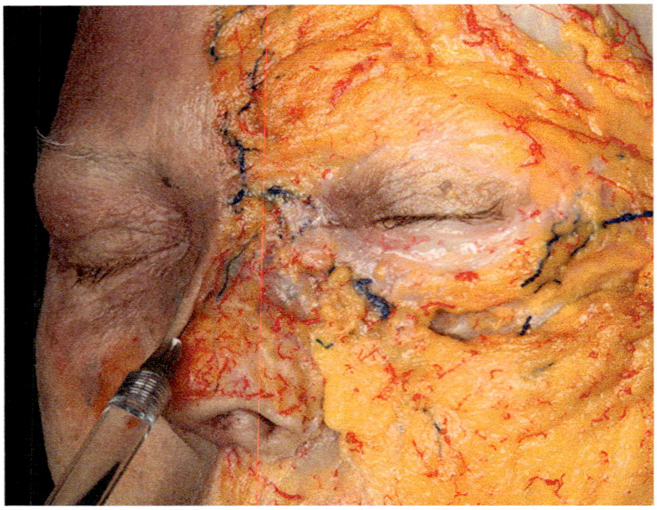

Figure 5.28 Depth of lower nasal dorsum deep injection.

deformity from the forehead to the hump should be avoided. Then augment the area of the dorsum below the hump. You can proceed with the tip if needed. Infradomal injection gives the illusion of cephalic tip rotation. A supra-tip break has to be preserved by filling this area as a last step, so the injection sequence is Na, Nd, Nt, St.

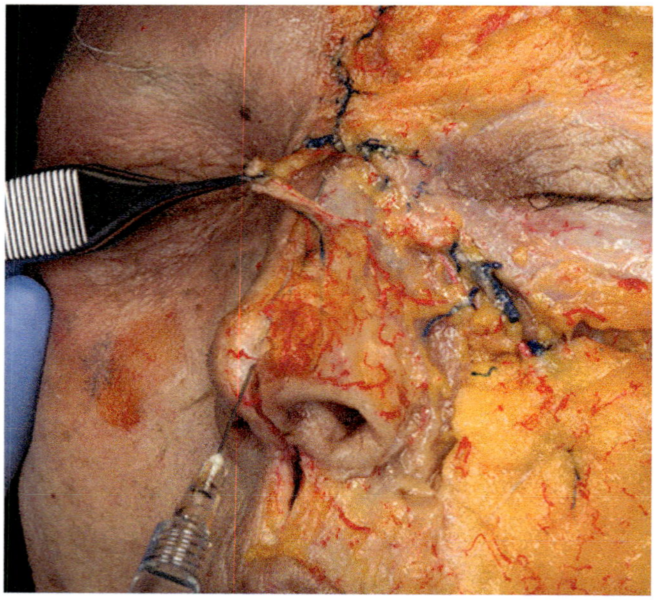

Figure 5.29 Depth of nasal dorsum injection with cannula (deep) injection.

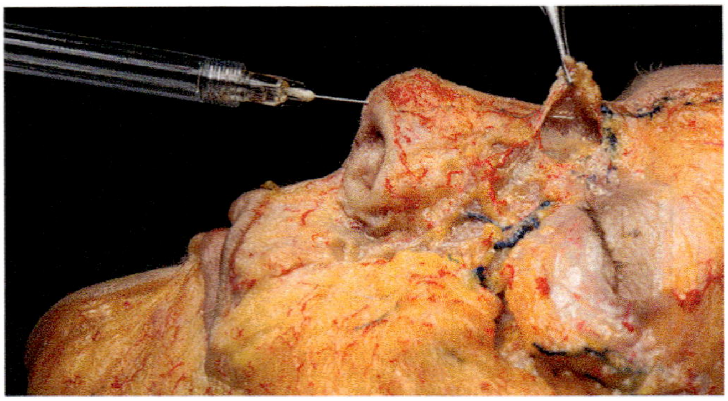

Figure 5.30 Depth of nasal dorsum injection with the cannula visible on the profile view.

Saddle nose: This is usual in Asian patients. If a CT scan shows a structural connection of the nasal dorsum anatomy, the shape can be corrected by filling the saddle area, which should be treated in multiple steps if the sagittal dorsal defect is more than 3 mm. First, define the tip projection, then filling runs from nasion to dorsum. So the injection sequence is Nt, Na, Nd, St.

Deprojected nose: The nasal spine, septum, and nasal base work as a scaffold that give support to the nasal tip. Subnasal injections that place HA anterior

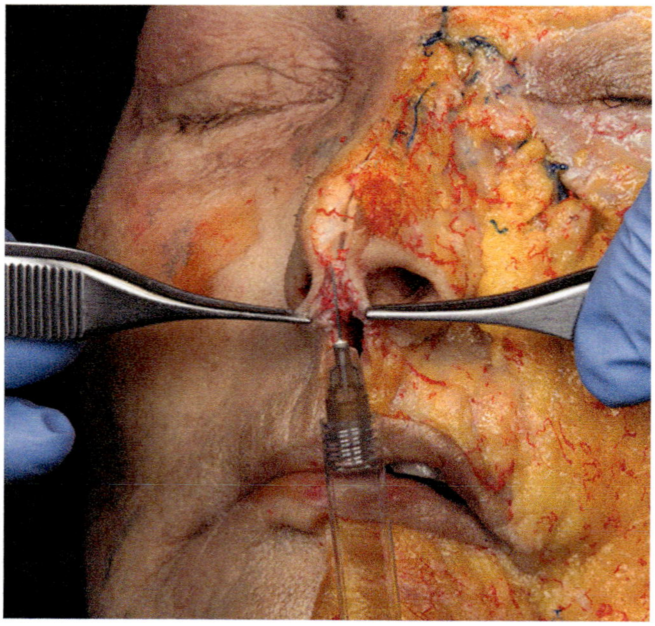

Figure 5.31 Depth of nasal columellar deep injection.

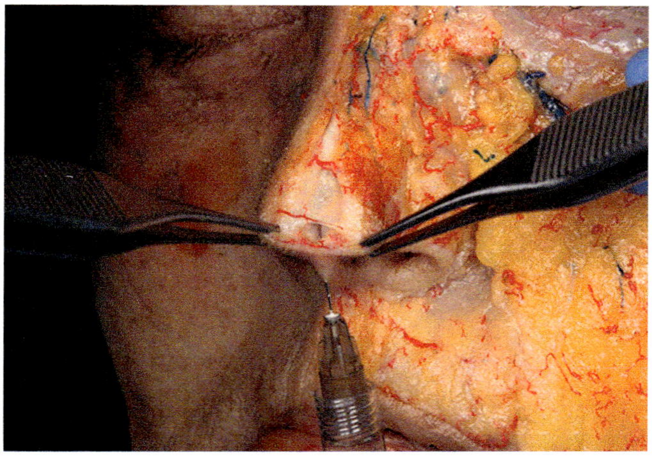

Figure 5.32 Depth of nasal tip deep injection.

to the nasal spine produce an opening of the nasolabial angle and an illusion of tip cephalic rotation. Then, augment the nasal tip. Proceed with Na and Nd, setting a straight line from the height of the new nasal radix to the dorsum; set the sagittal projection of the tip and avoid an undesirable fullness of the supra-tip. So the injection sequence is Sn, Rnb, Lnb, Nt, Na, Nd, St.

Nasolabial angle and columella: A defined nasolabial angle is vital to achieve a harmonious and balanced relation between tip and lip. Columellar retraction gives the illusion of tip caudal rotation. Perform a subnasal injection that places HA anterior to nasal spine, increasing columellar projection when needed. The second step is to support the lateral ala; then, perform a glabellar injection that should be carried out slowly and carefully to avoid ophthalmic artery embolization, deep to the bone. Next, perform tip injections and, only at the end, proceed to the nasal dorsum for refinement. So the injection sequence is nasal base, Nt, Ng, Nd.

Secondary Defects

Crooked nose deformity: Usually, the goal is to fill the concavities. The key point is the need to avoid the lateral nasal artery: the needle must enter on the midline; once the periosteum or perichondrium is reached, slide laterally deep to the defect or inject medially and mold laterally. The injection sequence is thus: Sn, Rnb or Lnb, Nt, Na, Nd, St.

Saddle nose deformity: This can be a consequence of aggressive primary surgery. If a CT scan shows a structural connection of the nasal dorsum anatomy the shape can be corrected by illing the saddle area. First, define the tip projection; then filling runs from nasion to dorsum. The injection sequence is Nt, Na, Nd, St. If there are dorsal structural voids, such as exaggerated scarring or mucosal defects, filler should not be injected because of the deficiency of the structural integrity of the scaffold. The only procedure that can solve this complication is a secondary rhinoplasty.

Alar retraction or collapse: This can be reshaped with Rna and Lna injections. This should be undertaken by expert injectors—nasal surgeons or injectors that have more than two years of experience in full facial rejuvenation—because of the high risk of skin necrosis. Filling is done in the deep subdermal layer; as soon as skin blanching is detected, injecting has to be stopped.

Checkups

Nasal reshaping with fillers requires regular maintenance. Results usually last 4–12 months once the desired result has been achieved. Maintenance of these results would require one or two treatments the first year, followed by treatment once a year. This means that a non-surgical nasal correction should be proposed as a treatment protocol, not based on the amount of the material used.

Although injectable facial fillers can offer an efficacious alternative to surgery for the aging face, they also have their limitations. It is important to recognize specific circumstances that may be best managed with an alternative to fillers.

COMPLICATIONS

Danger Zones

To avoid vascular complications, it is better to **stay in the midline** because all the "major" vessels (columellar arteries, angular arteries, lateral nasal arteries [Figure 5.33] and nasal dorsal arteries) normally lie away from the midline. The **plane of injection** is somewhat controversial, but **deep to periosteum and deep to perichondrium is our recommendation. Constantly holding the treatment area between two fingers during slow injection can avoid lateral filler displacement.** It has been possible to inject deep in the midline and to displace hyaluronic acid with molding. This technique has been useful to correct lateral nasal defects where there was an increased risk of intravascular injection. At the end of every injection, palpation and smoothing out of the skin with wet gloves helps to avoid undesired "bumps." The upper lateral cartilages are continuous with the nasal bones. The lower lateral cartilaginous vault comprises the medial, middle, and lateral crura. The anatomic dome is the junction of the medial and lateral crura. Depending upon the intrinsic relationship of these structures, the tip of the nose can be normal, bulbous, or boxy. Tip support is basically a combination of skin, ligaments, and cartilage. The depressor septi nasi is the most important muscle that acts on the tip and lip complex. It shortens the upper lip and drops the tip when smiling. Surgical resection or blocking with BoNT-A may be necessary to enhance the result of fillers, although this is not the rule. When reshaping the nose with fillers, the angles with the lips and the forehead are important. The former is the nasolabial angle and should be between 90° and 100° in men and between 100° and 110° in women. The latter is the nasofrontal angle, which is between the forehead and the nasal dorsum.

Clinical Considerations

It is important that all patients have realistic expectations for these procedures and understand that fillers can restore balance, enhance appearance, and minimize defects. Follow-up procedures a few weeks after the initial treatment may optimize results and lengthen the duration of the effects of these products which varies from about 3–12 months.

Non-surgical rhinoplasty is a safe procedure but complications may occur. Inexperienced injectors, improper patient selection, and defect/filler mismatch likely play an integrated role in the onset.

Although most complications of facial fillers are transient and minor in nature, it is important to discuss them with patients prior to injection. Common complications include bleeding, swelling, irregularity, erythema, bruising, and discoloration. Rare complications can include infections, lumps, the Tyndall effect, vascular compromise, necrosis and blindness.

Fillers should be resorbable to avoid undesired complications such as granuloma, nodules, dislocation, allergies, and long-term palpability. Currently high G′

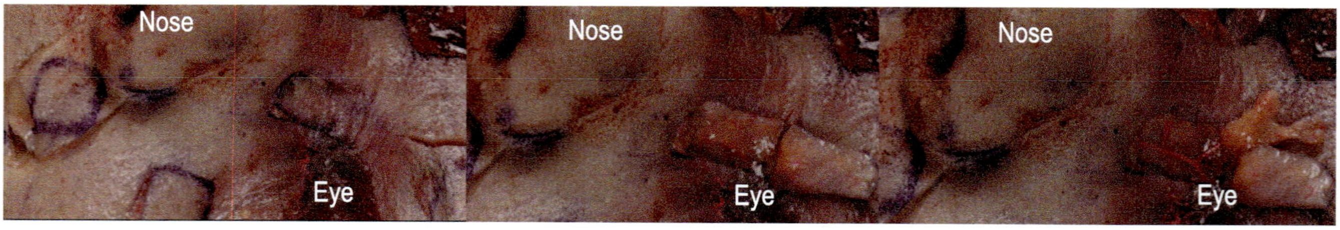

Figure 5.33 After skin removal, the fat is exposed. The lateral nasal artery is also visible.

HA is the "gold standard." Other materials can be palpable under the relatively thin nasal skin. Semi-permanent filler such as calcium HA or permanent soft tissue filler such as silicone or acquamid can also dislocate and produce severe granulomatous reactions with resulting nasal cellulitis, nodules, or ulcers that are difficult to be treated. Moreover, clinicians cannot correct injection imperfections because of a lack of an equivalent to hyaluronidase.

Immediate Complications

Bleeding is associated with patient anticoagulation due to concurrent and/or recent use of aspirin, NSAIDs or blood-thinning medications. The use of large-bore needles and injection into highly vascular areas, such in the nose, can worsen the bleeding.

Irregularity may be common. In cases with a deviated nose, the best method is to inject small amounts of filler, slowly, in a multiple-step procedure.

CAUTION

Embolization can involve the ophthalmic artery which can lead to blindness. Embolization can be a consequence of direct injection of the internal external carotid network, particularly in the facial danger zones. Simptoms can be Immediate (the majority of cases) or rarely delayed between 10 minutes and 1 hour. The dose of hyaluronidase differs among reports; however, we suggest 300–1500 IU of hyaluronidase repeated at frequent intervals (every 2–4 hours). The worst potential event is embolization of the ophthalmic artery, which can lead to blindness [1,7]. Should this occur, the clinician has the possibility of retro-bulbar injection of hyaluronidase with a 25G cannula within a timeline of 90 minutes. Options can be injecting hyaluronidase through a cannula either 8 mm below the inferior tarsal strip, following the orbital floor with a downward curved direction at a depth of 3 cm from the bony orbital rim or with entry 1 cm above the medial canthus directed 30° medially following the medial orbital wall.

Embolization can produce necrosis of down-stream structures. If this were to occur, injection of hyaluronidase (Hase) is mandatory. Inject as soon as possible and distribute Hase around the injected area at least 300 U/hour for at least 5 or 6 injections. Hot packs, soft massages, and application of nitroglycerin paste help promote vasodilatation but are less necessary if hyaluronidase has been injected. Low molecular weight heparin may be used to decrease thrombosis.

Delayed Complications

(See Chapter G.)

Bruising may be caused by needle injury. Avoid further injection unless essential; compress with gauze and apply ice packs to minimize bruising.

Infections are rare; however, patients with a susceptibility to or a history of herpes simplex may be candidates for prophylactic antiviral therapy.

Erythema accompanied by pruritis and fever may be related to hypersensitivity. In severe circumstances, corticosteroids are necessary.

Lumps are usually related to nodules or to a granulomatous reaction mediated by an inflammatory response. Treatment options include corticosteroid injection, hyaluronidase, and surgical removal.

The *Tyndall effect* denotes a bluish discoloration due to superficial product placement. Placement of the correct product in the proper plane may limit the likelihood of the Tyndall effect. Hyaluronidase may be needed for reversal.

References

1. Fedok FG. *Curr Opin Otolaryngol Head Neck Surg.* 2008;16:359–68.

2. Kurkjian TJ et al. *J. Plast Reconstr Surg.* 2014;133:121e–6e.
3. Raspaldo H et al. *J Cosmet Dermatol.* 2010;9:11–5.
4. Humphrey CD et al. *Aesthet Surg J.* 2009;29: 477–84. Erratum in: *Aesthet Surg J.* 2010;30:119.
5. Bertossi D et al. *Eur J Dermatol.* 2013;23:449–55.
6. Sundaram H et al. *Plast Reconstr Surg.* 2016;137:518e–29e.
7. Bertossi D et al. *Esperienze Dermatologiche Minerva Editions.* 2016;18(1):1–13.
8. Rodman R & Kridel R. *JAMA Facial Plast Surg.* 2016;18:305–11.
9. Jasin ME. *Facial Plast Surg Clin North Am.* 2013;21:241–52. Review.
10. Moon HJ. *Clin Plast Surg.* 2016;43:307–17. Review.
11. Saban Y et al. *Arch Facial Plast Surg.* 2008;10:109–15.
12. Carruthers A et al. *Dermatol Surg.* 2010;36:2121–34.
13. Nocini PF et al. *J Oral Maxillofac Surg.* 2011;69:716–23.
14. Thomas WW. *Facial Plast Surg Clin North Am.* 2016;24:379–89.
15. Rohrich RJ & Pessa JE. *Plast Reconstr Surg.* 2012;129(5S):31–9.
16. Rohrich RJ et al. *Plast Reconstr Surg.* 1995;95(5):795–9; discussion 800–1.
17. Tansatit T et al. *Aesthetic Plast Surg.* 2017;41(1):191–8. Epub 2016 Dec 28.

Further Reading

Andre P. *J Cosmet Dermatolo.* 2008;7:251–8.

Beer KR. *J Drugs Dermatol.* 2006;5:465–6.

Bertossi D et al. *Plast Reconstr Surg.* 2019; 143(2):428–39.

Botti G & Pelle Ceravolo M. *Acta Medica Edizioni.* 2012; vol 1.

Braccini F & Dohan Ehrenfest DM. *Rev Laryngol Otol Rhinol (Bord).* 2013;134(4–5):251–7.

Choucair RJ & Hamra ST. *Semin Plast Surg.* 2009;23:247–56.

Cosmetic Surgery National Data Bank Statistics. *Aesthet Surg J.* 2015;35(Suppl 2):1–24.

de Maio M. *Aesthetic Plast Surg.* 2018;42(3):798–814.

Donald WB 2nd et al. *J Plast Reconstr Aesthet Surg.* 2009;62:11–8.

Douse-Dean T & Jacob CI. *J Drugs Dermatol.* 2008;7:281–3.

Downs BJ & Wang TD. *Curr Opin Otolaryngol Head Neck Surg.* 2008;16(4):335–8.

Goldman A & Wollina U. *Clin Interv Aging.* 2010;5:293–9. Review.

Humphrey CD et al. *Aesthet Surg J.* 2009;29(6):477–84. Erratum in: *Aesthet Surg J.* 2010;30:119.

Humphrey CD et al. *Aesthet Surg J.* 2009;29:477–84. Erratum in: *Aesthet Surg J.* 2010;30:119.

Lazzeri D et al. *Plast Reconstr Surg.* 2012;129:995–1012. Review.

Raspaldo H et al. *J Cosmet Dermatol.* 2010;9:11–5.

Rootman DB et al. *Ophthal Plast Reconstr Surg.* 2014;30:524–7.

Stupak HD et al. *Arch Facial Plast Surg.* 2007;9(2):130–6.

Sundaram H et al.; Global Aesthetics Consensus Group. *Plast Reconstr Surg.* 2016;137:1410–23.

Sung MS et al. *Ophthal Plast Reconstr Surg.* 2010;26:289–91.

Youn SH & Seo KK. *Dermatol Surg.* 2016;42(9):1071–81.

Zenker S. *Prime J.* 2012:40–48.

6 NASOLABIAL REGION

Berend van der Lei, Jinda Rojanamatin, Marc Nelissen, Henry Delmar, Jianxing Song, and Izolda Heydenrych

ANATOMY

Although the terms "crease" and "fold" are often used interchangeably, they depict two discrete entities [1,2]. The nasolabial crease (sulcus) is a sharp, linear crease defining the border between the upper lip and the cheek. The fold is observed lateral to the crease as a distinct bulge which extends from the nasal ala to the cheilion area. Although the depth and density of the nasolabial crease may vary according to race, sex, age, and weight, the fold itself mostly starts slightly lateral to the nasal ala and ends 1–2 cm lateral to the angle of the mouth. Despite the widespread concept of the nasolabial fold as a pure cutaneous fold, it is documented to be a true anatomical border between the cheek, which has a generous layer of subcutaneous fat, and the lip, where the skin is firmly attached to the orbicularis muscle with no interposed fascia [2,3].

The nasolabial crease can thus be defined as the sharp line demarcating the start of the more laterally placed nasolabial fold. Softening of the crease optically reduces the severity of the nasolabial fold, while a deeper nasolabial crease, accompanied by a more bulging fold, contributes to a more aged appearance.

The nasolabial crease is also significant in portraying facial expression.

BOUNDARIES

There are two conflicting theories as to the formation of nasolabial crease: a muscular and a fascial theory. **The muscular theory** states that the nasolabial crease is formed predominantly by the musculodermal insertions of the upper lip levators. **The fascial theory** claims that the nasolabial crease is formed largely due to dense fibrous tissue and the firm fascial attachments into the fascia of the lip elevator muscles.

Beer et al. [4] found evidence for the muscular theory: They dissected and harvested the nasolabial creases from 14 facial halves and found numerous skeletal muscle fibers in the dermis. In addition, dermal muscle fibers were present 4 mm medial and 4 mm lateral to the nasolabial crease, but in amounts significantly less than directly in the crease. They subsequently demonstrated that the use of low doses of intradermal botulinum toxin placed directly in the nasolabial crease could minimize or even eradicate the crease, and thereby the fold, because of relaxation of the local muscle fibers around the crease.

Sandulescu et al. [5] recently found support for the fascial theory: After careful dissection, sophisticated three-dimensional reconstructions of the histological structures were performed together with scanning electron microscope (SEM) analysis of the nasolabial fold. They found that there is a NLF SMAS, which is a fibromuscular, three-dimensional meshwork bolstered with fat cells. Two SMAS structure types were identified adjacent to the NLF. The cheek SMAS structure demonstrated a regular, vertical, and parallel alignment of fibrous septae, creating a three-dimensional meshwork of intercommunicating compartments. It altered in morphology by condensing while transiting over the NLF to form an irregular structure in the upper lip region. SEM analysis demonstrated the connection between the fibrous meshwork and the fat cells. SMAS blood circulation expanded subcutaneously without perforating the fibromuscular septae.

There is an additional osseous aspect to the nasolabial fold. Several years after his first presentation, Pessa studied computed tomographic scans of patients of different ages and found that skeletal maxillary/orbital height changes indicated a deeper nasolabial fold [6].

Lastly, the skin also plays a role in the nasolabial fold appearance. In the older patient, the amount of skin excess above the fold accentuates it. This skin excess may be either true excess or pseudo-excess due to facial fat atrophy in especially the midface area.

In summary, the nasolabial fold divides an area with a fair amount of subcutaneous fat (cheek) and an area with minimal fat (Figure 6.1). The fold is caused by multiple factors, including muscular activity, SMAS, fat, bone, and skin. For this reason, there is no single approach to treatment of the nasolabial fold.

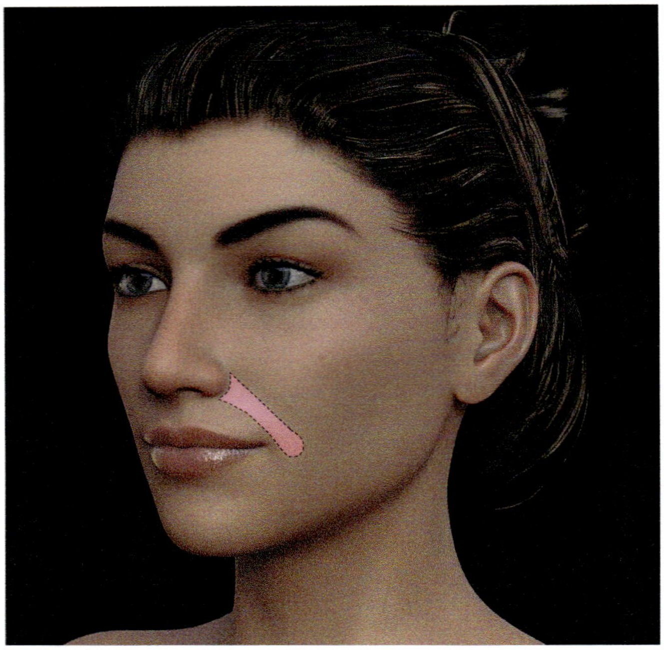

Figure 6.1 Nasolabial fold boundaries indicated in pink.

THE AGING NASOLABIAL FOLD

Facial aging is the recombinant result of atrophy, loss of facial fullness, progressive bone resorption, decreased tissue elasticity, and gravity (Figure 6.2). The gradual loss of underlying soft tissue support is responsible for descent and relative skin excess which manifests as deepening of the nasolabial folds. In elderly patients, the sagittal diameter of the upper third is smaller than the lower third, creating an appearance of overall hypertrophy of the lower part of the malar fat pad due to ptosis and caudal migration of fat tissue. These changes create deepening of the nasolabial fold.

It is important to first address the causative lateral facial vectors, thereby reducing gravitational sagging, before volume restoration of this area is attempted.

SKIN

The skin in the nasolabial area is rich in sebaceous glands and has a good vascular supply (Figure 6.3).

This area is prone to conditions such as seborrhoeic dermatitis and acne and should be carefully evaluated, with possible pretreatment before treatment with fillers is attempted.

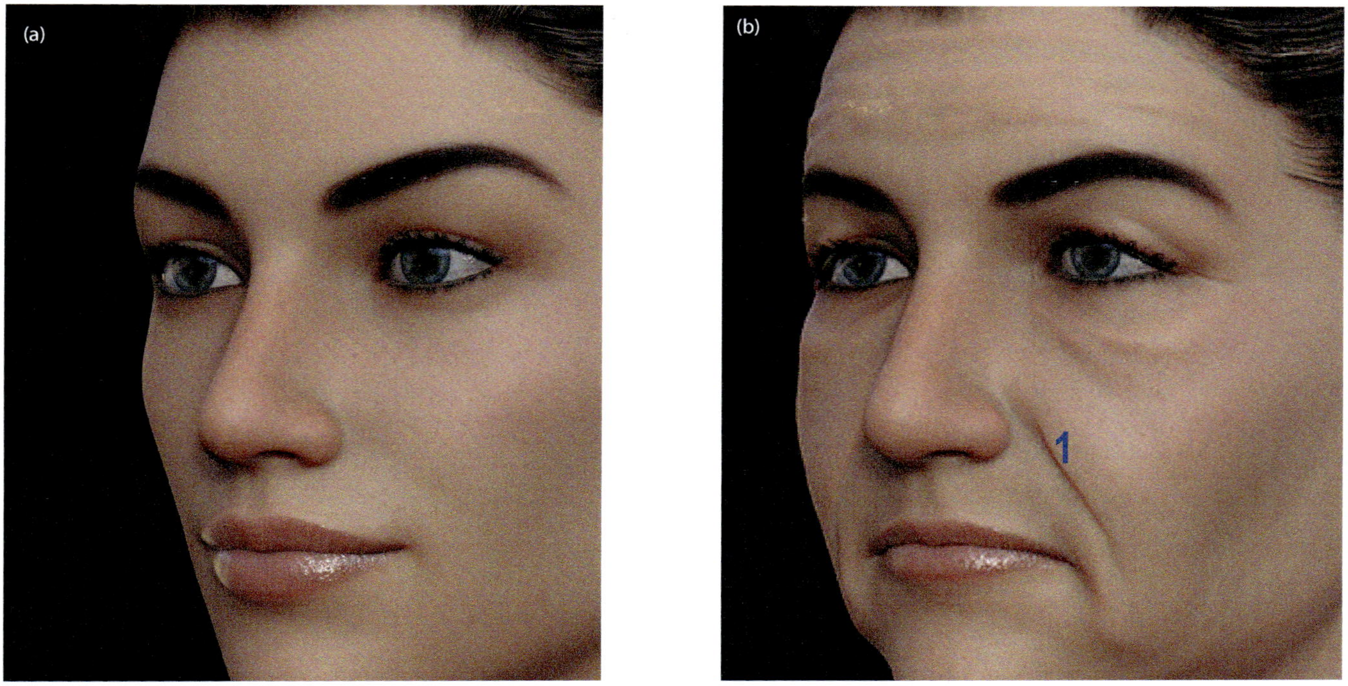

Figure 6.2 (a) Youthful appearance and (b) clearly defined nasolabial fold (1) in a middle-aged woman. The fold starts slightly lateral and above the nasal ala and ends 1 cm lateral to the corner of the mouth. Note the slight asymmetry of the left and right NLF.

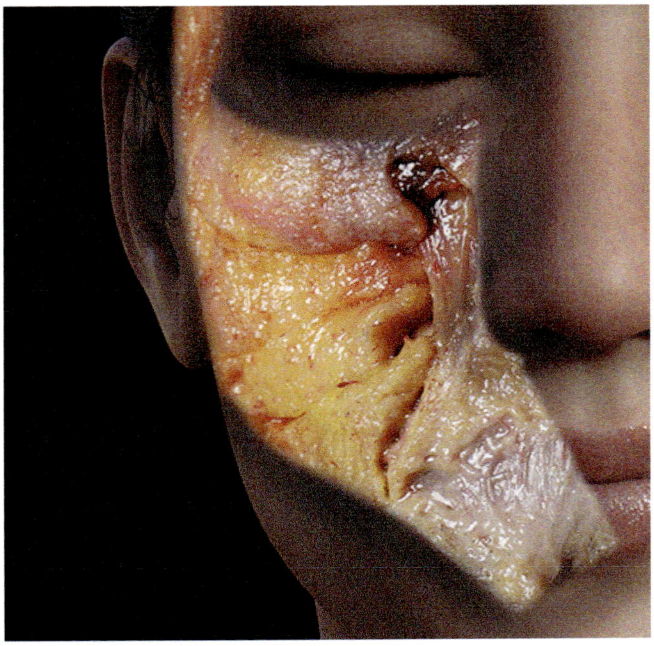

Figure 6.3 Dissection of nasolabial fold: skin.

FAT

The midface comprises several fat compartments (four superficial and two deep), of which two (nasolabial and deep medial cheek fat compartment) are connected to the nasolabial fold. These compartments have been extensively described elsewhere (see Chapter 4 and the key reference article of Rohrich and Pessa [7]).

The **superficial** nasolabial fat compartment joins medially to the nasolabial fold and laterally to the midcheek groove (Figures 6.4–6.6). The upper border of this compartment forms the lower edge of the tear trough and the medial border forms the lateral border of the nasolabial fold. The NLF is formed and separated from the upper lip by SMAS fibers (termed the

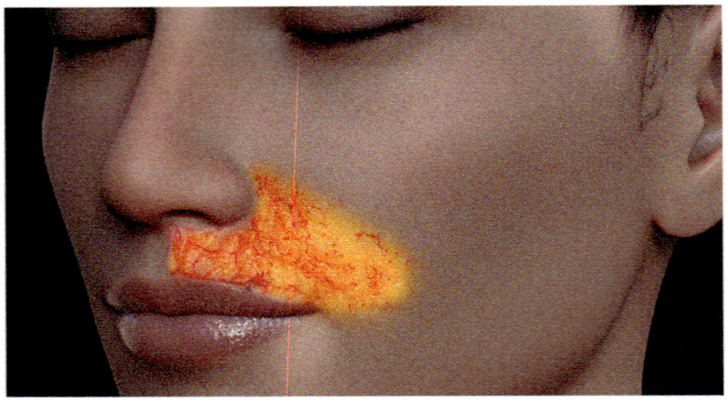

Figure 6.4 The superficial nasolabial fat compartment.

nasolabial septum). This border also contains perforating vessels that reach the skin.

The deep medial cheek fat compartment is located below and medial to the suborbicularius oculi fat pad (SOOF) and below the mid-cheek groove. It is thus located deeper than the medial and middle superficial fat pads. In the upper portion, the zygomaticus muscles define the posterior border of the fold, whilst in its lower portion the levator anguli oris muscle borders the anterior aspect of the fold.

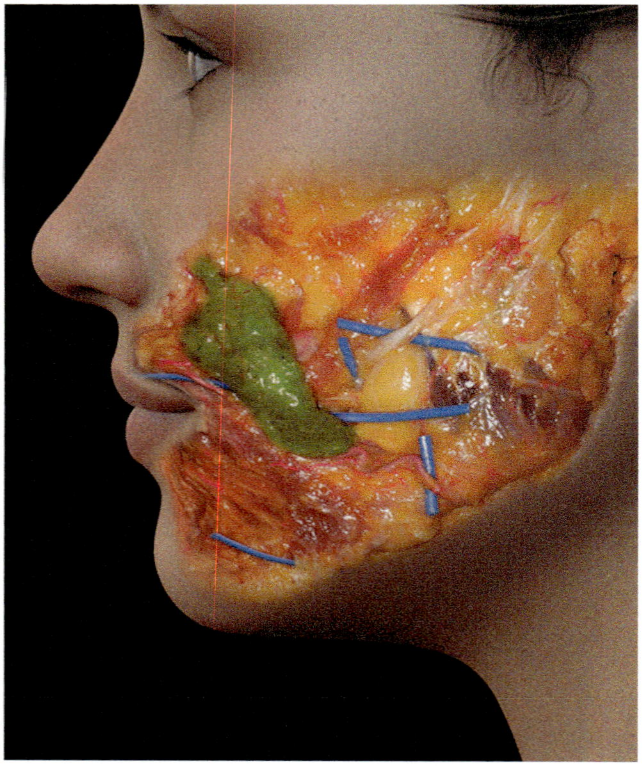

Figure 6.5 Nasolabial fat compartment (indicated in green) medially joined to the nasolabial fold and laterally to the mid-cheek groove.

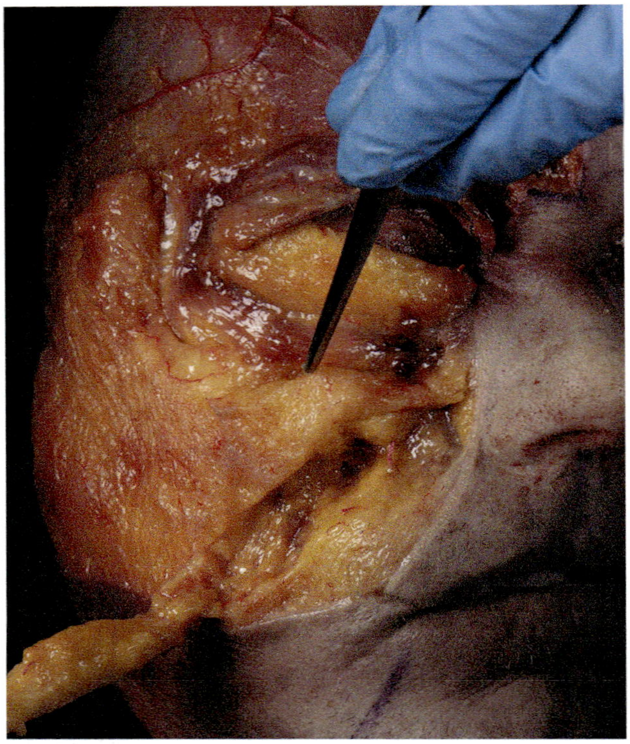

Figure 6.6 Nasolabial fat compartment laterally elevated from the nasolabial fold, exposing the deep structures: muscles and vessels.

MUSCLES

Snider et al. [8] elegantly dissected and described the anatomy of the muscles in relation to the nasolabial fold and discovered a "new" muscle, the so-called malar levator muscle. The following muscles will be described because of their relationship to and effect on the nasolabial fold (Figure 6.7):

- Levator labii superioris alaeque nasi (LLSAN)
- Levator labii superioris (LLS)
- Nasalis (1)
- Orbicularis oris muscle (OOrM) (2)

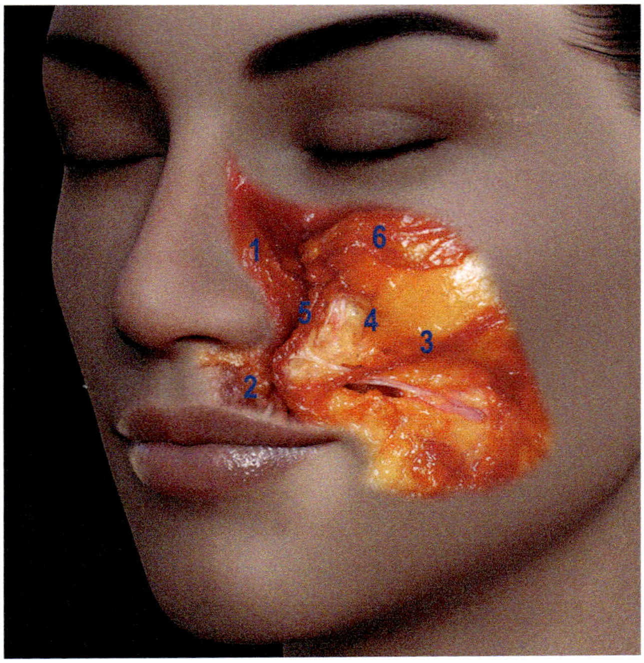

Figure 6.7 Muscles of the nasolabial fold.

- Zygomaticus major (ZM) (3)
- Malar levator muscle (MLM) (4)
- Levator labii superioris (LLS) (5)
- Orbicularis oculi muscle (OOM) (6)

The LLSAN is a long, thin muscle originating from the upper frontal process of the maxilla. It adheres to the lateral nasal wall, and curves around the lateral ala [8]. Superiorly it runs deep to the medial orbital orbicularis oculi, and inferiorly it is superficial to the LLS. The LLSAN inserts into the medial nasolabial fold and alar base before extending into the orbicularis oris, with an average width of 3.1 mm at its insertion site into the medial nasolabial fold. The broadest portion of the superior aspect of the muscle, a point located away from the LLS, is on average 8.4 $\pm$ 0.9 mm inferior and 4.6 $\pm$ 0.8 mm medial to the medial canthus. Contraction elevates and rotates the lateral ala, engraves the nasolabial angle, causes the lateral bunny lines, and enhances the medial nasolabial fold (Figure 6.8).

The LLS is a fan-shaped muscle located in a deeper plane relative to the LLSAN. It is widest superiorly at its origin on the maxilla near the infra-orbital foramen and has a broad insertion into the middle third of the nasolabial fold before extending into the orbicularis oris. Its central portion is on average 4.5 $\pm$ 0.4 cm inferior and 5.9 $\pm$ 0.8 mm lateral to the medial canthus [8]. The LLS has an average width of 12 $\pm$ 0.8 mm at its insertion into the middle nasolabial fold. Contraction of the LLS elevates the middle third of the nasolabial fold and is the principle elevator of the upper lip (Figure 6.9).

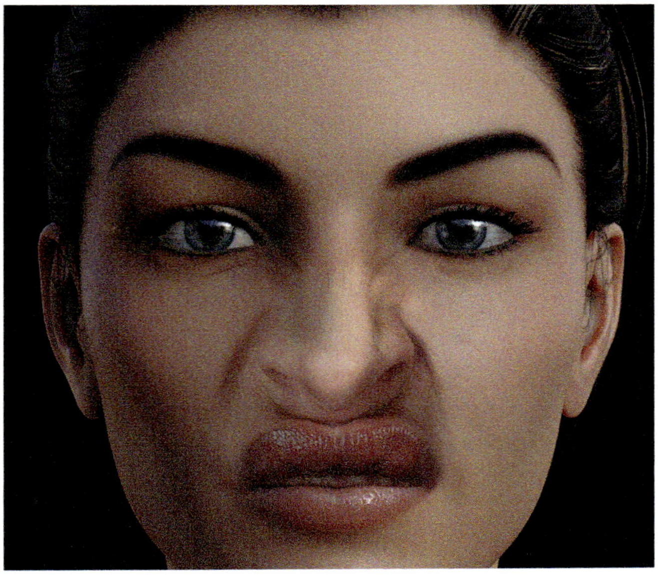

Figure 6.8 Snarled or angry appearance, primarily dominated by the LLSAN. Note elevation and external rotation of the lateral ala, acute nasolabial angle, enhanced medial nasolabial folds, and prominent lateral bunny lines.

The nasalis is a transverse muscle originating from the maxilla and lateral nasal sidewall. It traverses the bridge of the nose to meet the contralateral muscle [8]. The nasalis is deep and nearly perpendicular to the vertically oriented LLSAN.

The OOM lies superficial to its adjacent musculature. It is a circular, sphincteric muscle that covers the upper and the lower eyelids. It is a continuation in the same level as the frontails muscle but is separated from the forehead by the orbicularis retaining

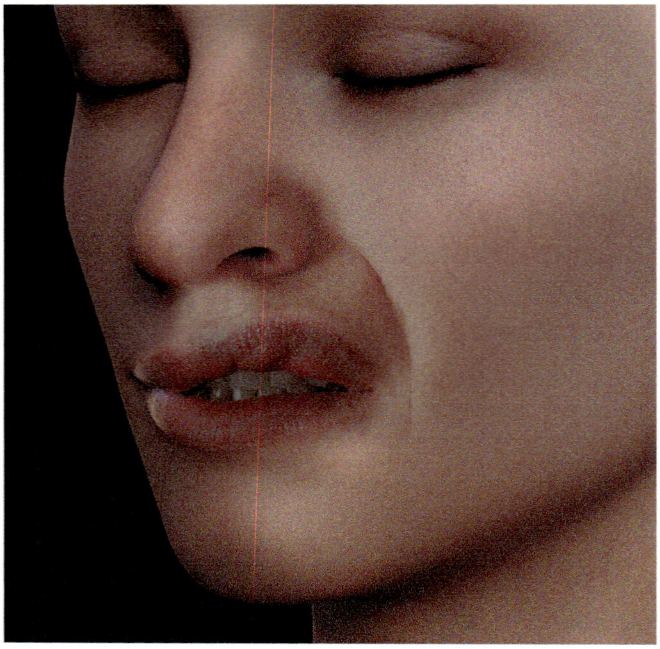

Figure 6.9 The levator labii superioris (LLS) elevates the middle third of the nasolabial fold and is the principle elevator of the upper lip.

ligament. In the lower eyelid, the ORL forms the deep boundary between the orbital rim and the cheek. The orbital portion of the OOM is thicker and darker, covering the frontal process of the maxillary-bone, the upper, medial portion of the deep medial cheek fat compartments (DMCF), and the origin of the LLSAN.

The ZM originates from the zygomatic bone and continues with orbicularis oculi on the lateral aspect of the levator labii superioris before inserting into the outer aspect of the upper lip. It draws the upper lip backward, upward, and outward and is used in smiling, thus exerting a dynamic influence on the position and shape of the nasolabial fold.

The "newly" discovered MLM (Snider et al. [8]) is a tubular muscle located obliquely between the orbital orbicularis oculi and the LLSAN and separated by individual fat compartments. It is positioned deep to the orbicularis oculi and superficial to the LLSAN in all specimens. It differs in both color and form from the adjacent musculature. Its cephalad origin is somewhat continuous with the LLSAN on the upper frontal process of the maxilla, and it inserts into the malar fat pad inferolaterally. The MLM diverges from the LLSAN on average 8.7 mm Inferior and 2.8 mm lateral to the medial canthus. It has an average length of 4.7 cm and a width of 5 mm. A distinct facial nerve branch innervates this muscle. The name "malar levator muscle" is associated with the vector of pull of the malar fat pad. Snider et al. [8] were able to identify this muscle in living patients and observed its implications on medial periorbital rhytides and the tear trough deformity. The MLM produced fullness just below the tear trough in repose, and tenting of the skin with a crepe-paper effect during animation (Figure 6.10).

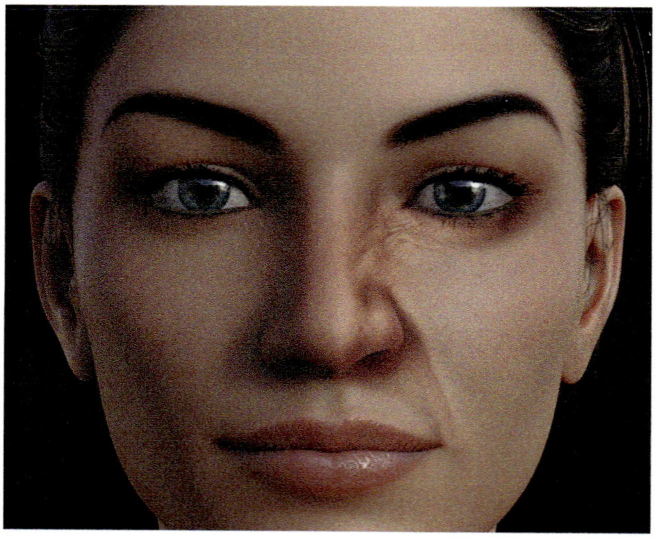

Figure 6.10 MLM activation forming dynamic medial periorbital rhytides which are enhanced depending on the level of activation. Rhytides are subtle during the natural smile as the malar fat pad is elevated, and enhanced with more forceful midfacial animation to produce a crepe-paper effect in the periorbital region without activation of the orbicularis oculi. The MLM also changes the nasolabial fold and its position.

VASCULARIZATION

The facial artery arises from the external carotid artery, after which it travels superoanteriorly from the premasseteric area to the adjacent portion of the nasion. Many studies have found that the facial artery branches to form the inferior and superior labial, inferior alar, lateral nasal, and angular arteries. It pursues a tortuous course and presents an extremely intricate and varied branching pattern (Figure 6.11).

The facial vein gives rise to the angular vein, which is sometimes accompanied by the cephalic branch of the infraorbital artery, duplexed angular artery or a detoured facial artery which may all travel in the tear trough channel. The infraorbital artery contributes to the blood supply along this crease, as do branches from the transverse facial artery and the infra- and supraorbital arcades (Figure 6.12).

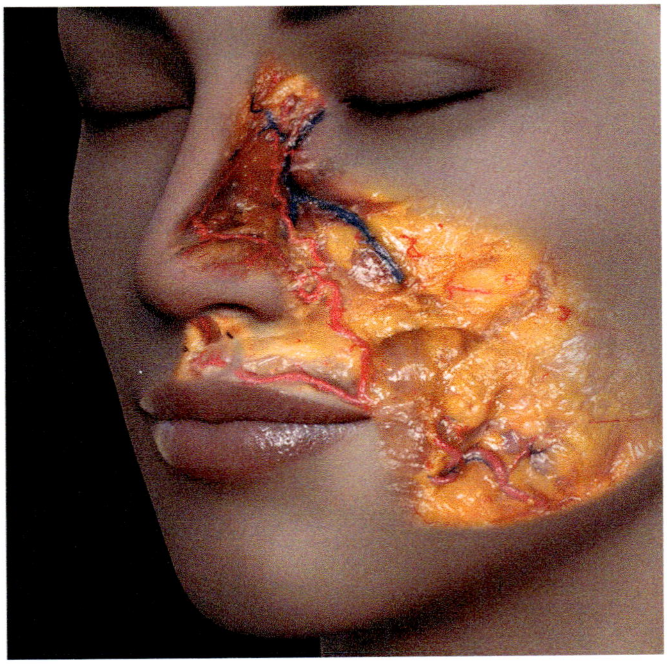

Figure 6.11 Vascularization of the nasolabial area. Facial artery indicated in red. Note the superficial labial, inferior alar and lateral nasal branches.

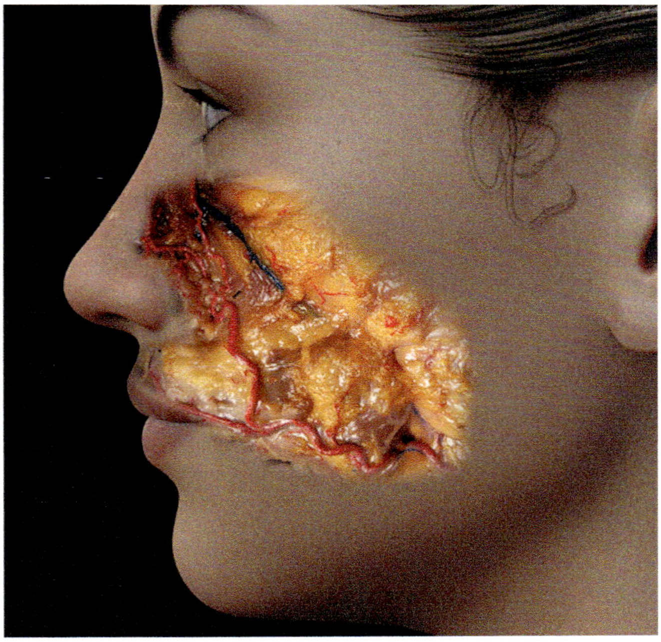

Figure 6.12 Vascularization of the nasolabial area. Note the facial vein giving rise to angular vein indicated in blue.

Detailed anatomy knowledge of the facial artery and its branches relative to the nasolabial fold is of crucial importance in preventing intravascular incidents in this region. Direct arterial injury and occlusion by injected filler may lead to arterial occlusion with subsequent soft tissue ischemia and/or blindness [9]. Three key reference articles are those of Yang et al. [10], Pilsl and Anderhuber [11], and Kim et al. [12].

Yang et al. describe in detail the course of the facial artery in relation to the nasolabial fold and the course of the detoured facial artery, a branch of the facial artery emerging into the inferior palpebral and infraorbital areas and merging to the angular artery (Figure 6.13).

They dissected 60 specimens from 35 embalmed cadavers (24 male and 11 female cadavers; mean age, 70.0 years) and one fresh male cadaver (age, 62 years) and found the following crucial findings: in 56 cases (93.3%), the branches of the facial artery were observed in the vicinity of the nasolabial fold.

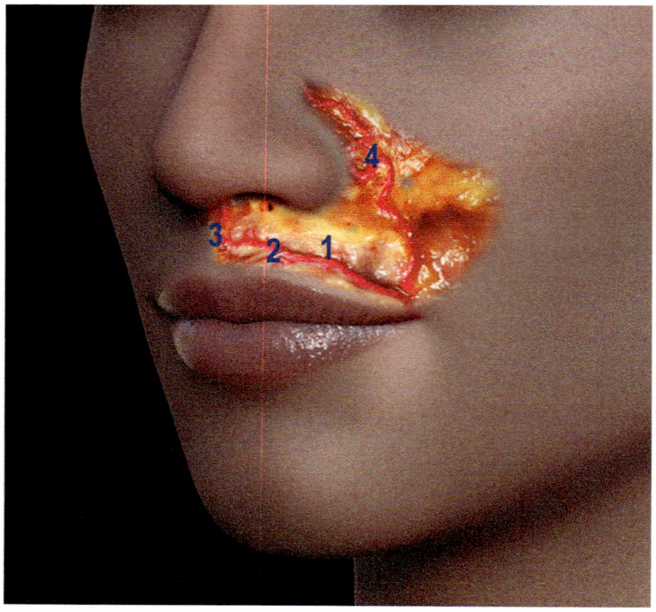

Figure 6.13 Specimen where skin and superficial fat and muscles have been removed: Detoured (superficial) branch of the facial artery. (1) OOM, orbicularis oris muscle; (2) SLA, superior labial artery; (3) CoA, columellar artery; (4) AA, angular artery.

The facial artery was located 3.2 ± 4.5 mm (mean ± SD) lateral to the ala of the nose and 13.5 ± 5.4 mm lateral to the oral commissure. From the cheilion point to the alar point, the facial artery ascended medial to the nasolabial fold within 5 mm in 42.9% of specimens and lateral to the nasolabial fold in 23.2%. In the remaining cases ($n = 19$ [33.9%]), the facial artery crossed the nasolabial fold. The facial artery and detoured (superficial) branches were found in 18 cases (30.0%). In the cases with detoured branches, the facial artery turned medially over the infraorbital area at 39.2 ± 5.8 mm lateral to the facial midsagittal line and 35.2 ± 8.2 mm inferior to the plane connecting the medial epicanthi of both sides. The nasojugal portion of the detoured branch traveled along the inferior border of the orbicularis oculi and then ascended toward the forehead, to form the angular artery.

Pilsl and Anderhuber [11] dissected 96 facial halves in 48 adult specimens to study the arteries of the outer nose, doing three-dimensional computed tomographic reconstructions and horizontal sections. They found three main types of blood supply to the external nose associated with the different types of facial arteries. Moreover, they found a deep course of the nasal arteries in relation to the nasolabial fold and a very superficial course in relation to the nasolabial groove. Therefore, the often-used injection area for nasolabial fold augmentation, located in the upper third of the nasolabial fold, a few millimeters lateral to the nasal wing, appeared to be a danger zone. Here the arterial arcades to the nose cross the injection area, making injury of the vessels with a consecutive intravascular filler injection an easy possibility. They recommended that filler injections into the nasolabial groove be performed deep to the arteries, either by a percutaneous injection very close to the bone (supraperiosteal) or better by an intraoral approach with a very low risk of injuring the arterial arcades.

Very recently, Kim et al. [12] studied the topographic anatomy of the infraorbital artery in relation to the nasolabial fold and its implications for nasolabial augmentation. The IOA was divided into three main branches—palpebral (IOAp), nasal (IOAn), and labial (IOAl) branches—in 34.7%, 100%, and 100% of the specimens. Analysis of the bilateral facial artery (FA) topography revealed that its vascular dominance was observed in 19.4% (7/36). The IOA was thicker and had a wider distribution on the nondominant side of the FA, while the IOAn anastomosed with the FA in the lateral nasal region in 57.1% (4/7).

INNERVATION

The nasolabial area has sensory and motor innervations:

- **Sensory**: Provided by the infraorbital nerve which is a branch of the trigeminal nerve. Innervation is bilateral up to the midline.

- **Motor**: Provided by the buccal branch of the facial nerve which exits from the parotid gland and proceeds together with Stenon's duct toward and behind orbicularis oris. The buccal branch is found below zygomaticus major, above risorius and anterior to the masseteric fascia (Figures 6.14 and 6.15).

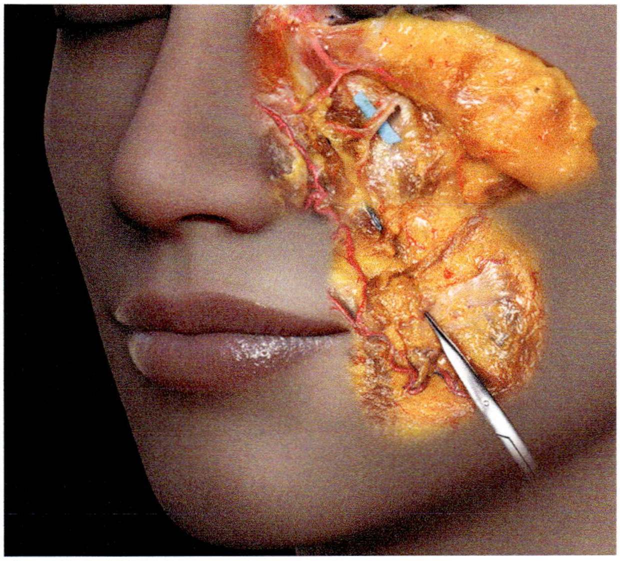

Figure 6.14 Note scissor tip indicating the course of the buccal branch of the facial nerve.

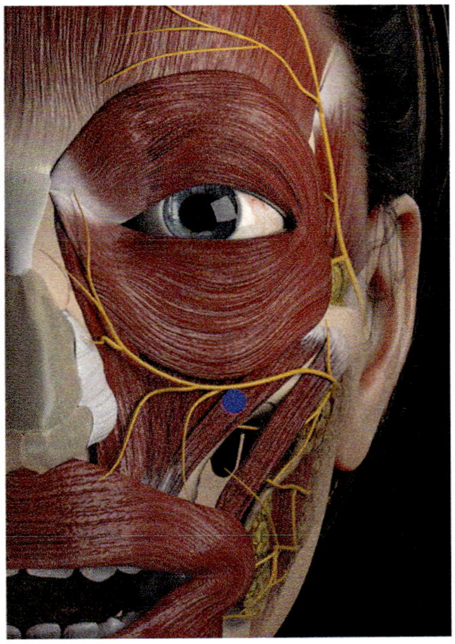

Figure 6.15 Blue dot: The buccal branch of the facial nerve.

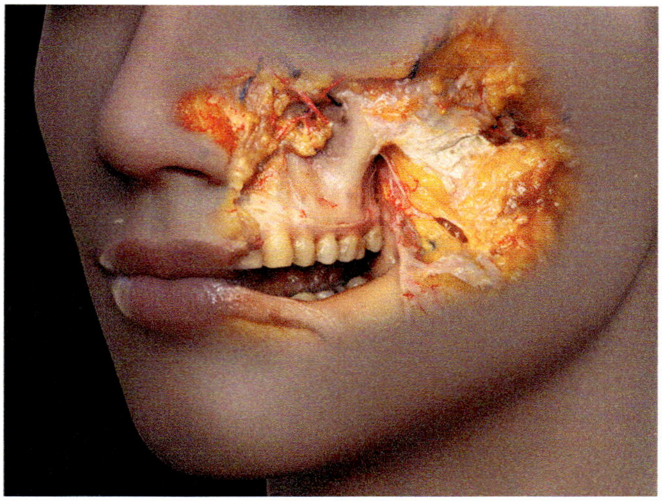

Figure 6.16 The maxillary bone supporting the nasolabial fold.

BONE

Facial bones undergo morphological changes with aging [6]. Bone resorption with widening of the orbital apertures results in a changing appearance of the overlying soft-tissue envelope. Likewise, maxillary resorption impacts the nasolabial fold. Cumulative bone resorption and fat loss from the centrofacial fat compartments result in pseudoptosis of the midface, with increased prominence of the nasolabial fold (Figure 6.16).

HOW I DO IT: BOTULINUM TOXIN

Gertrude Beer [4] demonstrated that botulinum toxin injected intradermally in the NLF reduces its depth, likely due to the effect on adjacent medial and lateral dermal muscle fibers.

Michel Kane [13] described the use of botulinum toxin by injecting into muscles associated with the dynamic behavior of the NLF. In certain patients, mimetic muscles around the NLF have cutaneous insertions in the fold, making it prominent by their early to mid-thirties. In the early 30s to late 50s, botulinum toxin can thus be used to weaken muscles (such as the LLSAN), thereby improving the NLF. A canine or gummy smile may also be improved in this manner. However, in case of ptosis of the soft tissues, botulinum toxin in the mimetic muscles is of limited use.

HOW I DO IT: FILLERS

Conduct a careful full-face assessment to evaluate underlying bone and soft tissue factors contributing to sagging. Always address causative factors and lateral facial vectors before refining the nasolabial area. Critically assess the upper, mid-, and lower third of the nasolabial fold when planning treatment.

In the nasolabial region, the facial artery runs in the middle tissue layer and needs to be meticulously avoided by injecting either in the superficial reticular dermis or deep on the bone.

Upper Nasolabial Fold: DEEP (Pyriform Fossa) with Needle (Figure 6.17)

- Cleanse meticulously and maintain stringent aseptic technique.
- Aim down from the nasal ala toward the opposite oral commissure, staying on the pyriform bone.
- Aspirate.
- Do not inject if not on bone.

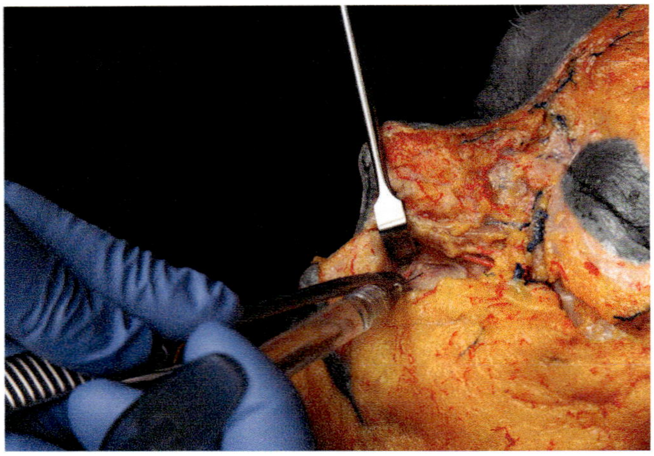

Figure 6.17 Filler injection technique on upper nasolabial fold deep pyriform fossa with needle.

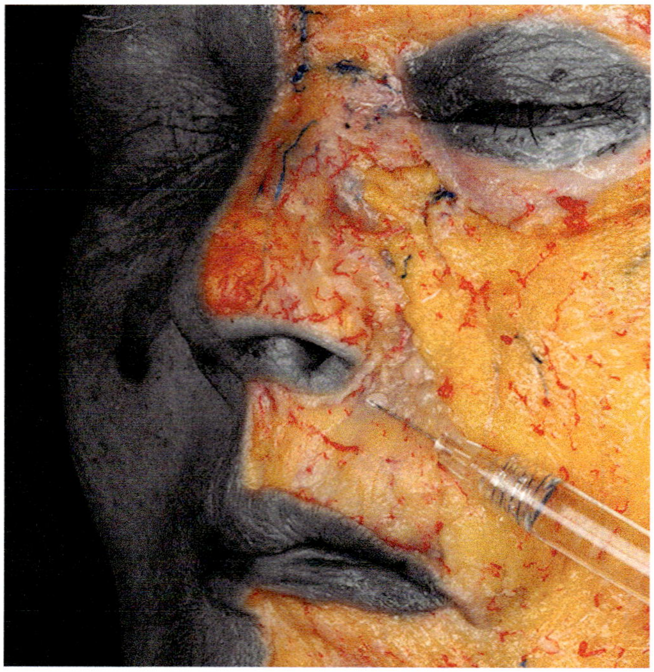

Figure 6.18 Dissection showing superficial injection technique on upper nasolabial fold (arteries seen in red).

Upper Nasolabial Fold: SUPERFICIAL (Needle or Cannula) (Figures 6.18–6.20)

- Placement should be in the reticular dermis or immediate subcutis.
- The angular artery runs at a depth of ~5 mm, and it crosses the nasolabial fold at the junction of the proximal with the middle third.
- Use a superficial fanning technique with cannula or needle.

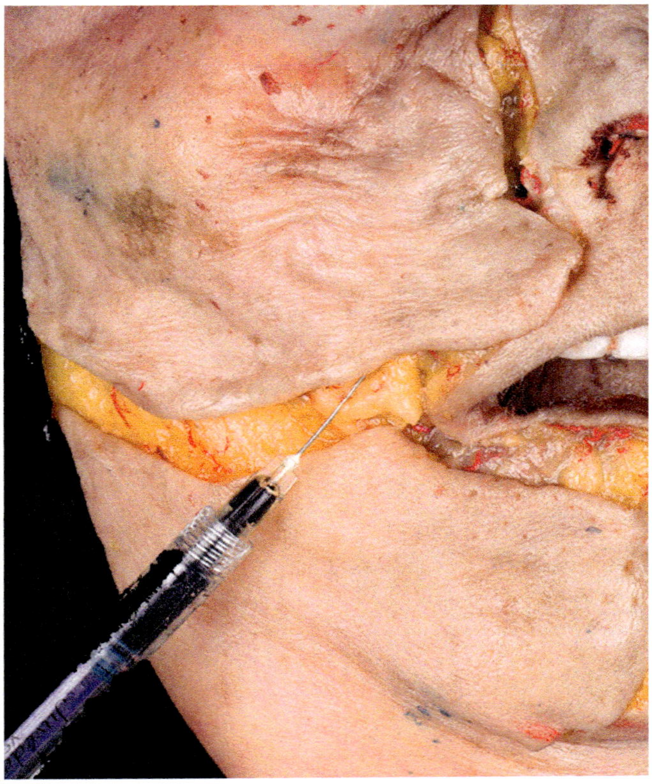

Figure 6.19 Dissection showing skin and superficial fanning injection technique.

Middle and Inferior Thirds

Inject in the superficial plane, being vigilant of the facial artery, using linear threading or fanning technique.

Tips

- The facial artery generally travels medial to the fold, starting 1.7 mm medial from the fold in the lower portion and crossing beneath the fold at a depth of 5 mm at the superior third of the fold, eventually reaching a point 3.2 mm lateral to the nasal ala [10].
- LLSAN, LLS, and zygomaticus minor insert into the nasolabial fold, with the facial artery traversing from medial to lateral within these fibers.

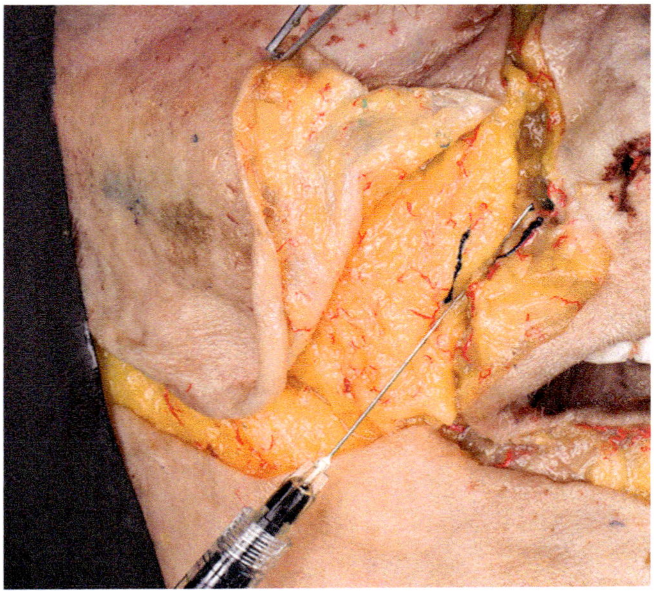

Figure 6.20 Dissection showing placement in the immediate subcutis.

COMPLICATIONS

For general complications and the concept of "safety by depth," see Chapter G.

Seckel divided the face into seven functional danger zones [14]; the nasolabial region includes danger zone 4.

Specific Considerations

- The facial artery poses a major safety risk in this area. Fillers should be injected either in the superficial subdermal plane or deep on the bone in the piriform fossa, with avoidance of the middle lamella.
- Inject medial to the fold to avoid creating heaviness in the midface.
- Be careful not to create irregularities that are unnatural in animation.

- Injecting deep on the bone in the pyriform fossa acts as a mechanical block to the LLSAN, which may be useful when treating a gummy smile. Be careful not to lengthen the upper lip in older patients with a long upper lip and insufficient dental support.

References

1. Pessa JE et al. *Plast Reconstr Surg.* 1998;101:482–6.
2. Wassef M. *Aesthetic Plast Surg.* 1987;1:171–6.
3. Barton FE Jr & Gyimesi IM. *Plast Reconstr Surg.* 1997;100:1276–80.
4. Beer GM et al. *Clin Anat.* 2013;26:196–203.
5. Sandulescu T et al. *Ann Anat.* 2018;217:11–17.
6. Pessa JE et al. *Plast Reconstr Surg.* 1999;103:635–44.
7. Rohrich RJ & Pessa JE. *Plast Reconstruct Surg.* 2007;119:2219–27.
8. Snider CC et al. *Aesth Plast Surg.* 2017;41:1083–90.
9. DeLorenzi C. *Aesth Surg J.* 2014;34:584–600.
10. Yang HM et al. *Plast Reconstr Surg.* 2014;133:1077–82.
11. Pilsl U & Anderhuber F. *Plast Reconstruct Surg.* 2016;138:830e–5e.
12. Kim HS et al. *Plast Reconstr Surg.* 2018;142(3):273e–80e.
13. Kane MAC. *Plast Reconstruct Surg.* 2003;12:66S–72S.
14. Seckel B. *Facial Danger Zones*, 2nd ed. Thieme; 2010.

Further Reading

Barton FE Jr & Meade RA. The "High SMAS" face lift technique. In: Aston SJ, Steinbrech DS, Walden JL, eds. *Aesthetic Plastic Surgery*. London: Elsevier; 2009, p. 133.

Scheuer JF et al. *Plast Reconstruct Surg.* 2017;139:103–8.

Seckle BR, Facial Danger Zones. *Avoiding Nerve Injury in facial Plastic Surgery*. St Louis, Missouri: Quality Medical Publishing Inc.; 1994.

Stenekes MW & Van Der Lei B. *J Plast Reconstr Aesthet Surg.* 2012;65:1618e–21e.

Van Eijk T & Braun M. *J Drugs Dermatol.* 2007;6:805–8.

7 LIPS

Ali Pirayesh, Raul Banegas, Per Heden,
Khalid Alawadi, Jennifer Gaona, and Alwyn Ray D'Souza

INTRODUCTION

The Lip region is one of the aesthetically most important areas for facial enhancement. The lips and eyes have eternally been highlighted as the two most beautiful regions of the human face [1].

Not only are the lips an important part of the central facial triangle, but they also play an essential role in sensual attraction and facial expression, articulation, and masticatory competence. The lips also maintain the oral seal and define the soft tissue boundaries for the teeth. The shape and thickness of the upper and lower lips differ, and there is significant individual and ethnic variation. In youthful Caucasians, the upper lip is usually narrower than the lower, with a lip ratio of approximately 60:40, whereas in those of African ethnic origin, this ratio is 50:50 [2].

BOUNDARIES

Cosmetic lip augmentation consists of the enlargement and reshaping of otherwise normal upper or lower lips. The aim is to improve the three-dimensional relationship with the nose, teeth, and surrounding facial structures at rest, as well as during animation and speech.

An in-depth understanding of the anatomy of the lip and perioral region is mandatory for successful and safe lip rejuvenation (Figure 7.1).

- The upper lip extends from the base of the nose superiorly and laterally to the nasolabial folds and inferiorly to the free edge of the vermilion border.
- The lower lip extends superiorly from the free vermilion edge, laterally to the commissures, and inferiorly to the mandible.
- The circumferential vermilion-skin border is a fine line of pale skin accentuating the color difference between the vermilion and normal skin.

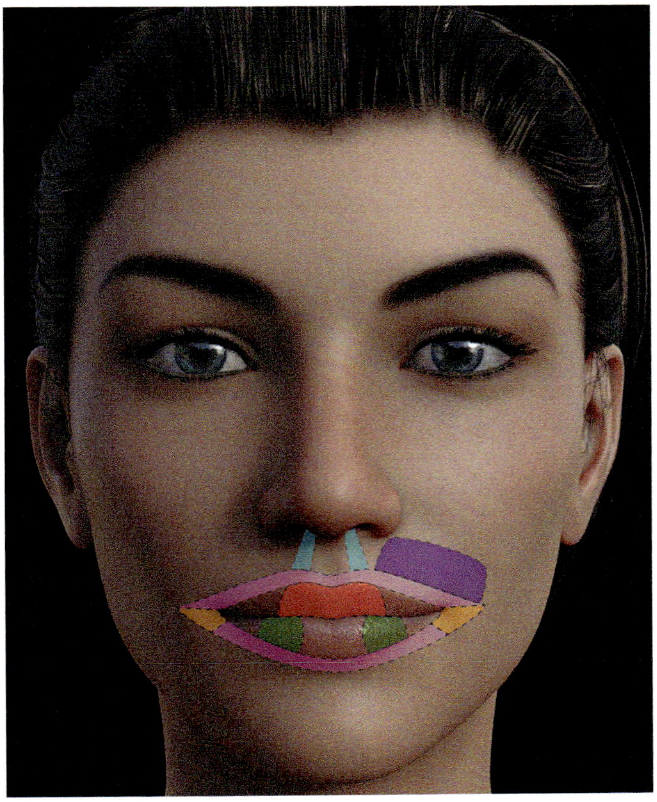

Figure 7.1 Boundaries of the lips.

- The Cupid's bow is formed by two paramedian elevations along the upper vermilion-skin border.
- The philtrum comprises two raised vertical philtral columns adjacent to a midline depression.

Aging, photodamage, hereditary factors, and smoking contribute to volume loss, perioral rhytides, and prominence of mentolabial folds.

Genetically thin lips and cosmetic asymmetry can be treated by soft tissue augmentation.

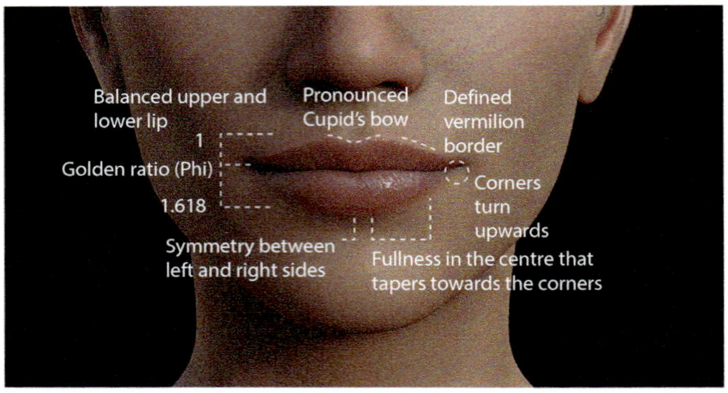

Figure 7.3 Features and dimensions of attractive female lips.

AGING

Features of the youthful lip include

- Smooth skin without visible rhytids immediately above the vermillion border
- Sharply defined philtral columns
- A well-defined central cupid's bow
- Upper lip with a prominent medial tubercle with bilateral depressions
- Lower lip with a corresponding small depression centrally
- Two lateral protrusions (Figure 7.2) [1]

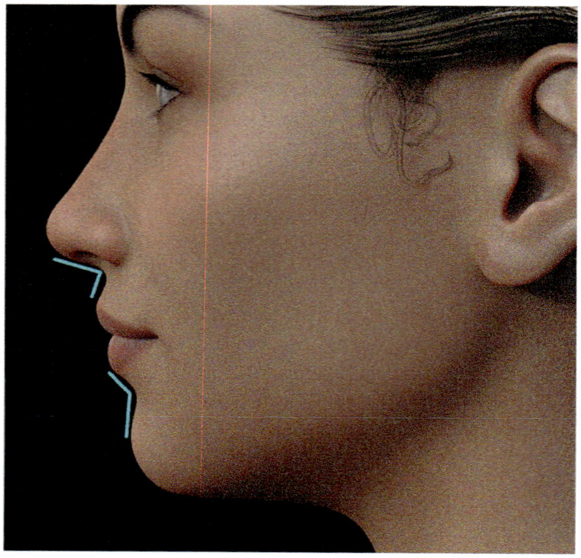

Figure 7.2 Features of the youthful lip.

On lateral profile, the upper cutaneous "white" lip should be short with a concavity approaching the "red" lip. The upper lip should project slightly further than the lower (around 2 mm). Attractive female lips tend to have an increased vermillion height, an increased nasolabial angle and an increased mentolabial angle (Figure 7.3) [2].

Aged skin shows thinning of the upper and lower lip, elongation of the upper lip, and perioral wrinkles (Figure 7.4).

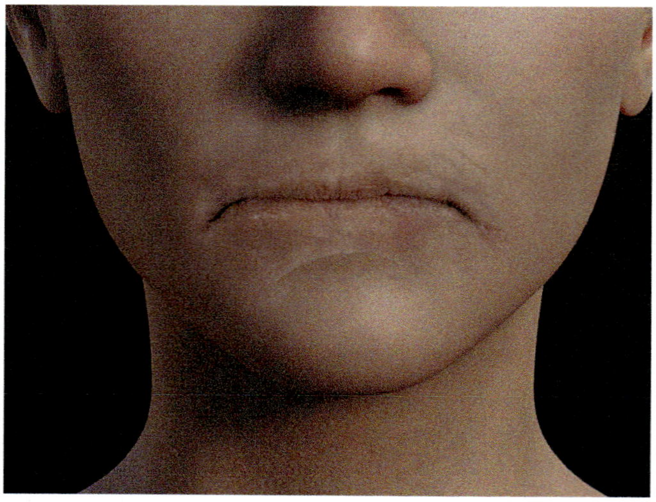

Figure 7.4 Aged lips with elongation of upper lip, thinning, and perioral rhytides.

SKIN

The skin of the lip is supremely exposed to the exposome, with triggers such as sunlight, infrared, and pollution playing a major role in the aging process of this cosmetically sensitive and highly animated region. Women tend to develop more and deeper wrinkles in the perioral region than men, with their skins exhibiting significantly smaller numbers of appendages than men. Although the number of hair follicles does not significantly differ between genders, lip skin in males has a significantly higher number of sebaceous glands, sweat glands and blood vessels, with a higher ratio between the vessel and connective tissue area in the dermis. Cadaver studies have also found the orbicularis oris muscle to be anchored 1.5 times closer to the dermis in women than in men [3] (Figure 7.5).

FAT

In the lip, as in the rest of the face, adipose units are based on the underlying blood supply and its membranous fixation to the skin. The overlying skin folds and creases are likewise determined by underlying vascular arcades, with the relationship between perioral wrinkles and fat loss described in the literature.

- The upper-lip fat compartments are defined as central (superior and inferior), superior, lateral, and lateral inferior.
- The lower-lip compartments are divided into central and lateral compartments (Figure 7.6).
- The lower-lip as an anatomic unit has thinner subcutaneous tissue than the chin (which is one reason for the lip-chin crease).
- The major wrinkles of the lower lip define superficial anatomic fat compartments that need to be

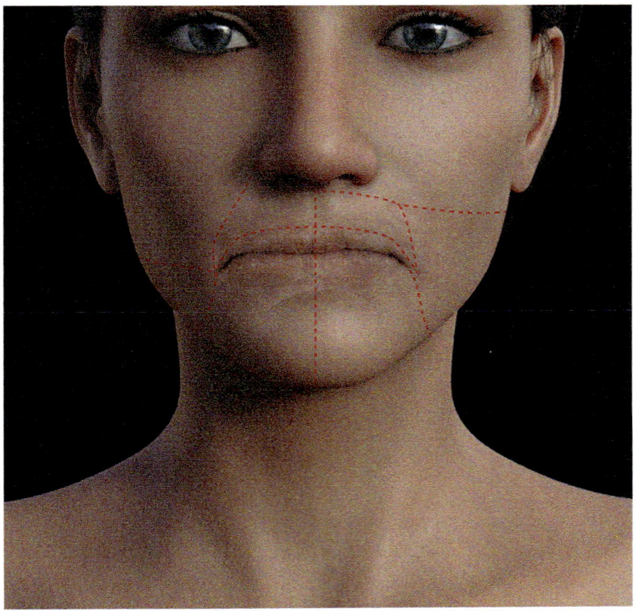

Figure 7.6 Upper-lip fat compartments: Central (superior and inferior), superior, lateral, and lateral inferior. Lowerlip compartments: Central and lateral compartments.

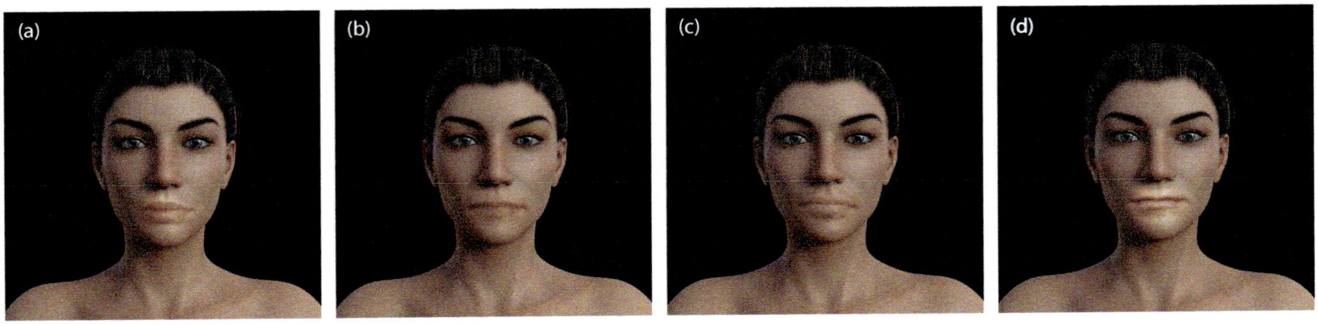

Figure 7.5 (a) Thick lip skin. (b) Thin lip skin. (c) Fatty lip skin. (d) Dry lip skin.

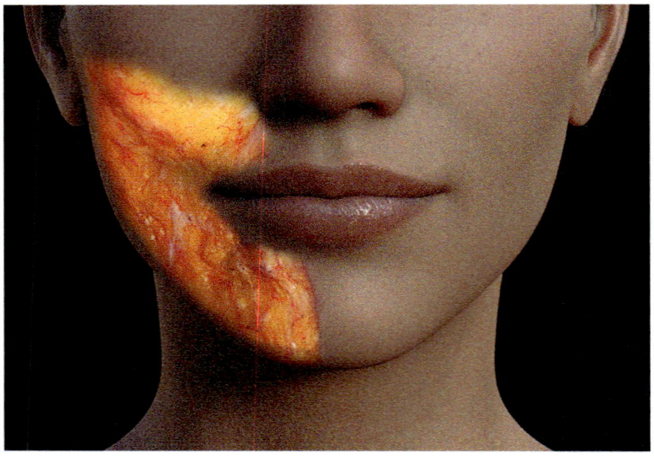

Figure 7.7 Subcutaneous fat superficial to orbicularis oris beneath both the vermilion and cutaneous lip.

individually addressed with fillers unless treating in the submuscular plane.

- The suborbicularis fat is located immediately deep to the muscle and is found beneath both the vermilion and cutaneous lip (Figure 7.7).
- Augmentation of suborbicularis fat of the vermilion lip may improve projection, shape, and contour.
- Augmentation of the vermilion lip diminishes vermilion rhytides resulting from collapse of the supporting deep fat.
- Augmentation of the deep fat of the upper cutaneous lip improves anterior projection, thus recreating a youthful convexity.
- Volume augmentation of the vermilion-cutaneous junction effaces perioral rhytides and imparts a slight youthful flare to the upper lip.

MUSCLES

The muscles of facial expression function as perioral and periocular dilators and sphincters which, in the lips, demonstrate an intricate three-dimensional arrangement of muscle slips capable of sophisticated movements and expressions (Figure 7.8).

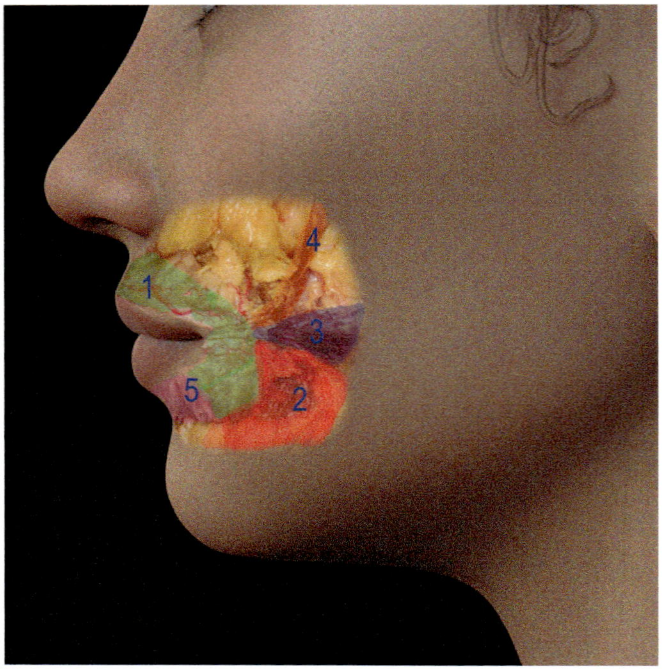

Figure 7.8 Muscles inserting around the lip: (1) orbicularis oris; (2) depressor anguli oris; (3) risorius; (4) zygomaticus major; (5) depressor labii inferioris.

Multiple perioral muscles coalesce to form the **modiolus**, which is a dense, compact, mobile fibromuscular mass, lateral to the lips. The size and shape of the modiolus has been proved to vary with age, ethnicity, and gender.

There are four distinct perioral muscular layers, from deep to superficial:

1. Deep: Orbicularis oris, deep slip of LLSAN, Z Maj, buccinator
2. Middle: Depressor labii inferioris, deep slip of platysma
3. Superficial: Upper-lip group (LLSAN, LLS), modiolus group (LAO, Zyg Maj, DAO), malar group
4. Most superficial: Upper-lip group (malaris and Zyg min), modiolus group (risorius)

The complex three-dimensional muscle anatomy allows sophisticated movement and positioning of the lips, with the **malaris muscle inserting more superficially** and the **buccinator in the deep perioral layers.** This allows closure of the oral cavity in addition to protrusion of the lips.

Muscles Inserting at the Lower Lip

There are three muscles within this group:

1. **Mentalis:** Runs inferiorly from the lower lip to its origin at the incisive fossa of the mandible
2. **Depressor labii inferioris:** Located superficial and lateral to mentalis with its origin laterally to mandibular surface between the symphysis menti and the mental foramen
3. **Platysma:** A thin sheet-like muscle stretching from its origin in the upper pectoral and deltoid fascia to its insertion in the lower lip

Muscles Inserting at the Angle of the Mouth (Modiolus)

The modiolus is an anatomic structure of closely intertwined fibrous tissue and muscle located lateral and superior to the angle of the mouth.

It contains six muscles:

1. **Orbicularis oris:** Sphincter muscle surrounding the mouth interdigitated with adjacent muscles. It has two parts:
    i. **Pars marginalis:** Located in the vermillion and acts as a sphincter and in front of the pars peripheralis, which gives the lips its curved shape.
    ii. **Pars peripheralis:** Located in the cutaneous lip and has a dilatory function.
2. **Buccinator:** Originates out of the alveolar processes of the mandible and maxilla and converges towards the modiolus.
3. **Risorius:** Thin muscle difficult to identify. Its origin and insertion are superficial to the masseter within the dermis. The muscle has no bony origin.
4. **Levator anguli oris:** Runs superiorly from its insertion to the origin in canine fossa of the maxilla.
5. **Depressor anguli oris:** Courses inferiorly from modiolus to the origin at oblique line of the mandible lateral to depressor labii inferioris.
6. **Zygomaticus major:** Anterior to the parotid duct where it pierces the buccinator and runs laterally and obliquely in the cheek region to its origin on the zygomatic arch.

Muscles Inserting at the Upper Lip

Three muscles insert in the upper lip:

1. **Levator labii superioris:** Originates at the inferior margin of the orbit cranial to the infraorbital foramen and lies deep to orbicularis oris and superficial to levator anguli oris.
2. **Levator labii superioris alaeque nasi:** Courses superiorly from the upper lip and located more medially to levator labii superioris, with its origin on the frontal process of the maxilla.
3. **Zygomaticus minor:** Tracks obliquely in cheek region and originates on the zygomatic arch. It has a more anterior origin site and more cranial orientation in the cheek compared to zygomaticus major.

VASCULARIZATION

Blood supply to both lips stems from the external carotid system.

The superior labial artery originates from the facial artery and is mostly superior to, or at the same level

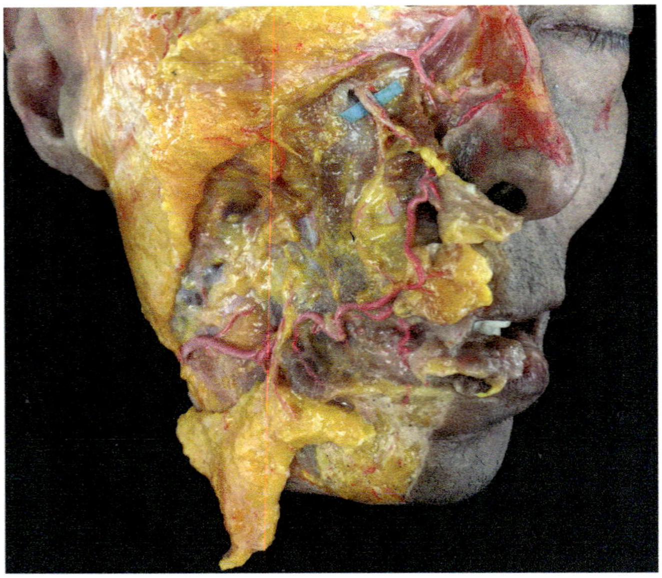

Figure 7.9 Facial artery gives rise to the superior and inferior labial arteries.

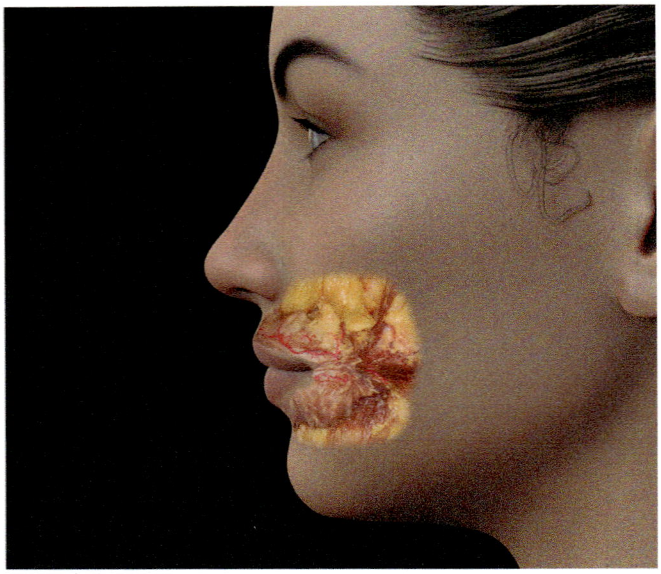

Figure 7.11 Course of the superior labial artery branching from facial artery.

as, the labial commissure. It can occasionally be inferior. The diameter of the superior labial artery at its origin ranges from 1 to 1.8 mm [5–9]. The superior labial artery travels forward to the upper lip, passing deep to the zygomaticus major muscle. The superior labial artery is usually larger and more tortuous than the inferior one. It enters the orbicularis oris muscle and travels between the muscle and the mucosa, along the edge of the upper lip (Figures 7.9–7.12) [10].

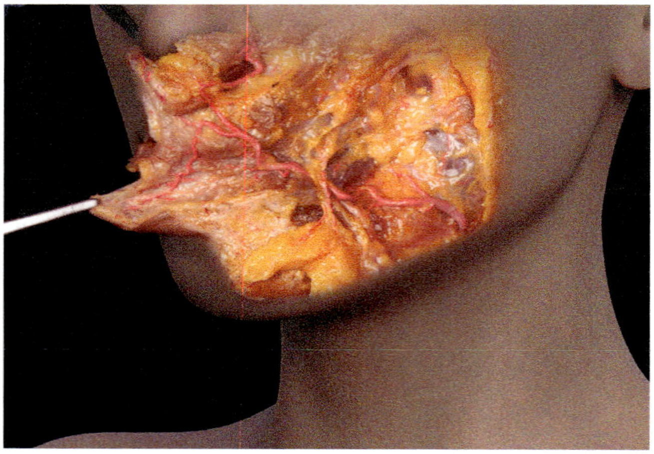

Figure 7.10 Labial artery runs deep to depressor anguli oris.

The **inferior labial artery** is also a branch of the facial artery and generally arises below or at the level of the labial commissure, seldom above it. Its mean diameter ranges **1.2–1.4 mm**. As with the superior labial artery, the point at which the inferior labial artery branches from the facial artery and the distance between its origin and the labial commissure exhibits a high variability ranging from 0.5 to 4 cm, with a mean distance of **2–2.5 cm**. After branching from the facial artery, it runs tortuously upward to the lower lip, deep to the **depressor anguli oris muscle**. The artery penetrates the orbicularis oris muscle and runs tortuously along the edge of the lower lip, lying between the muscle and the mucous membrane [10].

INNERVATION

The facial epidermis is richly endowed with unmyelinated sensory fibers as well as perifollicular dermal myelinated fibers. Sensation varies across the face and generally increases from lateral to medial, with the vermillions being the most sensitive region (Figure 7.13; see further [11]).

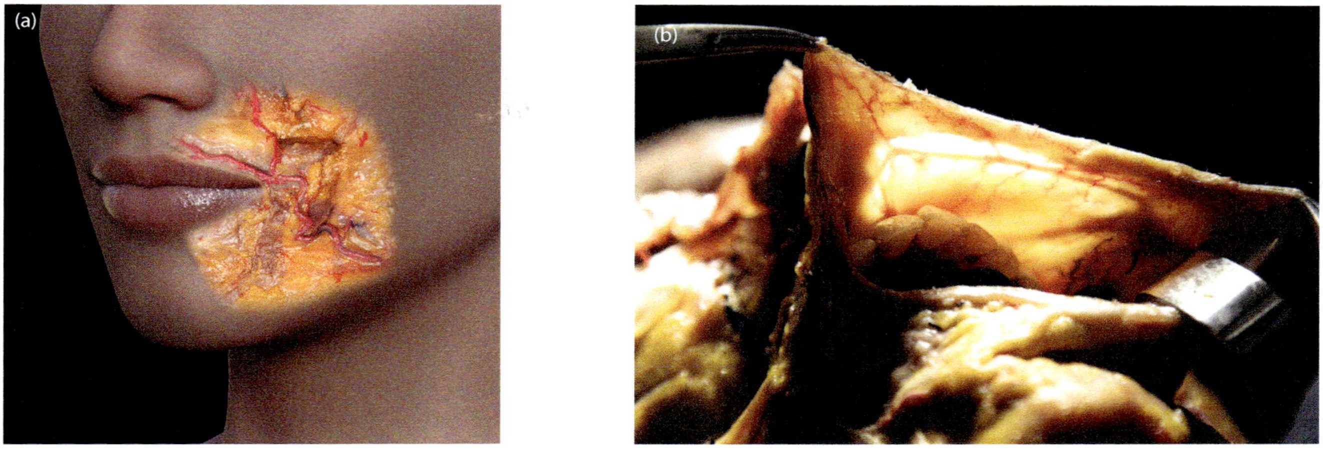

Figure 7.12 (a) Ascending philtral artery. (b) Transection through lip.

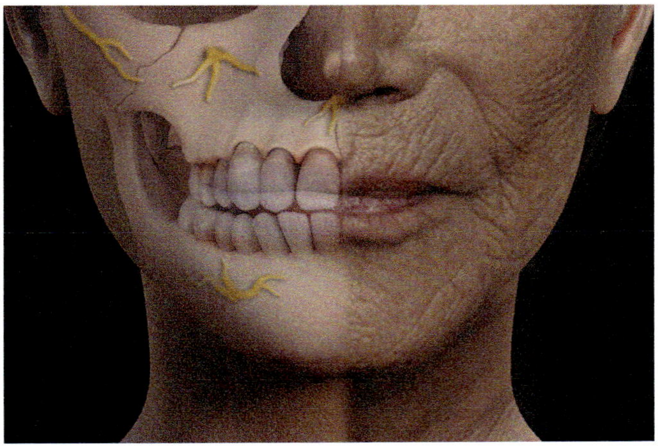

Figure 7.13 Sensory innervation: Infraorbital nerve (upper lip) and mental nerve (lower lip).

Sensory Innervation

The skin of the upper lip is innervated by branches of the infraorbital nerve (ION), which is a purely sensory terminal branch of the maxillary nerve. The main sensory supply is via the superior labial branch, which has two sub-branches: the medial branch supplying the central upper lip and the lateral branch innervating the lateral upper lip. This sensory supply to the upper lip may overlap with the external nasal branch.

A small area of the philtrum may be supplied by the internal nasal branch.

Cutaneous sensory supply to the lower lip is provided by the mental nerve, which is one of the two terminal branches of the inferior alveolar nerve. The mental nerve exits through the mental foramen, which is located below the second mandibular bicuspid and has 6–10 mm of lateral variability. The mental nerve divides into a medial and lateral inferior labial, angular (corner of mouth), and mental branches.

The skin overlying the corner of the mouth may also receive sensory innervation from terminal rami of the long buccal nerve.

Motor Supply

The lip and perioral muscles are innervated primarily by the buccal and mandibular branches of cranial nerve VII.

Motor supply: Buccal and mandibular branches of facial nerve (CN VII).

BONE

Bone support for lips is a fundamental anatomic area that influences lip shape (Figure 7.14).

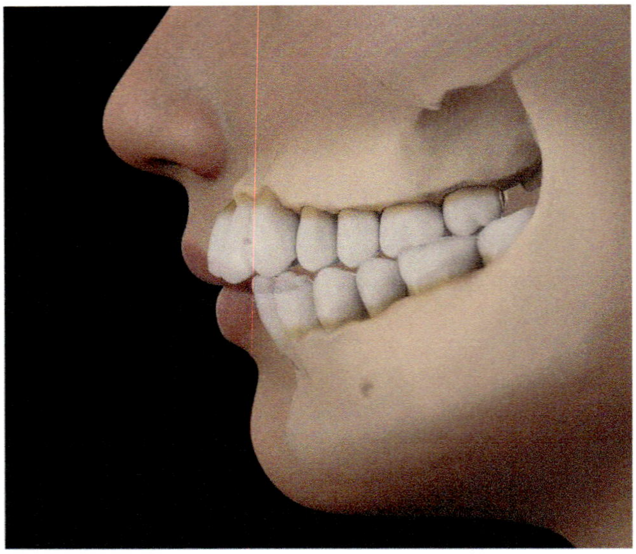

Figure 7.14 Relationships between bone and soft tissues.

It can vary due to ethnicity, language, and environmental factors, as well as personal habits (thumb sucking or other personal habits).

As a general rule we distinguish teeth relationships by looking at the two dental arches—the upper and the lower—that are hosted in the upper and the lower jaws (Figure 7.15a–c).

Class I occlusion occurs where the upper and lower jaw are accompanied by perfect contact for upper and lower teeth (Figure 7.15d).

Class II occlusion occurs where the lower jaw is in a more posterior position and is sometimes contained deeply within the palatal arch, creating an inversion of the lower lip (Figure 7.15e).

Class III deformity occurs where the lower jaw is projected forward in a more anterior position with regard to the upper jaw (Figure 7.15f). In extreme cases, the lower lip does not touch the upper lip.

As a general rule, the upper lip should not cover the upper incisors that may be visible in the lip relaxed position—1.8 mm in male and 2.4 mm in females.

Another factor to take into account should be the overjet, which means how much the upper and the lower incisors axis is projected forward. The greater

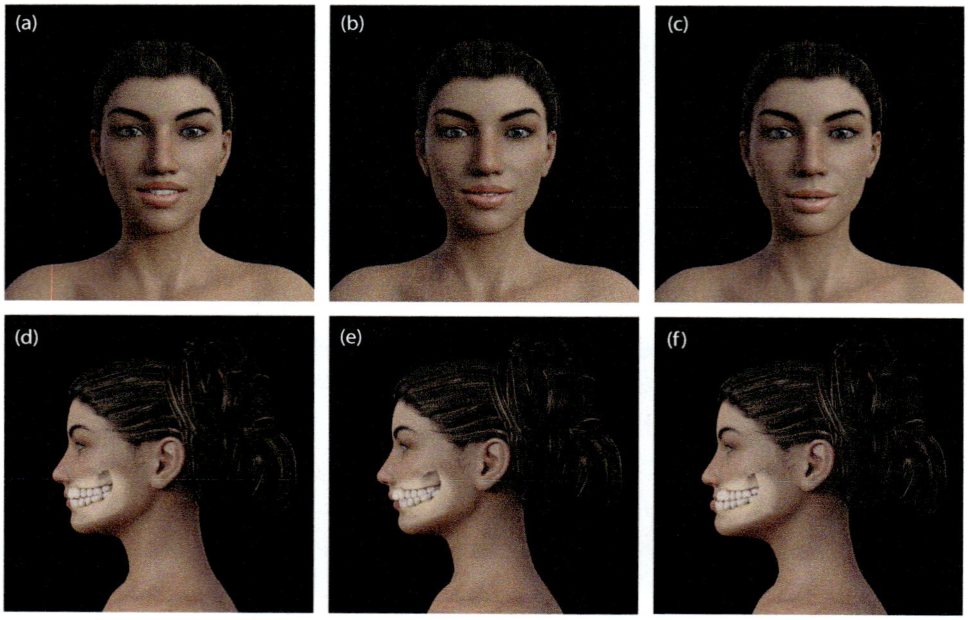

Figure 7.15 (a) Class I relationships. (b) Class II relationships. (c) Class III relationships.

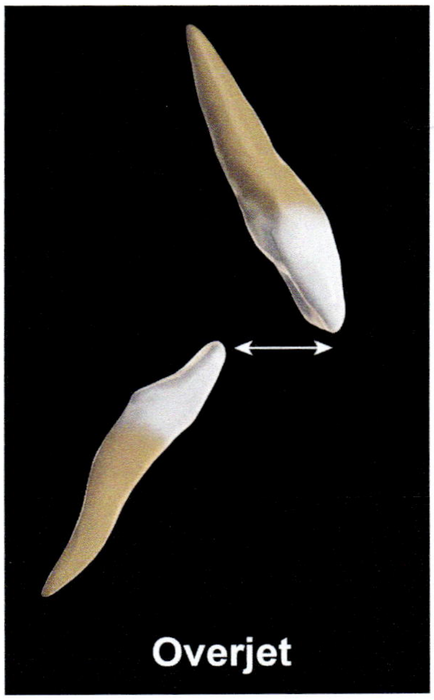

Figure 7.16 Overjet relationships.

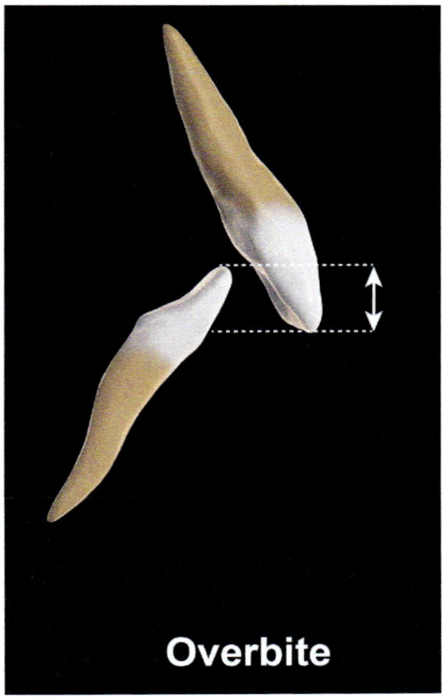

Figure 7.17 Overbite relationships.

the overjet value, the more upper lip protrusion we will observe (Figure 7.16).

The overbite refers to how much the upper incisor edge covers the lower incisors. The higher the overbite value, the more the lower teeth are covered by the upper teeth, creating a shorter lower third height and redundancy of lip contact (Figure 7.17).

LIPS: HOW I DO IT BOTULINUM TOXIN

- Ensure realistic patient expectations: Toxin treatment will soften functional radial perioral lines but not remove resting lines.
- Additional improvement can be achieved with a combination of fillers and energy based devices.
- Start with incremental doses so as not to influence phonation and articulation, especially in singers and public speakers, etc.
- Consider double diluting the toxin to have additional control over the small number of intended units.
- Mark 2–4 symmetrical points on the upper and two on the lower lip (Figure 7.18).
- Inject precise, superficial aliquots (0.5–1 U) just adjacent to the vermillion to prevent spreading to adjacent musculature (Figure 7.19).

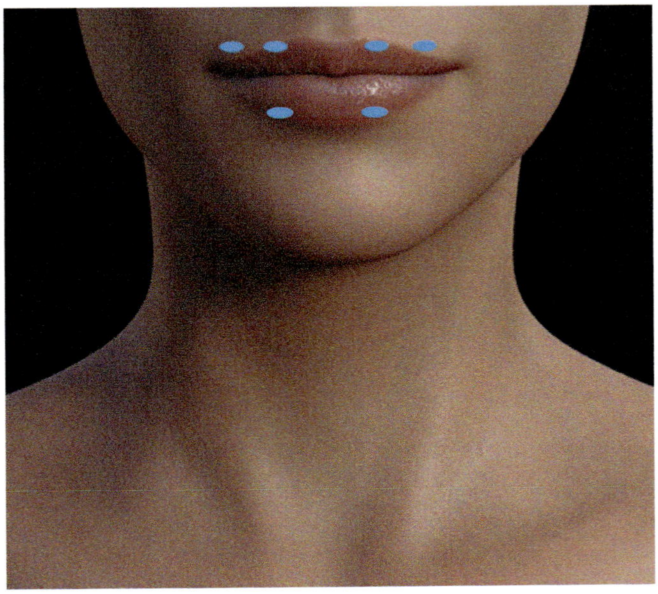

Figure 7.18 Toxin injection at the vermillion border: 2–4 symmetrical points on the upper and 2 on the lower lip.

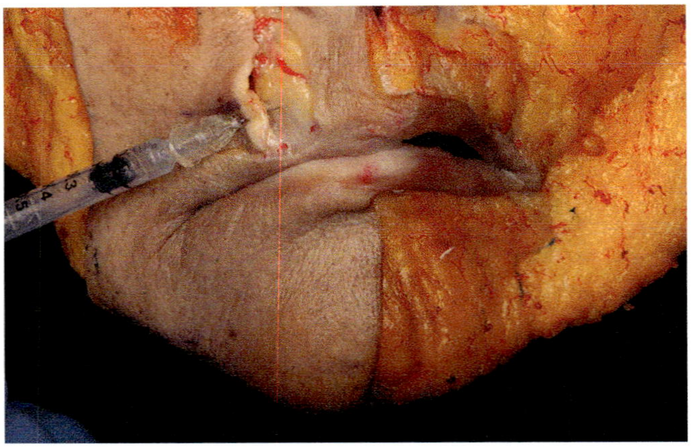

Figure 7.19 Toxin injection: Superficial aliquots (0.5–1 U) adjacent to the vermillion; 4–6 U of onabotulinum toxin is recommended for the upper and lower lips.

- A cumulative dose to 4–6 U of onabotulinum toxin is recommended for the upper and lower lips.
- Ice, topical anesthesia, or vibration may dull the pain with injection.

HOW I DO IT: FILLERS

Linear Threading Technique

Linear threading technique is usually accomplished in a retrograde manner, with filler being injected on withdrawal of the needle or cannula. Anterograde technique refers to filler extrusion while advancing the needle. This method may be safer than other techniques because the filler, flowing ahead to the needle tip, pushes vessels out of the way, thus minimizing tissue trauma and avoiding potential intravascular injection.

The main injected sites for this technique are

- **The vermilion border:** Retrograde threading technique. The cutaneous skin should not be injected in order to avoid a sharp and over-defined lip contour, which may result in unnatural fullness of the vermilion border and further elongation of the cutaneous upper lip.
- **The perioral rhytides:** Retrograde threading with a 30G needle placed directly in the line. With this technique, it is possible to correct both static and dynamic lines.
- **The philtral columns:** Insert the needle at the top of the two humps formed by the Cupid's bow, toward the nasal septum, using a slow retrograde threading technique and pinching the skin with the non-dominant hand during the injection to prevent lateral splaying. At the end of the retrograde injection, a small amount of gel can also be deposited to produce a lift of the cupid's bow and support the projection of the central upper lip.

Fanning Technique

This technique is similar to linear threading as it involves lengthwise insertion of the needle and extrusion of filler while the needle is withdrawn. However, the needle is not fully removed but changes its direction toward a new filling area. The filler is thus injected along multiple short lines with the advantage of fewer access points and less tissue trauma.

The main injected site using this technique is

- **The vermilion body**, starting the treatment from this area minimizes the risk of overcorrection and improves the appearance of associated perioral radial rhytides. In this site, injection should be performed from the mucosal side of the lip by inserting a needle at a 45° angle or using a cannula to reduce the possibility of post-treatment bruising and swelling. The injection should then be directed toward the center at a 20° angle, changing direction every time to provide a homogeneous and complete filling (Figures 7.20–7.29).

Serial Puncture Technique

The serial puncture technique involves multiple, closely placed injections. It is helpful to pull the skin

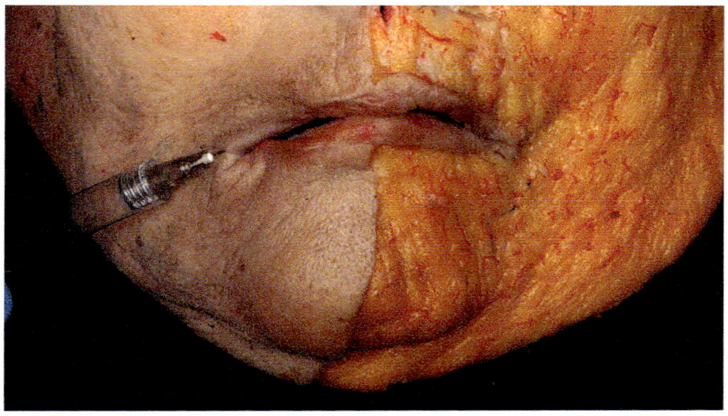

Figure 7.20 Linear threading technique: aspirate before injection.

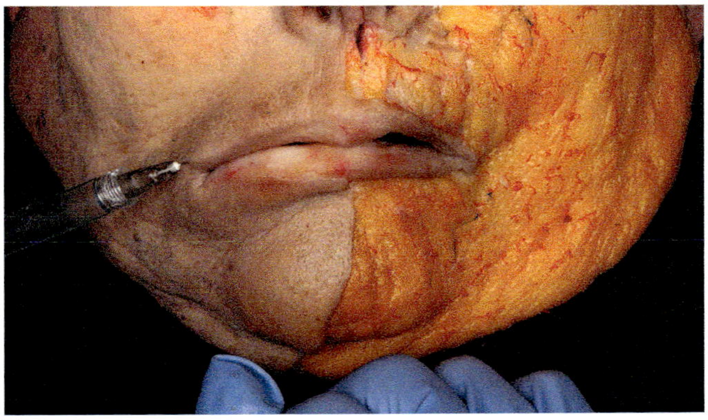

Figure 7.21 Linear threading can be retrograde or antegrade (antegrade being regarded as a safer option).

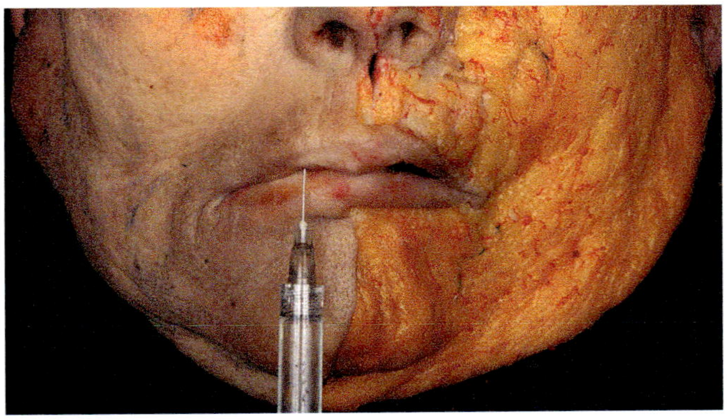

Figure 7.22 The serial puncture technique involves multiple, closely placed injections.

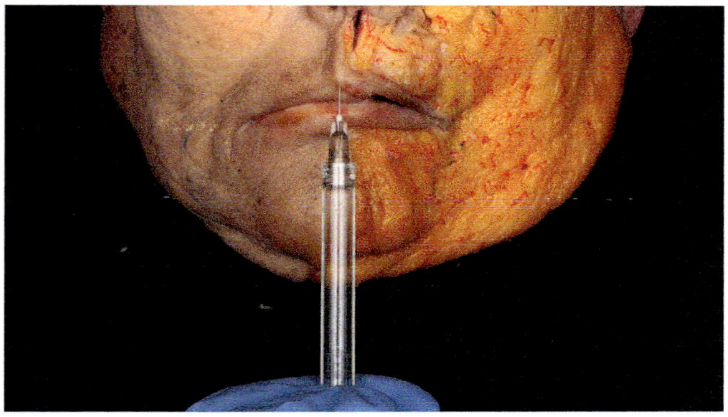

Figure 7.23 Philtrum enhancement by retrograde injection of microaliquots of filled slightly increasing from nasal sil to lip tubercle.

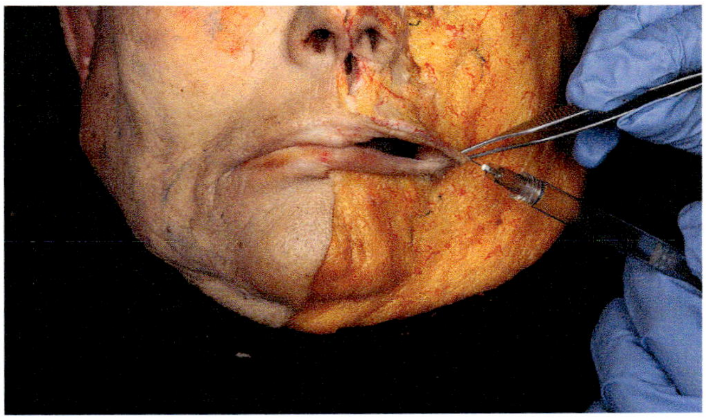

Figure 7.24 Fanning technique: Lengthwise insertion of the needle and extrusion of filler but the needle is not fully removed and changes its direction toward a new filling area.

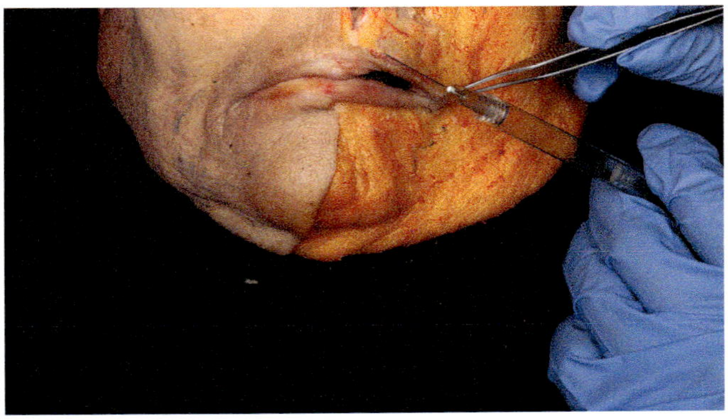

Figure 7.25 Microdroplets of filler retrograde.

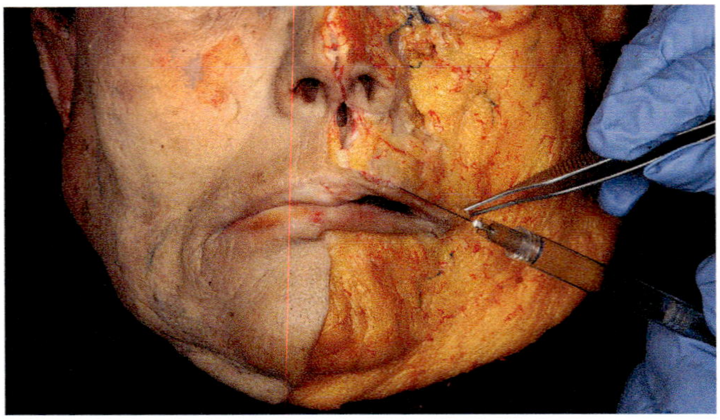

Figure 7.26 Aspiration before injection and change of direction adds safety.

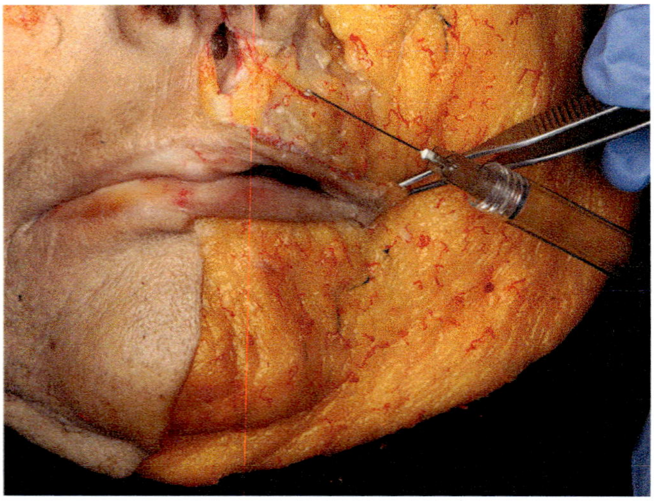

Figure 7.27 Fanning technique: The filler is injected along multiple short lines with the advantage of fewer access points and less tissue trauma.

slightly away and out in order to keep the skin taut while injecting. Multiple deposits of closely spaced gel should be placed, and in the case of post-injection gaps, soft massage should be performed to blend the filler. This technique allows for tight control and more precise filler placement. However, the possibility of increased bruising and swelling due to increased tissue trauma remains controversial [7].

The main injection site for this technique is

- **The vermilion border**, injecting at a third of the height of the cutaneous upper lip to enhance the site and correct some short perioral rhytides.

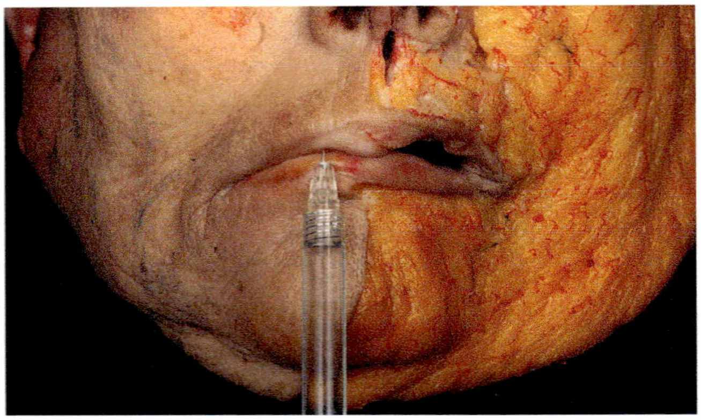

Figure 7.28 The perioral wrinkles: Retrograde threading with a 30G needle placed directly in the line. With this technique, it is possible to correct both static and dynamic lines.

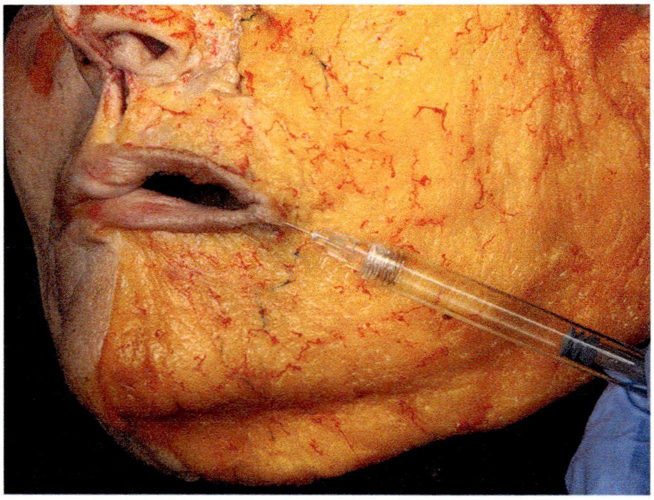

Figure 7.29 Filler injection into modiolus region for corner of the mouth elevation.

Treatment Choices

Today's facial surgeons have more options than ever to rejuvenate the perioral area and increase lip fullness; there are both non-surgical and surgical options for treating the lip region. Non-surgical treatment is ideal for patients seeking lip augmentation with minimal downtime and no surgically related risks. Accurate patient selection, history, and a detailed consultation—outlining the benefits, limitations, and adverse events of lip reshaping—is critical to obtaining good results. It is important to respect realistic and rational patient desires; unrealistic expectations should be discussed. Patients should also be informed that injecting fillers is a sculpting process and not a single treatment.

Patients requesting lip augmentation tend to fall into three groups:

- Patients with good lip shape who desire more fullness
- Patients wishing to enhance atrophic lips caused by aging or genetics
- Patients with poor definition of the vermilion border, often associated with advancing age or a history of cigarette smoking

The patient should be medically fit and well. If there is a history of herpes simplex, pretreatment antiviral medication should be prescribed, and treatment should not take place if herpes simplex lesions are visible. Awareness of medications that predispose to bruising is essential (pain relief medication, nonsteroidal anti-inflammatory drugs, anticoagulant medication, vitamin E, etc.).

Informed written consent must also be signed, dated, and initialed on every page.

Preoperative and postoperative photographs in frontal and lateral views are critical. These photographs will highlight any asymmetry, which must be relayed to the patient prior to commencement of treatment.

Pretreatment considerations

- Accurate and careful anatomical evaluation of the lips is mandatory.
- Correct choice of filler (type and quality) and optimal technique is vital.
- Before and after pictures are useful to illustrate average treatment outcomes.

Anesthesia

Various topical anesthetics are effective and include combinations of lidocaine, prilocaine, tetracaine, and phenylephrine. Topical anesthetic is applied approximately 30 minutes prior to treatment. Infraorbital and mental nerve blocks, either intraoral or transcutaneous, may also be utilized. It is critical not to distort the shape of the lips. Currently, it is easier to use a premixed HA with lidocaine as an add-on to reduce pain.

Several common injection techniques exist:

- **Linear threading technique:** (anterograde or retrograde): Full lengthwise insertion of the needle into the middle of a wrinkle, fold or lip with extrusion of filler along an imaginary seam.
- **Threading or fanning technique:** Injecting a continuous line of filler while keeping the syringe moving forward or backward.
- **Serial puncture technique:** Injecting separate beads or boluses of filler along the vermilion.

The desired instrument (cannula vs sharp needle) will depend on the preferred technique [5].

Cannulae have a hollow bore and rounded blunt end. The injection process may involve numbing the skin with ice, injecting a small amount of local anesthetic with a tiny needle and then puncturing the skin with a needle. The cannula is then threaded into the puncture site and advanced along the natural tissue planes, thus providing access to a large area for filler placement. Fanning technique with a cannula is useful as limited entry points are required.

The benefits of cannulae are:

- Less pain during the treatment
- Less risk of bleeding and bruising
- Safer option to avoid intravascular injections

Although cannulae offer many potential benefits, they may not be ideal for filling acne scars or injecting extremely fine superficial lines. When very small amounts are needed for touch-ups or injection of small areas such as the Cupid's bow of the upper lip, a needle remains the best option.

When multiple injection points are required, 27G or 30G needles are preferred. However, multiple injection sites increase the risk of vascular puncture, with the concomitantly increased risk of bruising. Sharp needles may also result in more tissue trauma and subsequent swelling, particularly in the lip area. Additional risks, although rare, include skin irregularities, infection at the injection site, and tissue necrosis, after inadvertent intravascular injection.

Where to Inject?

Since the lip does not have an organized epidermis-dermis complex, the injection is performed in the mid-dermis. When injecting in the correct mid-dermal plane, there is:

- No extreme skin blanching (indicating too superficial placement)
- No inability to see the filled area (indicating too deep placement)

If the goal is to increase the general lip volume, however, the needle is inserted deeper into the lip in approximately the outer one-third to one-half of the lip thickness.

What to Inject?

Ideal characteristics for lip fillers include

- Low to moderate G′ hyaluronic acid filler
- Gel particles with homogeneous diameter and shape [6]
- Low viscosity, low density

The correct rheological properties (elasticity, viscosity, hardness, and the ratio of viscosity to elasticity) facilitate ease of placement in the reticular dermis, thus helping to reduce the risk of bluish discoloration at the injection site (Tyndall effect). This allows the desired results with lower quantities of filler [7].

Product degradation usually occurs gradually over time as it is absorbed by surrounding tissue (isovolumetric degradation). During this process, each molecule continues to bind water, maintaining the final results over time. Complete degradation occurs at approximately 6–12 months, on average.

COMPLICATIONS

For general complications and the concept of "safety by depth," see Chapter G.

Seckel divided the face into seven functional danger zones [4]. The lips include danger zones 4 and 7: injury to danger zone 3 can lead to paralysis of the lower lip; 4 paralysis of the upper lip; 6 numbness of the upper lip, and 7 numbness of the lower lip.

SPECIFIC CONSIDERATIONS

Bruising and swelling are common side effects.

Other common complications include:

- Blanching/occlusion
- Infection
- Delayed nodules
- Palpable or visible material

It is important to remember that the labial artery mostly runs deep in the body of the lip. Thus, deep injections are more likely to cause bruising or intravascular placement.

Use the lowest possible needle gauge or blunt tipped cannula in danger areas to minimize bruising and swelling.

Using small aliquots of less than 0.1 or 1 mL in total during initial lip enhancement; re-treat at least two weeks later when deemed necessary [8].

The use of an ice pack after the procedure is optional and oral steroids may be useful for early swelling.

Bruising may be difficult to predict; when severe bruising does occur, resolution may be hastened by using a vascular laser.

Intravascular injection is an early, serious complication which may lead to tissue necrosis and potential scarring. To avoid this, it is helpful to

- Aspirate before injecting, ensuring the needle does not change position before injection.
- Inject very slowly.
- Use aliquots of under 0.1 mL of product per site.
- Actively check for signs of arterial compromise, especially in watershed areas such as the nasal tip and glabella, with the main signs being blanching, pallor, and pain.
- For intravascular injection, current best practice is the use of high-dose pulsed hyaluronidase (HDPH).

Other early complications include undertreatment, overtreatment, and asymmetry, which may cause varying degrees of patient dissatisfaction; dialogue with the patient is fundamental to finding an optimal solution.

- For overtreatment/cosmetically unacceptable filler: 10–15 U/0.1 mL HA used will usually suffice.

Causes of palpable product include

- Over-injection: Small, uninflamed palpable nodules may simply be massaged away.
- Infection should prompt early treatment with antibiotics.
- Hyaluronidase may be used to dissolve visible or cosmetically unacceptable HA filler.
- Uneven product placement: Injection into the body of the lip frequently causes unevenness, which may be technique related. It is presumed that muscular contraction of orbicularis oris may compound this problem by collecting the product into pockets.

References

1. Trevidic P. Ageing of the lips. In: Azib N & Charrier JB & Cornette de Saint-Cyr B et al., eds. *Anatomy and Lip Enhancement.* E2e Medical; 2013, p. 9.
2. Jacono AA. *Arch Facial Plast Surg.* 2008: 25–9.
3. Paes EC et al. *Aesthetic Surg J.* 2009;29(6): 467–72.
4. Seckel B. *Facial Danger Zones*, 2nd ed. Thieme; 2010.
5. Goldman MP. *Cosmet Dermatol.* 2007;20:14–26.
6. Glogau RG et al. *Dermatol Surg.* 2012;38(7 Pt 2): 1180–92.
7. Sundaram H. & Cassuto D. *Plast Reconstr Surg.* 2013;132(4 Suppl 2):5S–21S.
8. Kim JH et al. *J Korean Med Sci.* 2014;29(Suppl 3):S176–82.
9. Signorini M et al. *Plast Reconstr Surg.* 2016; 137(6):961–71.
10. Tansatit T et al. *Aesthetic Plast Surg.* 2014; 38(6):1083–9.
11. Von Arx T et al. *Swiss Dent J.* 2017;127(12): 1066–75.

Further Reading

Carruthers A et al. *Dermatol Surg.* 2008;34(Suppl 2): S161–6.

Park CG & Ha B. *Plast Reconstr Surg.* 1995;96:780–8.

8 PERIORAL REGION

Krishan Mohan Kapoor, Philippe Kestemont, Jay Galvez, André Braz, John J. Martin, and Dario Bertossi

INTRODUCTION

Our understanding of the processes integral to facial aging has extended beyond the loss of elasticity and sagging of facial skin; there is now far greater appreciation of the role of involutional changes in soft tissue volume, suspensory elements, and skeletal mass. The cosmetically sensitive perioral regions, including lips, jawline, chin, subnasale, and mandible, have previously been insufficiently analyzed regarding factors predisposing to perioral deflation and rhytides. The current, growing recognition of the need for volume, microaliquots of toxin, and effective methods for skin tightening is heralding a new rejuvenation chapter for the central lower face.

ANATOMY

The upper lip extends from the subnasale/subnasal point at the nasal base (cranially), to the nasolabial folds (bilaterally), to the lower edge of the vermilion border (caudally). The lower lip extends from its free vermilion edge (cranially), the oral commissures (laterally), and the labiomental crease (inferiorly). At the vermilion-cutaneous junction, a thin, pale line termed "white roll" highlights the color difference between the vermilion and the skin. In the upper central region, the white roll forms a V which, together with paramedian vermilion prominences, forms the Cupid's bow. Two vertical tissue columns (the philtral columns) form a midline depression (philtrum), which extends from lip border to the columella above (Figure 8.1). The labiomental crease passes horizontally in an inverted U shape across the lower lip, separating it from the chin.

AGING

The features of a youthful lip include upper lip eversion which results in 2–3 mm of upper tooth show. This reduces with age due to inversion secondary to loss of tissue volume and structural support. In youth the upper lip projects 1–2 mm ahead of the lower lip. With age, loss of structural volume leads to loss of upper lip projection with subsequent recession and flattening in the lateral view. The youthful, well-defined lip border/white roll loses definition with age.

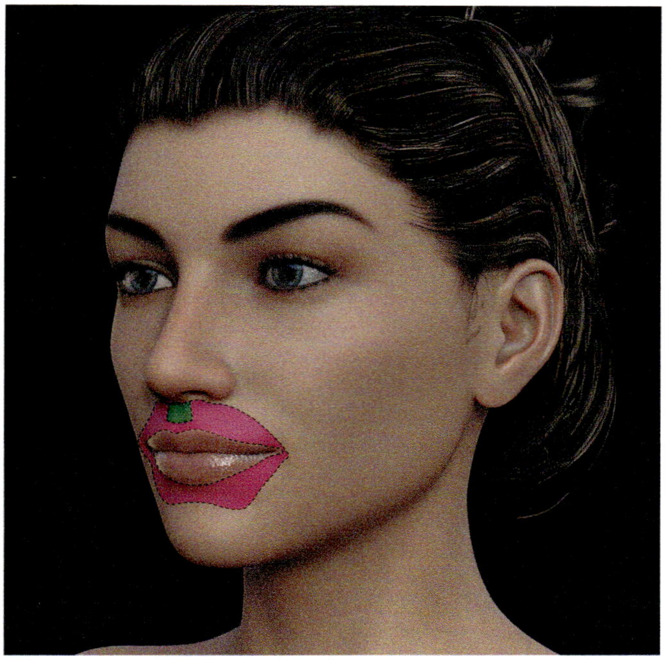

Figure 8.1 Boundaries of the perioral region. Green denotes the philtrum.

Youthful philtral columns are well defined, prominent, and cast a shadow zone in the philtrum.

In youth, lip eversion increases visibility of the wet–dry junction and in profile, the area from the nostril to the vermilion border forms a definitive concavity or ski slope. With loss of volume and structural support, this natural curve decreases (Figure 8.2).

SKIN

Traditional signs of aging rarely go unnoticed, and patients are frequently aware of subtle signs of perioral aging which may add years to estimated age and even impact resting facial expression. The perioral skin is thin in the females (Figure 8.3) and thicker in males, particularly in the chin area. The oral commissures and modiolus develop fullness and depressor anguli oris (DAO) action predominates. Down-turned oral commissures cause a serious and

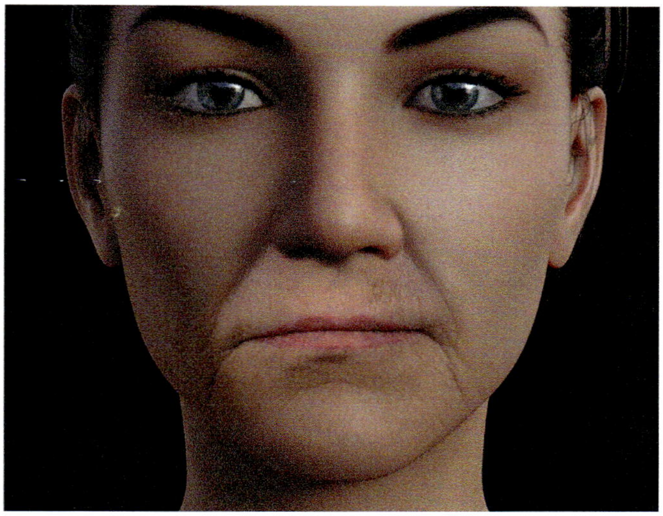

Figure 8.2 Loss of natural upper curve due to decreased tissue volume and structural support. Note skin changes, down-turned oral commissures and associated marionette lines.

sad appearance. The resulting downward forces create melomental rhytides or "marionette lines," vertical lines running from the corner of the mouth to the chin, thereby creating the unpleasant mouth frown. Flattening of the Cupid's bow and loss of definition of

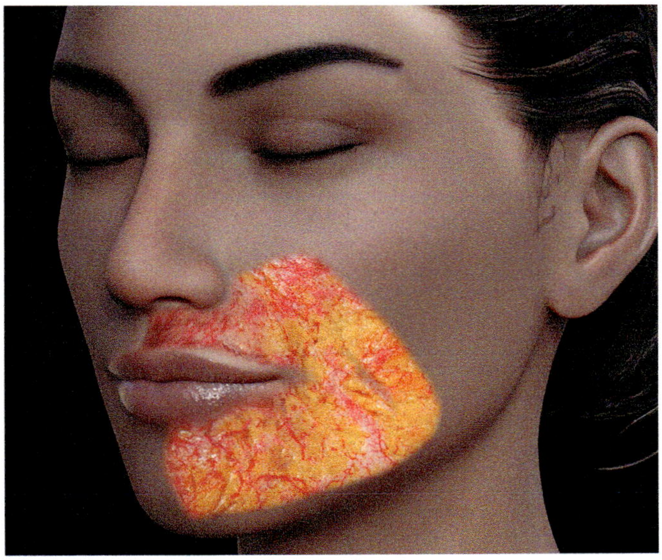

Figure 8.3 Superficial fat pads of the perioral region and jowl. Note the course of the superficial labial artery along the upper vermilion border with vertical branches.

the philtral columns contribute to the appearance of a thin and elongated upper lip. The skin around the vermilion border is particularly adherent to the underlying muscle, thus repetitive muscle contractions induce creating wrinkles or folds over time. Softening the perioral lines and shallow contours may restore a youthful fullness to the lower face.

FAT

The delineation of lower facial fat compartments is a relatively recent concept and includes identification of the superior and inferior mandibular fat compartments that extend over the inferior mandibular border. Soft tissue changes in this region accompany the slow resorption of bone. The lower face fat compartments exist in a superficial and deep layer. Superficial fat (Figure 8.4) overlies the orbicularis oris muscle, whilst the deep fat (Figure 8.5) lies deep to the orbicularis oris and mentalis muscles. The age-related deflation of the perioral fat compartments and fat malposition cause distortion of soft tissue and the mandibular border. Perioral fat atrophy leads to progressive deterioration of skin contour, while overt dimpling and shadowing is described as a peau d'orange. Jowling, marionette lines, and deepening prejowl sulci are common stigmata of aging. A "witch's chin" may result due to severe loss of volume and support.

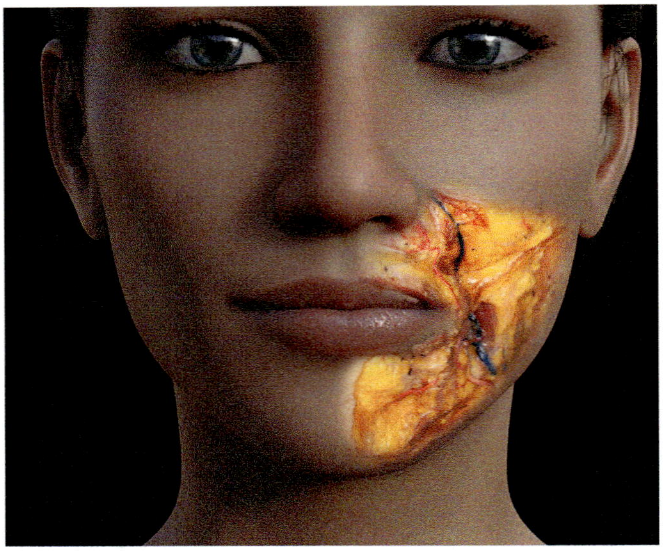

Figure 8.5 Deep perioral fat compartments lie beneath the orbicularis oris and mentalis muscles.

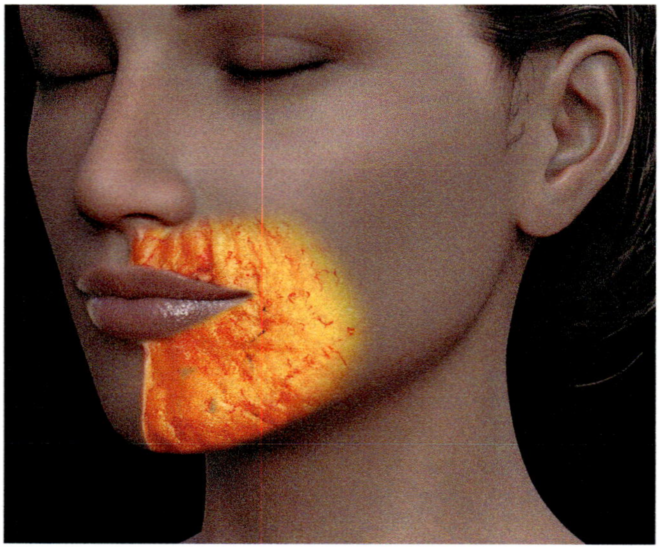

Figure 8.4 Superficial lip fat lies above the orbicularis oris muscle.

MUSCLES

Muscles Inserting in Modiolus

The modiolus lies lateral and slightly superior or inferior to the oral commissure. It forms a bilateral junction point for seven facial muscles of the mid and lower face which is held together by fibrous tissue. The facial muscles converge, interlace and appear like the spokes of a wheel around the modiolus (Figures 8.6 and 8.7). Its structure is critical to oral movement, facial expressivity and stability of the lower dentition. The modiolus receives its blood supply from branches of the facial and labial arteries and its motor nerve supply from the facial nerve.

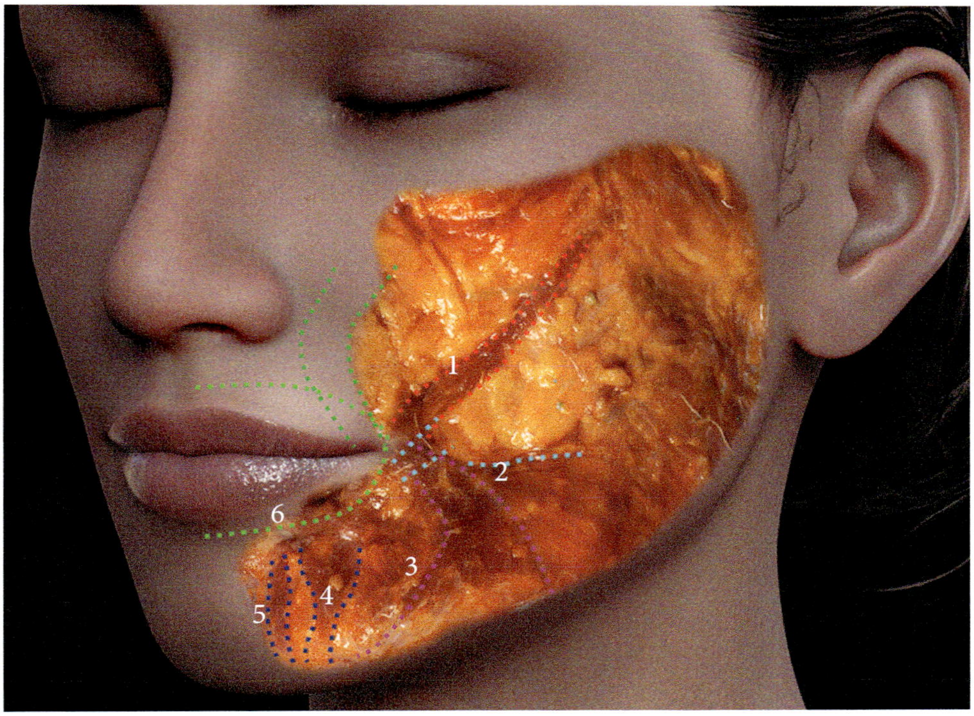

Figure 8.6 Important muscles of the perioral region: (1) Zygomaticus major; (2) risorius; (3) depressor anguli oris (DAO); (4) depressor labii inferioris (DLI); (5) mentalis; (6) orbicularis oris.

Orbicularis Oris

The orbicularis oris muscle (OOM) is a broad, ellipse-shaped muscle present around the mouth. The mouth seal remains intact due to tonic orbicularis sphincter contraction. Active or phasic contraction of the OOM is required to narrow the mouth during whistling or kissing. The lateral fibers insert on the modiolus on either side of the oral commissure. The OOM has two parts:

- **Pars marginalis:** Fibers in the vermilion region of lip
- **Pars peripheralis:** Fibers in the peripheral cutaneous part of the lip

Anatomically, pars peripheralis fibers have been found to decussate at midline level, inserting into the contralateral philtral ridge. Pars marginalis fibers, on the other hand, form a continuous band from one modiolus to the other.

Orbicularis oris blood supply is mainly from the superior and inferior labial arteries, which are branches of the facial artery. Additional blood supply is derived from the mental and infraorbital arteries, branches of the maxillary and transverse facial arteries and a

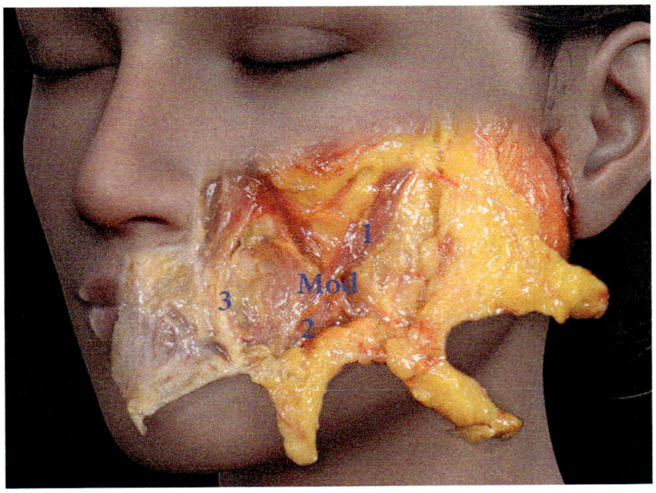

Figure 8.7 Muscles inserting into the modiolus (Mod): (1) Zygomaticus major; (2) DAO; (3) orbicularis oris.

branch of the superficial temporal artery. The motor innervation is via the buccal and marginal mandibular branches of the facial nerve.

Zygomaticus Major

The zygomaticus major originates from the zygomatic bone just in front of the zygomaticotemporal suture. It passes to the angle of the mouth, blending with the fibers of the orbicularis oris and the levator anguli oris, and merges with the modiolus. The zygomaticus major pulls the angle of the mouth upward and laterally, as seen during laughing. Its vascular supply is mainly via the superior labial artery, a branch of the facial artery. Muscle innervation is via the zygomatic and buccal branches of the facial nerve.

Levator Anguli Oris

The origin of levator anguli oris (LAO) is from the maxillary canine fossa, just caudal to the infraorbital oramen. Its fibers pass downward and laterally to insert into the modiolus. The infraorbital nerve and artery emerge from the infraorbital foramen between the origins of the LAO inferiorly and the levator labii superioris superiorly. The LAO elevates the angle of the mouth during smiling. Vascular supply is via the superior labial artery, a branch of the facial artery, and the infraorbital artery, a branch of the maxillary artery. Muscle innervation is by the zygomatic and buccal branches of the facial nerve.

Risorius

Morphologically the risorius ranges from being a slender collection of muscle fibers to a wide, thin, fan pattern. Its fibers may start from a wide area including the zygomatic arch, parotid fascia, masseteric fascia, and fascia over the mastoid process. These fibers converge at the modiolus. The risorius provides lateral pull to the angle of the mouth on contraction during various facial expressions including grinning and laughing. The risorius muscle is supplied mainly by the superior labial artery, a branch of the facial artery. Muscle innervation is via buccal branches of the facial nerve.

Buccinator

The buccinator originates from the outer surfaces of the alveolar processes of the maxilla and mandible, respectively, opposite the molar teeth. Its fibers converge toward the modiolus. The buccinator presses the cheek against the teeth and gums during mastication and expels the distended cheek air between the lips (an activity important when playing wind instruments). The buccinator is supplied by branches of the facial and buccal arteries. The latter is a branch of the maxillary artery. Muscle innervation is via the buccal branch of the facial nerve.

Depressor Anguli Oris

The depressor anguli oris (DAO) originates from the mental tubercle and oblique line of the mandible, inferior and lateral to the depressor labii inferioris (DLI). The muscle fibers converge into a narrow bundle that travels toward the angle of the mouth to insert into the modiolus, blending with fibers of the OOM and the risorius. The DAO is supplied by the inferior labial branch of the facial artery and the mental branch of the maxillary artery. Muscle innervation is via the buccal and mandibular branches of the facial nerve.

Platysma

The platysma, although considered a muscle of the neck, contributes to the perioral muscle complex. It has three parts: mandibular, labial, and modiolar. The pars mandibularis attaches to the lower border of the mandible body. The pars labialis lies between, and in the same plane, as the DAO and the DLI. The adjoining margins of all three muscles blend to form similar labial attachments. The fibers of the platysma pars modiolaris lie posterolateral to the DAO and travel deep to the risorius superomedially for modiolar attachment.

Muscles Inserting in Upper Lip

Zygomaticus Minor

The zygomaticus minor originates from the area of the zygomatic bone immediately lateral to the zygomaticomaxillary suture and passes downward medially to insert in the muscular substance of the upper lip. The zygomaticus minor is an elevator of the upper lip and reveals the maxillary teeth on contraction, with deepening of the nasolabial crease. The zygomaticus minor is supplied mainly by the superior labial artery, a branch of the facial artery. Muscle innervation is via the zygomatic and buccal branches of the facial nerve.

Levator Labii Superioris

The levator labii superioris (LLS) originates from the maxilla and zygomatic bone superior to the infraorbital foramen. Its fibers descend into the upper lip muscle tissue, between the zygomaticus minor and the lateral slip of the LLSAN. The LLS raises and everts the upper lip. It is supplied by branches of the facial artery and the infraorbital artery which is a branch of the maxillary artery. Muscle innervation is via the zygomatic and buccal branches of the facial nerve.

Levator Labii Superioris Alaeque Nasi

The levator labii superioris alaeque nasi (LLSAN) originates from the upper part of the frontal process of the maxilla, and its muscle fibers pass downward and laterally, dividing into medial and lateral slips. The medial slip merges with the perichondrium of the lateral crus of the alar cartilage of the nose. The lateral slip extends to the lateral part of the upper lip, where it blends with the LLS and the orbicularis oris. The lateral slip elevates and everts the upper lip and increases the curvature of the upper part of the nasolabial fold. The LLSAN is supplied by the branches of the facial artery and the infraorbital artery, a branch of the maxillary artery. Muscle innervation is via the zygomatic and superior buccal branches of the facial nerve.

Muscles Inserting in Lower Lip

Depressor Labii Inferioris

The depressor labii inferioris (DLI) originates from the oblique line of the mandible between the symphysis menti and the mental foramen. The muscle fibers pass upward and medially to insert into the skin and mucosa of the lower lip. The fibers also blend with its contralateral fellow and with fibers of the orbicularis oris, and it is continuous with the platysma inferolaterally. The DLI pulls the lower lip downward and laterally and helps in lower-lip eversion. The DLI is supplied by the inferior labial artery, a branch of the facial artery and the mental artery, a branch of the maxillary artery. Muscle innervation is via the marginal mandibular branch of the facial nerve.

Mentalis

The mentalis originates from the incisive fossa of the mandible, and its fibers descend downward to attach to the skin of the chin. The contraction of muscle fibers pull the chin skin up and deepen the labiomental crease. The mentalis raises the lower lip and causes wrinkling of the skin of the chin. The mentalis is supplied by the inferior labial artery, a branch of the facial artery, and the mental artery, a branch of the millary artery. Muscle innervation is via the marginal mandibular branch of the facial nerve.

VASCULARIZATION

Intravascular injection in an artery can pose serious complications after dermal filler injections (Figures 8.8–8.11), thus knowing the vascular anatomy of the facial areas to be injected can significantly reduce the risk of serious complications. The ability to visualize the path of the facial artery and its branches helps an injector to determine the correct placement and depth of injection.

Facial Artery and its Branches

The facial artery takes its origin from the external carotid artery in the neck. It initially runs under the platysma before passing to the face at the anterior border of masseter where its pulsation may be palpated as it runs around the mandible border. The artery initially travels deep to the skin and subcutaneous fat; during its upward course, it passes deeper to the zygomaticus major and risorius muscles and superficial to the buccinator and the LAO. It becomes superficial during its course along the nasolabial fold. It passes over or through the LLS and takes a tortuous course from the lateral side of the nose to the medial canthus. Near its termination, it may be embedded in fibers of the LLSAN.

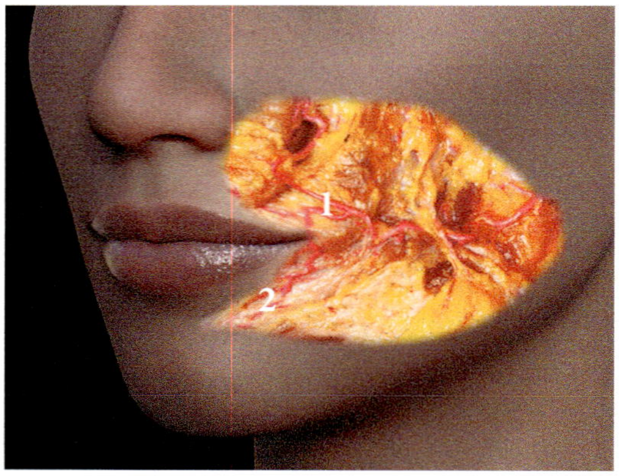

Figure 8.8 The superior labial artery (1) is larger in caliber and takes a more tortuous course than the inferior labial artery (2).

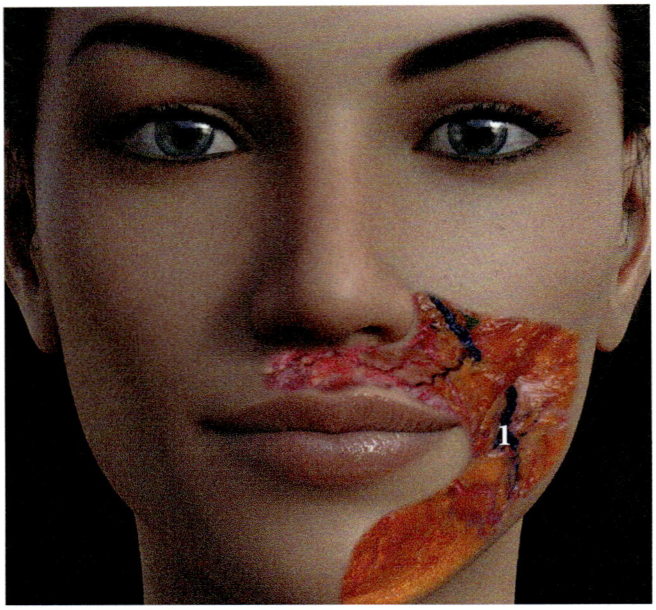

Figure 8.9 The facial vein (1) lies lateral to the facial artery and runs a more direct course than the tortuous facial artery.

The facial vein lies lateral to the artery and runs a more direct course on the face. At the level of the anterior border of the masseter, the two vessels are very close to each other, with the facial vein more

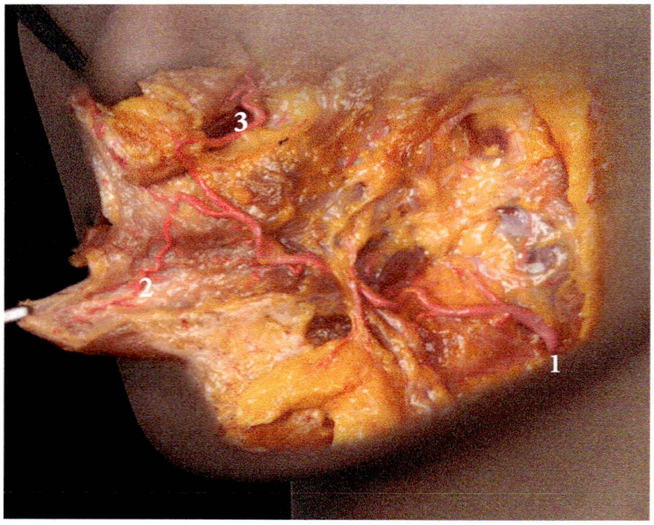

Figure 8.10 The facial artery and its branches in the perioral area: (1) Entering the face at the mandibular border 1 cm anterior to the anterior border of the masseter; (2) inferior labial artery; (3) superior labial artery.

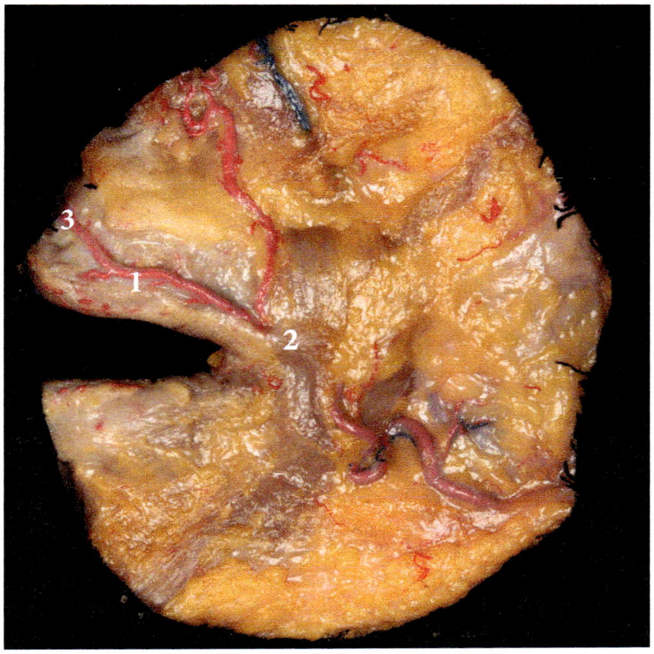

Figure 8.11 The SLA (1) runs deep to the zygomaticus major (2) and becomes more superficial as it becomes the ascending philtral artery (3) adjacent to the philtral column.

lateral, whilst in the neck the vein lies more superficial to the artery. During its course the facial artery supplies multiple branches to the facial muscles and skin. The perioral branches are the superior and inferior labial arteries and lateral nasal artery. The facial artery distal to the lateral nasal artery is called the angular artery.

Inferior Labial Artery

The inferior labial artery (ILA) arises from the facial artery before or near the angle of the mouth, passing superomedially beneath the DAO, and may run in the mental crease. The ILA or its branch may penetrate the orbicularis oris to run between the muscle layer and the mucosa. It supplies the inferior labial glands, mucosa, muscle layer, and skin in this area. It anastomoses with its contralateral artery and with the mental artery, a branch of the inferior alveolar artery, emerging from the mental foramen.

Superior Labial Artery

The superior labial artery (SLA) is larger in caliber and takes a more tortuous course in comparison to the inferior labial artery. It arises from the facial artery near the angle of the mouth and passes deeper to the zygomaticus major or the LAO. It penetrates the orbicularis oris to run between muscle and mucosa, anastomoses with its contralateral artery and supplies the mucosa, muscle layer, and cutaneous part of the upper lip. It gives off an alar branch and a columellar branch, which ramifies in the lower part of the nasal septum.

Submental Artery

The submental artery is the largest cervical branch given off by the facial artery before it enters the face. It originates from the facial artery as it curves around the submandibular gland and runs forward on the mylohyoid muscle below the mandible. It supplies branches to the overlying skin and muscles and anastomoses with the sublingual branch of the lingual artery and mylohyoid branch of the inferior alveolar artery. As it reaches the chin, it ascends over the mandible, dividing into superficial and deep branches. These branches anastomose with the inferior labial artery and ipsilateral mental artery. Together, these branches supply the chin and lower lip region.

Branches of the Internal Maxillary Artery in the Perioral Area

Mental Artery

The mental artery takes its origin from the first part of the maxillary artery as it emerges out of the mental foramen as the terminal branch of the inferior alveolar artery. After emerging on the face at the mental foramen, after traversing the mandibular canal, it supplies the muscles and skin in the chin area. It anastomoses with the inferior labial and submental arteries to form a network in the lower-lip and chin areas.

Infraorbital Artery

The infraorbital artery takes its origin from the third part of the maxillary artery. It emerges through the infraorbital foramen to supply the lower eyelid, cheek, lateral nose and ipsilateral upper lip. The infraorbital artery has extensive communications with the transverse facial artery and branches of the facial artery and the ophthalmic artery.

Perioral Venous Drainage

The facial vein supplies the main venous drainage of the face. It receives the supratrochlear and supraorbital veins and travels obliquely caudally along the lateral border of the nose, passing under the zygomaticus major, risorius, and platysma muscles. It descends to the anterior border of the mandible and runs downward in the neck, draining into the internal jugular vein. Its uppermost segment, the angular vein, joins the superior labial vein from upper lip tissue to form the facial vein. This provides communication between perioral venous drainage with the cavernous sinus through the angular vein. The facial vein receives venous drainage from superior and inferior labial veins, buccinator, parotid, and masseteric veins, in the perioral region.

INNERVATION

Sensory Innervation

Trigeminal Nerve

Three significant facial areas may be mapped to demonstrate the sensory nerve fields associated with the three branches of the trigeminal nerve. Embryologically, each branch of the trigeminal nerve belongs to a developing facial process which gives rise to a definitive area of the adult face: the ophthalmic nerve supplies the structures developing from the frontonasal process, the maxillary nerve supplies those from the maxillary process and the mandibular nerve supplies structures from the mandibular process. Hence, the sensory nerve supply in the perioral region comes from the infraorbital branch of the maxillary nerve and the mental branch of the mandibular nerve.

Infraorbital Nerve

The infraorbital nerve, the terminal branch of the maxillary nerve, enters the face through the infraorbital foramen where it lies between the LLS and the LAO muscles. It gives palpebral, nasal, and superior labial branches. The nasal branches supply sensation to the nose, ala, and columella. In the perioral area, it gives multiple, large-sized superior labial branches, which descend behind the levator labii superioris muscle to supply the skin of the anterior cheek and the upper lip.

Mental Nerve

The mental nerve, the terminal branch of the inferior alveolar nerve, enters the face through the mental foramen. It supplies the skin of the lower lip and the labial gingiva (Figure 8.12).

Motor Innervation

Facial Nerve and its Branches

The facial nerve emerges from the base of the skull at the stylomastoid foramen, then enters the parotid gland, to branch into superior (temporofacial) and inferior (cervicofacial) trunks (Figure 8.13). These

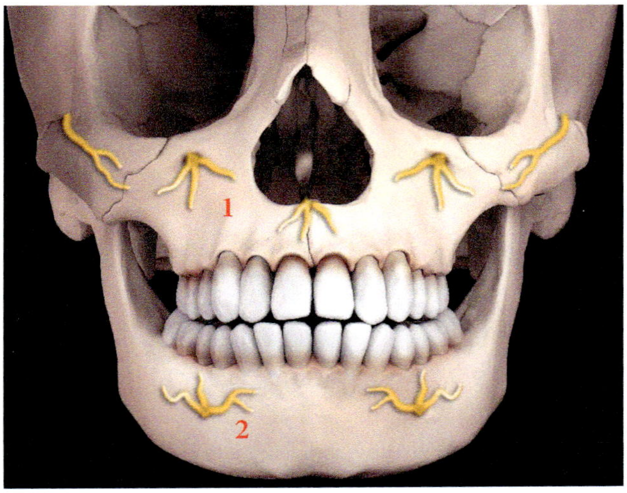

Figure 8.12 Sensory nerve supply in the perioral region comes from the infraorbital branch of the maxillary nerve (1) and the mental branch of the mandibular nerve (2).

trunks branch to form a parotid plexus, which gives rise to five main terminal branches, which exit the parotid at its anteromedial surface to supply the muscles of facial expression.

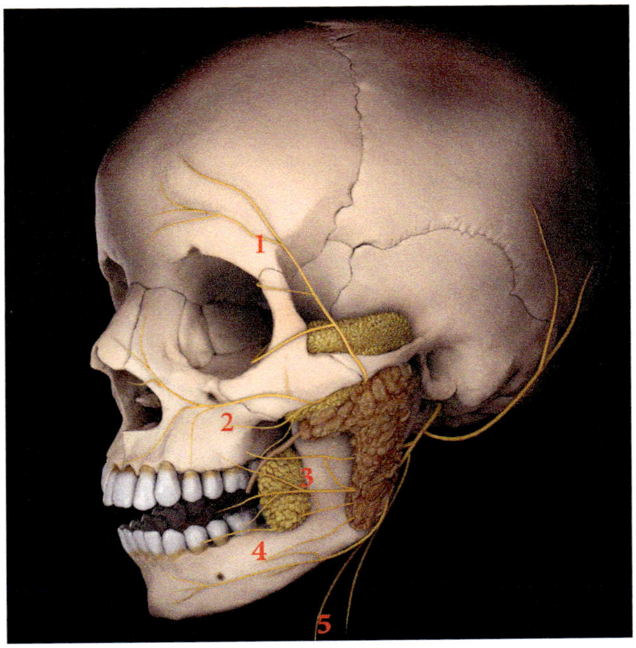

Figure 8.13 Facial nerve CN VII branches after exiting the parotid gland: (1) Frontal; (2) zygomatic; (3) buccal; (4) marginal mandibular; (5) cervical.

Upper and Lower Buccal Nerves

The buccal branch of the facial nerve runs in close relation to the parotid duct for about 2.5 cm after coming out from the parotid gland. Upper deep buccal branches supply the zygomaticus major and levator labii superioris muscles. These branches also provide motor nerve supply to the zygomaticus minor, LAO, LLSAN, and the small nasal muscles. Lower deep branches supply the orbicularis oris and the buccinator.

Marginal Mandibular Nerve

There usually are two marginal mandibular branches supplying muscles in the lower face. They run downward and forward toward the angle of the mandible in a plane deeper to platysma. These branches then run upward across the mandible to pass under the DAO. These branches supply the risorius and the muscles of the lower lip and chin.

Cervical Branch

The cervical branch exits the lower part of the parotid gland and runs in an anteroinferior direction under platysma to the anterior part of the neck. It supplies the platysma in this area.

BONE

Aging of the craniofacial skeleton is the cumulative effect of bone atrophy, bone expansion, and bone loss. Loss of teeth causes resorption of the mandibular alveolar ridge whilst maxillary resorption causes lack of support in the upper lip, thus contributing to perioral wrinkling (Figure 8.14).

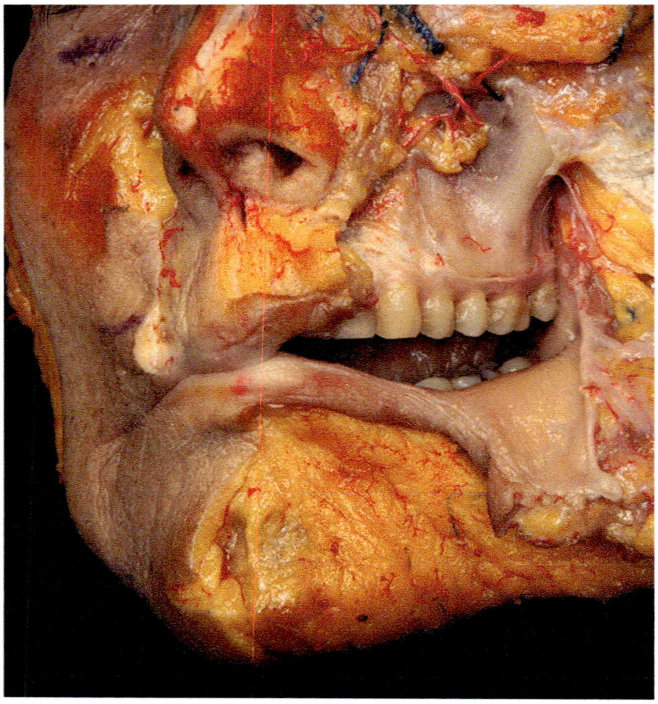

Figure 8.14 Loss of maxillary bone contributes to aging of soft tissues.

HOW I DO IT: BOTULINUM TOXIN

The perioral cosmetic unit extends superiorly from the base of the nose and extends laterally to the nasolabial folds, with the inferior border being formed by the labiomental sulcus. The upper lip comprises the upper cutaneous lip, the vermilion, and the philtrum, while the lower lip is subdivided into the cutaneous lower lip and the vermilion.

The important muscles for toxin treatment in this area are the orbicularis oris (OOM), DAO and LLSAN (discussed in Chapter 7).

OOM: May be treated by 2 superficial injections per quadrant of 1 unit of onabotulinum toxin each. Be careful not to overtreat or impede phonation or mouth closure.

DAO: May be treated with 2–4 units of onabotulinum toxin per side. Injections are performed adjacent a line drawn from the nasolabial fold to the jawline, placed 1 cm cephalad to the jaw, slightly posterior to the line.

LLSAN: May be treated in patients with a gummy smile by injecting 2 units of onabotulinum toxin per side at the lateral nose, into the bulk of the LLSAN. Be careful not to unduly lengthen the upper lip.

Pretreating the skin quality with energy-based devices (e.g., non-ablative fractional laser) may add great value to natural perioral filler treatments.

Practical Points

- Pretreat patients with a history of herpes simplex (HSV) with prophylactic oral antivirals (e.g., valaciclovir) from the preceding day, completing the full 5-day course, to prevent reactivation of HSV or subsequent eczema herpeticum.
- Carefully assess the area for underlying skin conditions requiring pretreatment such as acne, melasma, perioral dermatitis, angular cheilitis, and herpes simplex.
- Cleanse the skin meticulously, suggest pretreatment oral rinsing with chlorhexidine mouthwash and warn against habits such as lip licking and fiddling, which would compound infective risk.
- Be cautious when treating patients with a long upper lip or insufficient dental support.
- The perioral is an aesthetically important area which also provides vital lip support. This mobile area is extremely unforgiving and mandates great care in product choice, volume, and placement. Reversible HA derivates with optimal visco-elastic properties are most suitable for this delicate area, and product should be insightfully selected according to placement, aesthetic requirements, and individual expertise.

HOW I DO IT: FILLERS

- Individual rhytides may be treated with HA derivates injected as tiny intradermal or directly subdermal aliquots, with the needle held at 10° to the skin to ensure extremely superficial placement. Due to initial, slight blanching, this is sometimes termed the superficial blanching technique.
- An alternative method would be to inject a very low HA product symmetrically into the upper lip quadrants using a 25G/27G cannula and subdermal fanning technique.
- The layering of filler either over or under the perioral mimetic muscles may induce a myomodulatory effect (Figures 8.15 and 8.16). Care should thus be exercised in selecting the correct level of placement as this may temporarily alter phonation, as may large volumes in the perioral area or the chin.
- Layering product over the DAO or the orbicularis oris with a cannula will reduce muscle action by increasing tissue resistance. This effect may be consciously utilized when treating patients with facial palsy (see Myomodulation, Chapter D).

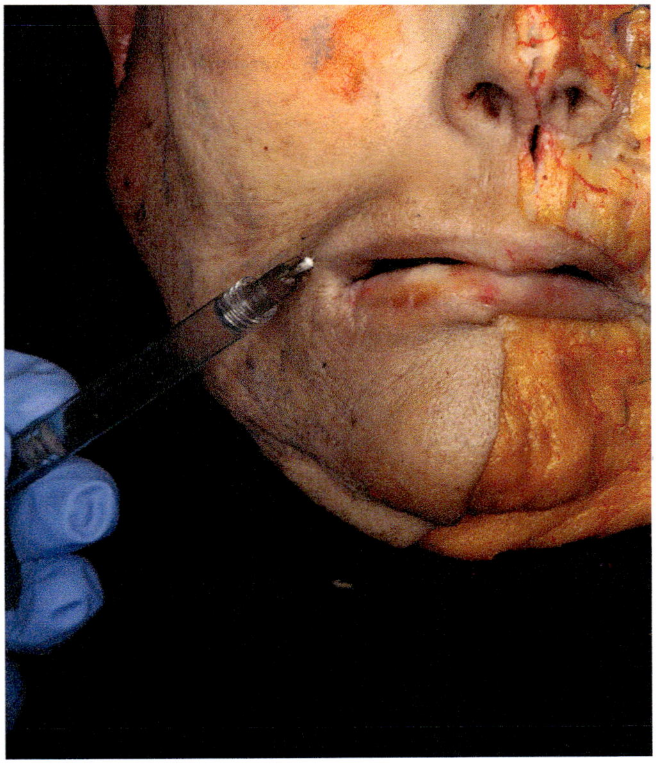

Figure 8.15 Low G′ fillers may soften perioral rhytides injected as tiny subdermal aliquots. The so called "blanching technique" may be used.

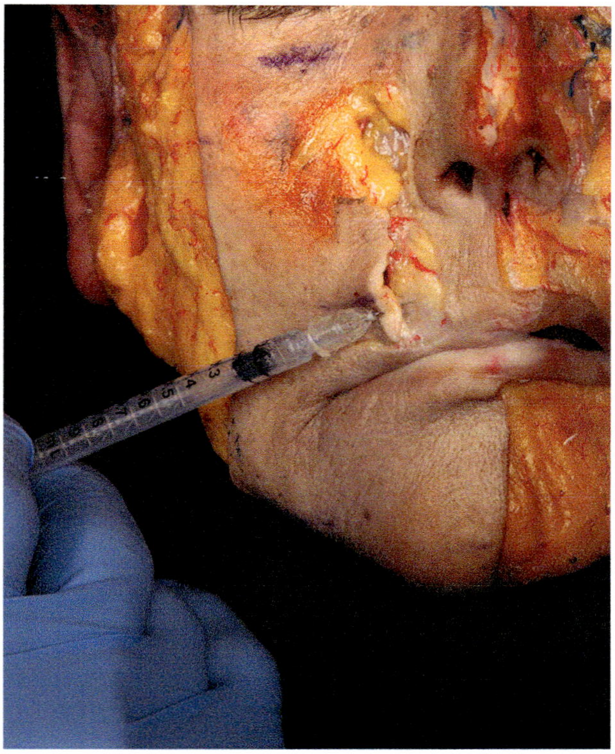

Figure 8.16 Toxin injection for softening perioral rhytides in mature perioral region and for sensual upward curl of vermilion and prevention of "smokers" lines in younger lips.

COMPLICATIONS

For general complications and the concept of "safety by depth," see Chapter G.

Seckel divided the face into seven functional danger zones [1]; the lips and perioral region include danger zones 4 and 7.

Pitfalls to Avoid with Fillers

- Intravascular injection of mental artery
- Bruising due to high density of veins in the area around the modiolus
- Palpable and visible nodularity due to product dislocation secondary to perioral muscular activity or too superficial mucosal injection

Reference

1. Seckel B. *Facial Danger Zones*, 2nd ed. Thieme; 2010.

Further Reading

Ehsani AH et al. *J Cosmet Dermatol.* 2019;18(6): 1632–4.
Ho TT et al. *Aesthet Surg J.* 2019, sjz108 Mar 15.
Lee KL et al. *Clin Anat.* 2019. Mar 25.
Linkov G et al. *Arch Plast Surg.* 2019;46(3):248–54.
Palomar-Gallego MA et al. *Dermatology.* 2019; 235(2):156–63.
Rauso R et al. *Aesthet Surg J.* 2019;39(5):565–71.
Samizadeh S et al. *Aesthet Surg J.* 2019;39(11): 1225–35.
Stojanovič L & Majdič N. *J Cosmet Dermatol.* 2019; 18(2):436–43.
Taylor SC et al. *Dermatol Surg.* 2019;45(7):959–67.
Vidič M & Bartenjev I. *Acta Dermatovenerol Alp Pannonica Adriat.* 2018;27(3):165–7.

9 CHIN AND JAWLINE

Ash Mosahebi, Anna Marie C Olsen, Mohammad Ali Jawad, Tatjana Pavicic, Tim Papadopoulos, and Izolda Heydenrych

INTRODUCTION

The chin and jawline are anatomically distinct regions which should be considered as independent but closely associated aesthetic units; they age simultaneously and treating one affects the appearance of the others. One should be mindful of this when considering injectable procedures in this region.

BOUNDARIES

Anatomically, the mandible comprises a "body," an "angle," and a "ramus." The two bodies from each side of the face fuse in the sagittal midline to form the mentonian symphysis.

The "mandibular line" is the term given to the area between the mentum (most protruding part of the chin) and the angle of the mandible (gonial angle). Melomental folds are also known as marionette lines and are the creases formed between the angle of the mouth and the area adjacent to the chin (Figure 9.1).

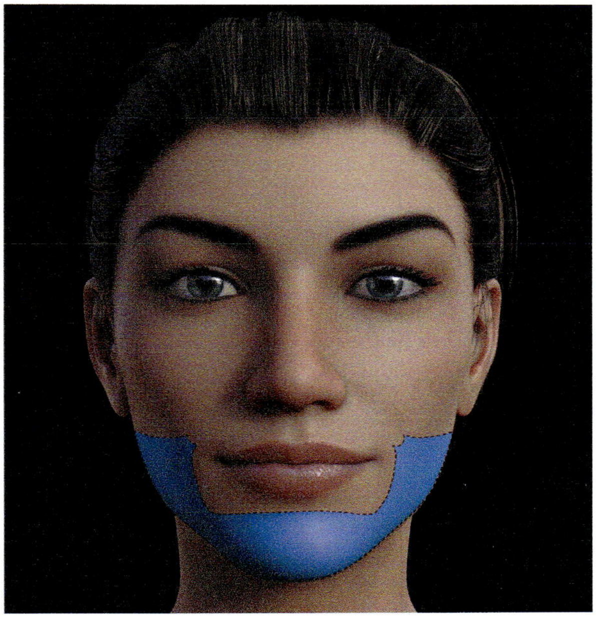

Figure 9.1 Boundaries of the chin and jawline indicated in blue.

CHIN

The chin is the region produced by the mentonian symphysis and overlying structures. The anatomical layers here are the skin, superficial fat compartment, mentalis muscle, deep fat compartment, and bone.

Chin topography can be further subdivided into six superficial anatomical subunits (Figure 9.2):

1. Mental crease (labiomental sulcus)
2. Apex
3. Anterior chin–soft tissue pogonion
4. Submental–soft tissue menton
5. Lateral lower chin
6. Pre-jowl sulcus [1]

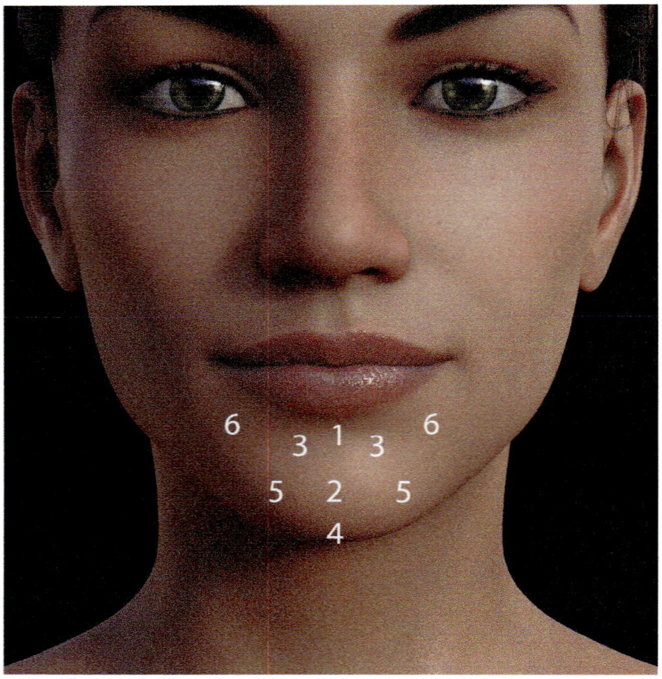

Figure 9.2 The six anatomical subunits of the chin indicated numerically as 1–6.

AGING

Progressive and unequal loss of skin elasticity, bone resorption, atrophy of fat compartments, and dehiscence of the mandibular septum cause caudal descent of the superior and inferior jowl compartments.

The melomental folds, also known as marionette lines, are creases formed between the angle of the mouth and the area adjacent to the chin. The creases traverse all the layers of the underlying facial architecture, namely skin, superficial fat compartment, DAO muscle, and bone [2]. Quantifying the severity of marionette lines has been undertaken by Carruthers et al. with the creation of a validated five-point photonumeric rating scale (Figure 9.3), which can determine the extent of injection volumization [3].

Aging of this area is related to gender, hormonal changes, alveolar bone, and teeth support.

Knowledge of anatomical layers is crucial in understanding injection safety and effective volumization. The pre-jowl sulcus is the area between the chin and the jowl (Figures 9.3 and 9.4). The jowl begins after the platysma mandibular ligament (PML) and mandibular osseocutaneous ligament (MOCL), and the anatomical layers are the skin, superficial fat compartment, platysma and fused DAO muscle, deep fat compartment, and bone. The mandibular line layers are skin, superficial fat compartment, platysma, deep fat compartment, and bone [2].

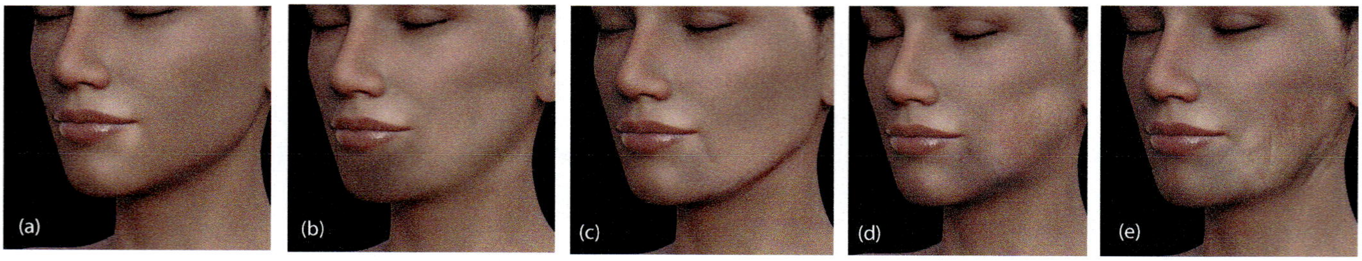

Figure 9.3 (a) Marionette lines grading scale: 0, No visible folds; continuous skin line. (b) 1, Shallow but visible folds with slight indentation. (c) 2, Moderately deep folds. (d) 3, Very long and deep folds. (e) 4, Extremely long and deep folds.

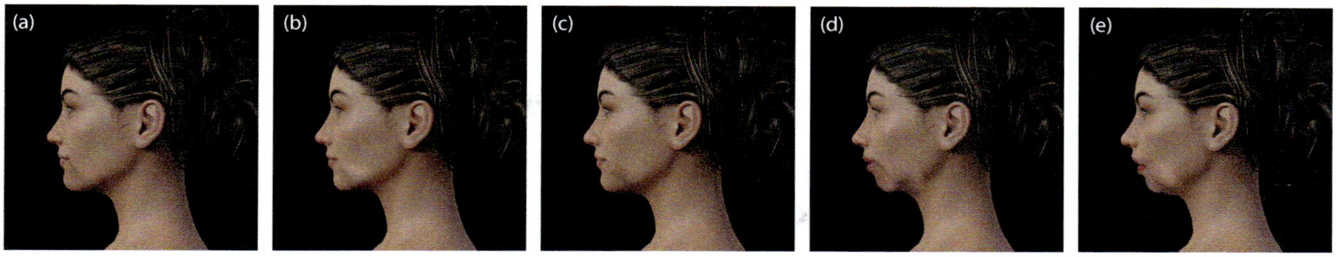

Figure 9.4 Progressive aging of the chin and jawline skin. (a) No visible folds; continuous skin line. (b) Shallow but visible folds with slight indentation. (c) Moderately deep folds. (d) Very long and deep folds. (e) Extremely long and deep folds.

SKIN

The chin is an area rich in sebaceous glands and prone to conditions such as acne, perioral dermatitis, and herpes simplex. Preexisting conditions should be pre-treated, with adequate time allowed for clearance and repair of barrier function (Figure 9.5).

FAT

Distinct chin and submental compartments are identifiable (Figures 9.6 through 9.8). While the chin compartment is well demarcated from adjacent compartments, the limits of the submental compartment vary [4].

- The labiomental crease forms the boundary between the lips and chin and is indicative of an underlying vascular arcade.
- There are discrete fat compartments extending from the vermilion to the lip-chin crease.
- The chin compartment is demarcated by the mentolabial groove superiorly, the submental ligaments inferiorly, and the labiomandibular grooves laterally.
- The submuscular fat of the chin is distinct from suborbicularis oris fat.

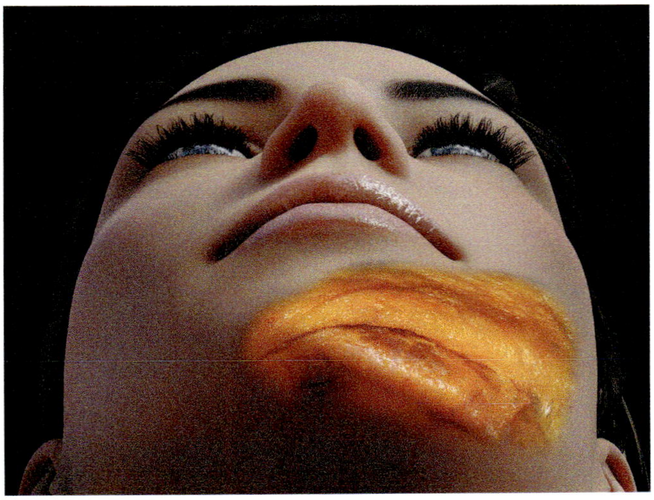

Figure 9.5 Superficial fat layer of the chin.

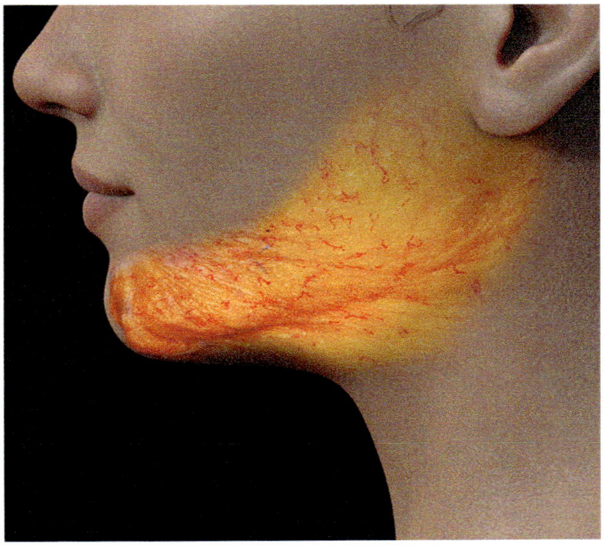

Figure 9.6 Superficial jowl and submandibular fat compartments.

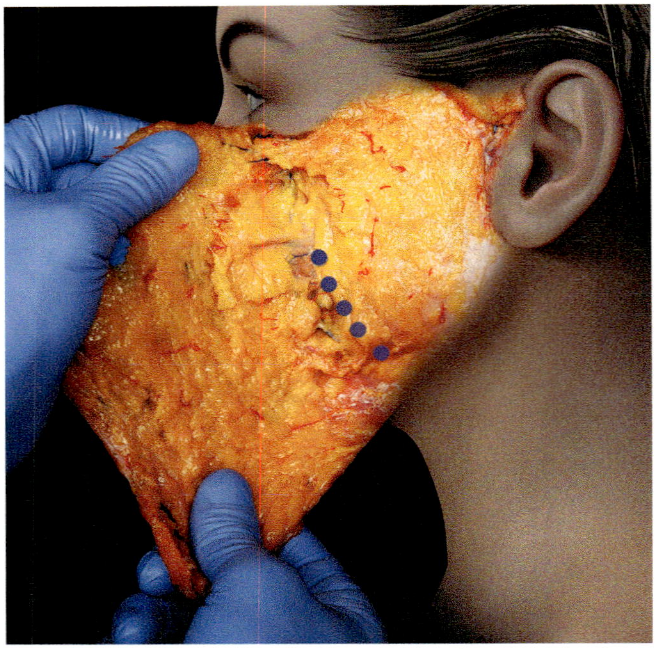

Figure 9.7 Dissection of facial fat compartments stretched out to show jowl fat (blue dots).

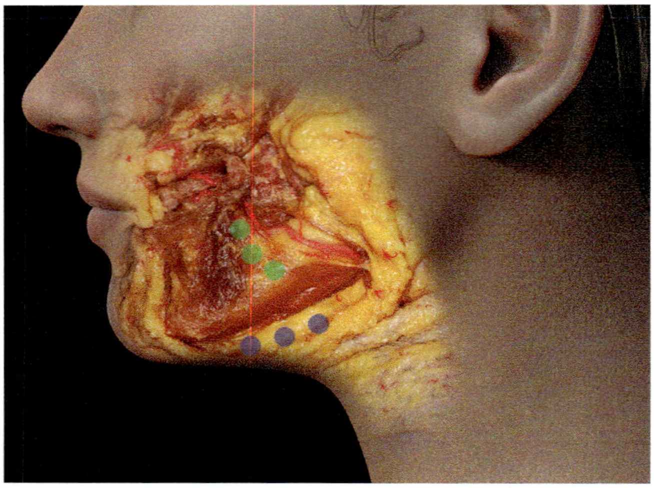

Figure 9.8 Deep jowl fat (green dots) and submandibular compartments (blue dots).

- Submentalis fat is found immediately deep to the mentalis muscle on either side of the midline and is not in continuity across the midline of the chin. The submental compartment is demarcated from the chin by the submental ligaments, laterally by the paramedian platysma-retaining ligaments, and inferiorly by the hyoid ligament.

LIGAMENTS

There are two key retaining ligaments in the chin and jaw (jowl). The superior and inferior superficial jowl compartments are separated from the more caudally located submandibular fat compartment by the PML. This osseomuscular septum is located approximately 5 cm from the angle of the mandible, just above the mandibular border. The PML is believed to retain the structure of the jowl and is also a nidus of muscular stability for platysma as it traverses the mandible. Over time, a reduction in the structural integrity of the PML leads to the descent of the jowl [5] (Figure 9.9). The MOCL is located more cranial to the PML, approximately 5.5 cm distal to the angle of the mandible and 1 cm above the mandibular border. The MOCL is approximately 3.5 mm wide with its distal fibers interdigitating with the depressor anguli oris (DAO) muscle, forming the inferior aspect of the marionette line [5]. Clinically, the MOCL can be palpated as the tethering point between the anterior jowl and marionette line. The importance of the MOCL in adhering the skin to the mandible can be seen during rhytidectomy after release of the MOCL

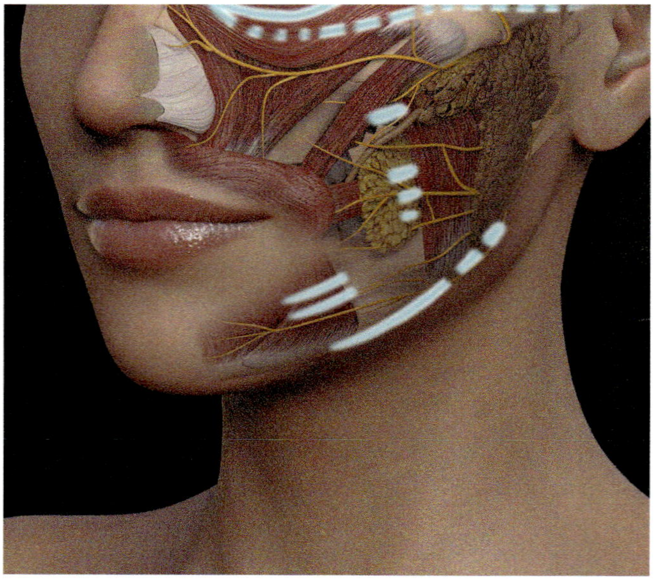

Figure 9.9 Ligaments of the chin and jawline.

to allow adequate mobilization of the skin and SMAS (superficial muscolar aponeurotic system).

The PML and MOCL are osseocutaneous ligaments. Non-osseous ligaments, called masseteric cutaneous ligaments, attach muscle to the overlying skin and are also important in maintaining integrity of the facial architecture.

MUSCLES

A significant understanding of muscular anatomy arises from generations of careful anatomical dissection and observation. More recently, Olszewski et al. have carried out an in vivo three-dimensional magnetic resonance imaging (MRI) isotope study to illustrate the uniqueness of muscular anatomy in this region [6].

The jowl and chin region contain three key muscles: the depressor labii inferioris (DLI), the DAO, and the mentalis. These three muscles interdigitate caudally with the platysma and are closely related to the orbicularis oris muscle.

Orbicularis Oris

This complex muscle comprises muscle fibers constituting the lips proper in addition to fibers from other facial muscles, which insert into the lips in different layers. The deep layer of orbicularis oris consists of fibers from the buccinator, with medial fibers decussating at the angle of the mouth. Buccinator fibers arising from the maxilla insert into the lower lip while fibers arising from the mandible insert into the upper lip. In contrast to these middle fibers, the most superior and inferior buccinator fibers traverse the lips from side to side without decussation.

Superficial to this is another layer of orbicularis oris formed by interdigitation with fibers from the

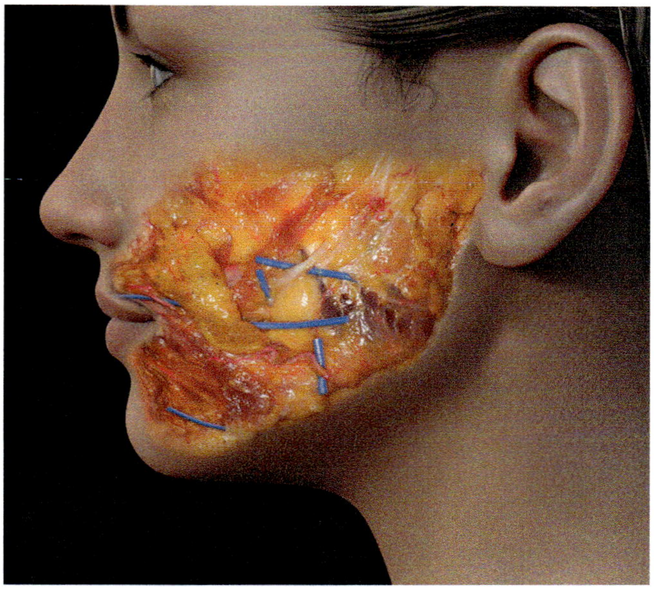

Figure 9.10 Dissection showing lateral view of chin and jawline muscles.

lip elevators and depressors. The levator anguli oris (LAO) and DAO cross each other at the angle of the mouth, with the LAO fibers passing to the lower lip and DAO fibers passing into the upper lip before inserting into the skin at the midline. Further contributing to this layer are muscle fibers from levator labii superioris (LLS) which lies adjacent to LAO, DLI, and zygomaticus major which is adjacent to the lateral edge of the vertical component of orbicularis oris. The fibers of these muscles travel predominantly in an oblique direction (Figure 9.10).

These interdigitations contribute to the muscle fibers of the lip and provide lip thickness from skin to mucous membrane. There is also a lamina propria within the lip sphincter which is located between the orbicularis oris muscle and the mucosa, thus adding additional structural integrity.

Orbicularis oris is innervated by the buccal branches of the facial nerve and functions as a sphincter of the mouth and as a projector of the lips. Over time, it contributes to perioral rhytides.

Depressor Labii Inferioris (DLI)

The DLI originates from the line of the mandible between the mentonian symphysis and the mental foramen and inserts on the orbicularis and the skin of the lower lip. It is innervated by the mandibular branch of the facial nerve and depresses the lower lip.

Depressor Anguli Oris (DAO)

The DAO originates from the oblique line of the mandible and mandibular tubercle where it is fused with platysma. It inserts into the modiolus angle of the mouth where it is fused with the orbicularis oris and the risorius. It is innervated by the mandibular branch of the facial nerve and depresses the corners of the mouth. For detailed discussion of the modiolus, see Chapter 15.

Mentalis

The mentalis originates from the upper mentonian symphysis and mental fat compartments. The muscular fibers spread cranially, fan outward, and insert into the orbicularis oris muscle and skin of the lower lip. It is innervated by the mandibular branch of the facial nerve and elevates and projects the lower lip outward.

It also causes wrinkles in the skin of the chin, and overuse, or hypertrophy, of the mentalis can result in the formation of a permanent fold and a "witch's chin" appearance [7].

The "v" shape of mentalis combined with the DLI on either side produces the "M" shape of lower lip and chin. Mentalis strain occurs where there has been atrophy of the mental fat pad as with aging or in individuals with Angle's class II jaw malocclusion [8].

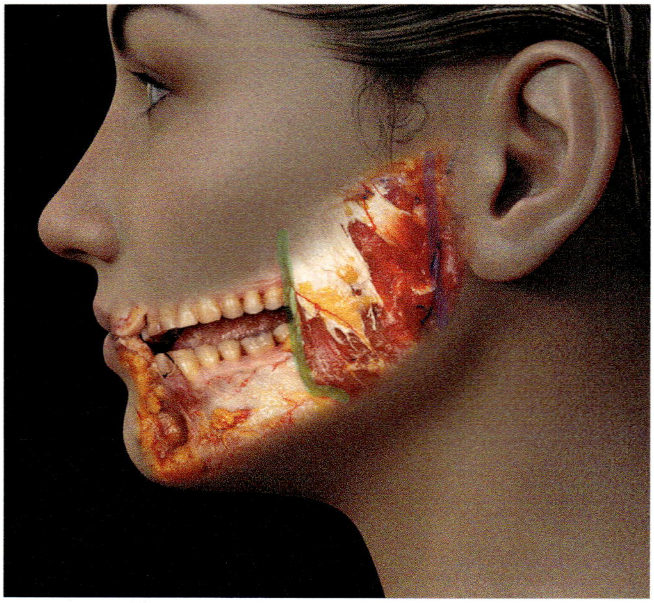

Figure 9.11 Lateral view of chin and jawline showing superficial part of masseter between blue and green lines.

Masseter

The masseter muscle is composed of superficial and deep parts: the superficial part originates from the zygomatic process and anterior two-thirds of the zygomatic arch and inserts into the angle and inferior ramus of the mandible; the deep part originates from the posterior one-third of the zygomatic arch and inserts in the superior part of the ramus of the mandible.

Anteriorly, the masseter projects over the buccinator muscle and posteriorly is covered by the parotid gland. From the parotid gland, Stensen's duct crosses over the masseter as it travels anteriorly and penetrates the buccinator to enter the oral cavity opposite the second upper molar tooth (Figure 9.11).

VASCULARIZATION

Understanding the vasculature in this region is of paramount importance in avoiding complications such

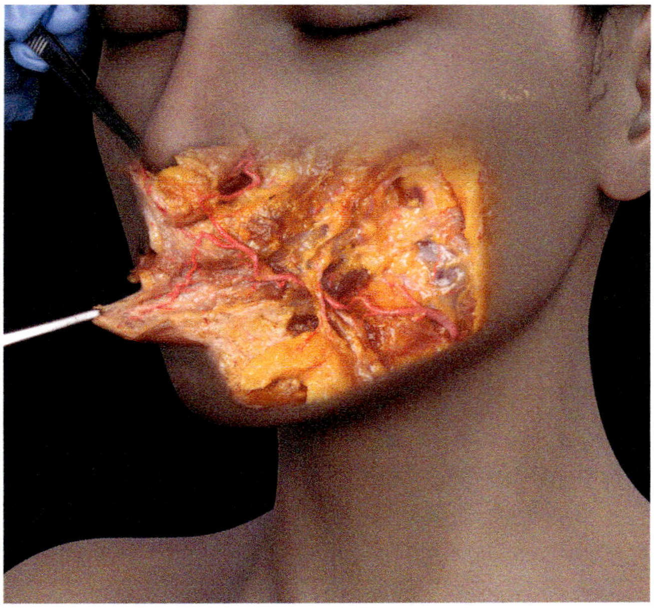

Figure 9.12 The facial artery ascends above the mandible, deep to the platysma muscle, approximately 3 cm distal to the angle of the mandible and is also identified in front of the anterior border of the masseter (0.3 mm–1 cm).

as inadvertent intravascular cannulation and occlusion. The facial artery (Figure 9.12) ascends above the mandible, deep to the platysma muscle, approximately 3 cm distal to the angle of the mandible and is also identified in front of the anterior border of the masseter (0.3 mm–1 cm) and can be identified by palpating its pulsation.

Anatomical variations in facial artery distribution are common and can complicate injections. Computer tomography angiography and cadaveric studies have illustrated how the facial artery originates in the neck from the external carotid artery, giving off the **submental artery** close to this origin. The dominance of the facial artery at this point is associated with respective presence or absence of an angular system on the ipsilateral side. Clinically, however, this is of little value in determining which patients would be suitable for deep injection.

Nevertheless, at the level of this vascular network, the **facial artery** has an average diameter of 2.3 mm and **is situated deep to the DAO and zygomaticus major muscles**. This allows safe superficial injections from the oral commissure to the nasolabial crease.

The facial artery branches into an inferior labial artery (ILA) and a superior labial artery (SLA) and continues past the angle of the mouth toward the nose as the angular artery. Studies have found that the ILA is more likely to be present or dominant on the right side than the left. The ILA passes deep to the platysma and often unites with the labiomental artery to form a common trunk. **The ILA originates approximately 2.5 cm from the labial commissure** and 2.5 cm superior to the inferior border of the mandible. The ILA has an average diameter of 1.3 mm [5]. The **ILA** continues in the **submucosal plane** on the anterior wall of the oral cavity just above the alveolar ridge. The inferior border of the buccinator can be used to estimate the level at which the ILA courses toward the midline. In most cases, the ILA runs as low as the labiomental crease and can run either within the orbicularis muscle itself or between its different layers formed by interdigitations with surrounding muscles (Figures 9.13 and 9.14).

The ILA gives off a branch that travels with the mental nerve and sends perpendicular perforators to the lower lip. In 11% of cases, the ILA and SLA will share a common trunk before bifurcating, and in these cases, the ILA will then run along the vermillion–cutaneous junction of the lower lip [5]. This produces an uncertain danger zone for injection along the vermillion–cutaneous junction and when placing boluses in the oral commissure. There is no definitive consensus on the depth of the ILA, but studies to date suggest that on average, the vessel is 4.7 mm deep at its origin and will transcend to 2.3 mm in depth upon reaching the midline [5].

Lying **deep** and **more lateral** to the facial artery is **the facial vein**.

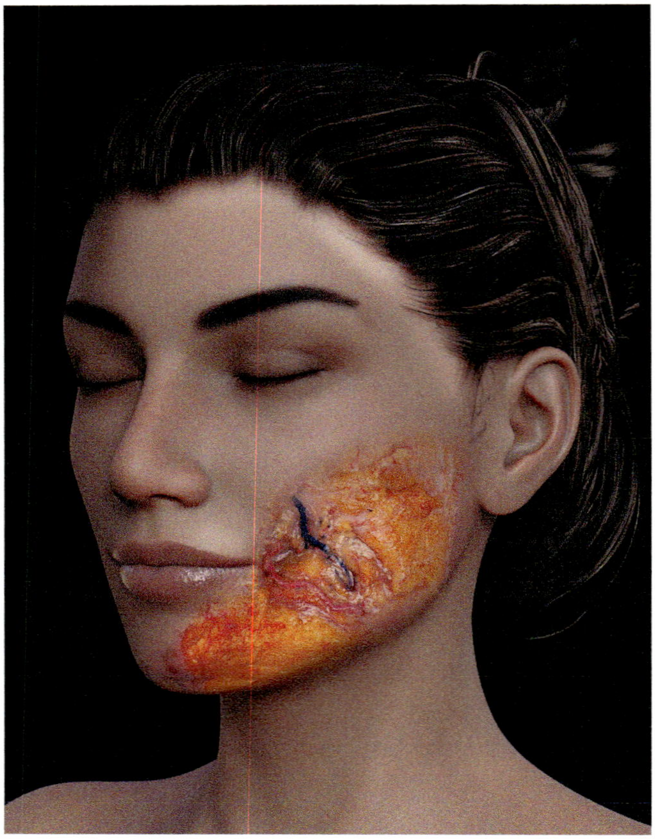

Figure 9.13 The ILA originates approximately 2.5 cm from the labial commissure and 2.5 cm superior to the inferior border of the mandible.

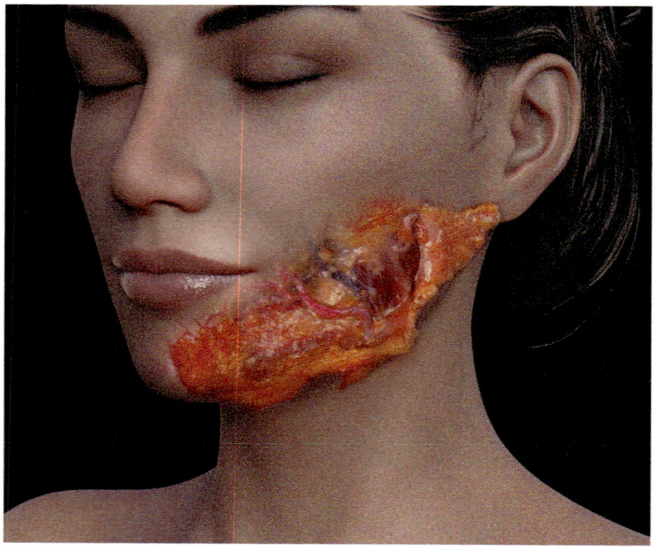

Figure 9.14 Lying **deep** and **more lateral** to the facial artery is **the facial vein**.

INNERVATION

The mental foramen allows passage of the mental neurovascular bundle into the face. It is situated on the bone, between the first and the second pre-molar teeth, halfway between the upper and lower borders of the mandible. The mental nerve provides sensory innervation to the lower lip, jowl, and chin regions (Figure 9.15).

Motor innervation of the face is predominantly from branches of the facial nerve, and in this region, the buccal and marginal mandibular branches are of paramount importance. The facial nerve divides into its five main branches in the parotid gland:

- Temporal
- Zygomatic
- Buccal
- Marginal mandibular
- Cervical

As the marginal mandibular branch exits the parotid-masseteric fascia, it travels under the SMAS and crosses approximately 3 mm superficial to the facial artery and vein [5]. The pulsations of the facial artery can, therefore, be used as a landmark to identify the marginal mandibular nerve at this point. It continues in this plane until the DAO, after which it transitions

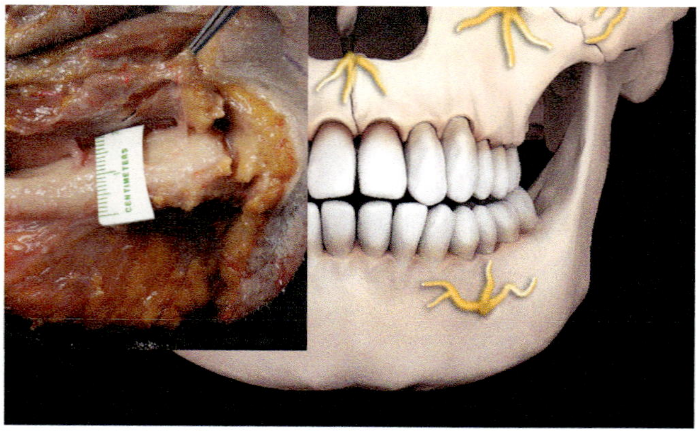

Figure 9.15 Sensory innervation of the chin and jawline: mental nerve.

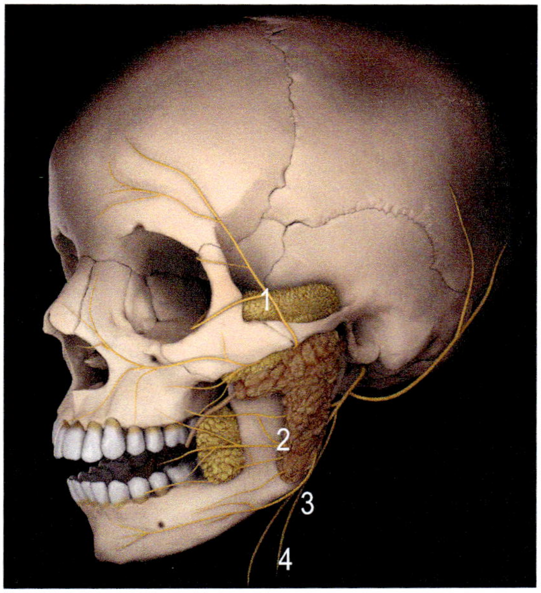

Figure 9.16 Motor innervation of the chin and jawline. Facial nerve: (1) temporal branch; (2) buccal branches; (3) marginal branch; (4) cervical branches.

superficially to terminate as two branches, with the dominant branch ending 1 cm superior to the MOCL (Figure 9.16).

The marginal mandibular nerve innervates the DLI, the DAO, and the mentalis. In 81% of cases, this nerve travels cranial to the mandibular border. Injections caudal to the labiomental crease and subperiosteal injections on the mandibular border, when carried out from a medial approach, are thus considered safe in avoiding nerve damage [5].

BONE

With age, both the projection and shape of the chin changes as a result of changes in the maxilla and the mandible and a slight increase in facial width and depth. In the mandible, loss of teeth leads to marked resorption of the alveolar ridge. Ptosis of the chin pad occurs secondary to resorption of the bony mandible. There is a general coarsening of mandibular bony protuberances at the points of insertion of

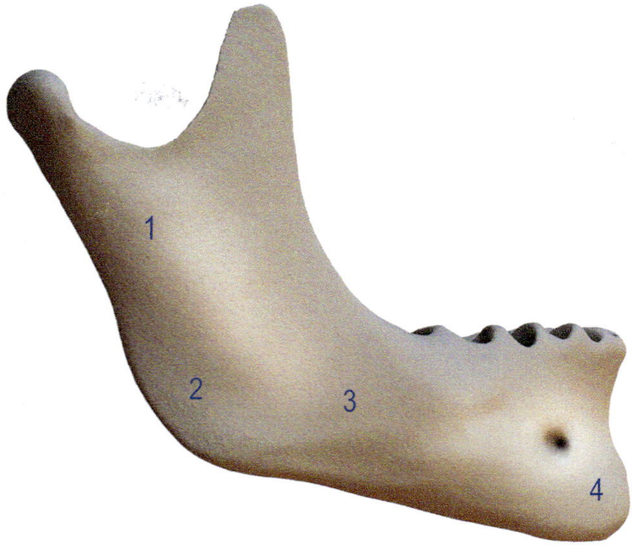

Figure 9.17 The mandible or jawbone: (1) ramus; (2) angle; (3) body; (4) chin.

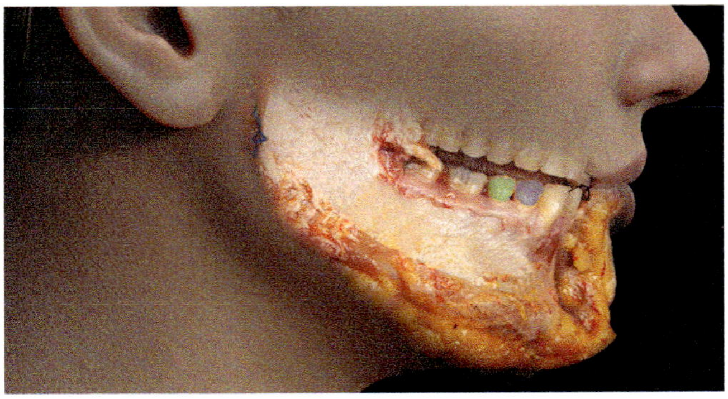

Figure 9.18 Lateral view of mandible and teeth. Blue dot is first pre-molar, green dot is second pre-molar.

masticatory muscles (e.g., the gonial angle and inferior edge of the zygomatic eminence) (Figures 9.17 and 9.18) [9].

HOW I DO IT: BOTULINUM TOXIN

DAO

There are various described methods for toxin treatment of the DAO. When using lower-face toxins, the

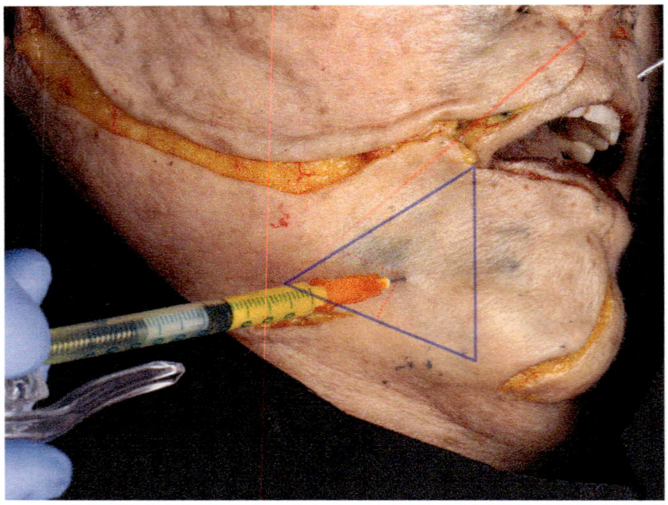

Figure 9.19 Toxin treatment of DAO showing injection technique: DAO blue triangle, inject 1 cm anterior to the red line or posterior margin of DAO and 1 cm above the mandibular margin.

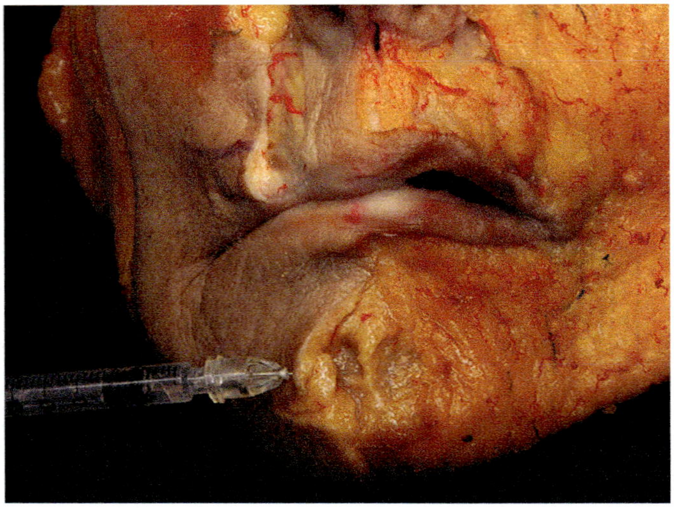

Figure 9.20 Toxin treatment of mentalis showing perpendicular injection technique.

effects are subtle, but side effects may be unforgiving. The safest method entails the following:

- Extend an oblique line from the nasolabial fold to the mandible.
- Inject 2–4 U of onabotulinum toxin at the jawline, 1 cm anterior to this line and 1 cm superior to the jawline (mandibular bony margin) with the 32G 4 mm needle perpendicular to skin and 4 mm deep (Figure 9.19).
- Additional treatment of the platysma and the mentalis facilitates synergistic effects.
- Be careful not to allow medial migration of product into the DLI and request that the patient not manipulate the area directly after treatment.

Mentalis

- Place one central or two adjacent areas at the mentum in the inferior mentalis.
- Inject perpendicular to the skin and deep into the bulk of the muscle (Figure 9.20).
- The average dose is 4 U units per side of onabotulinum toxin.

Masseter

- Trace a line from the tragus to the oral commissure and mark the anterior margin of the masseter.
- Inject perpendicular to the skin and deep (13 mm needle) into the bulk of the muscle (Figure 9.21).
- The average dose is 20–30 U of onabotulinum toxin per side in 3, 4, or 5 points.

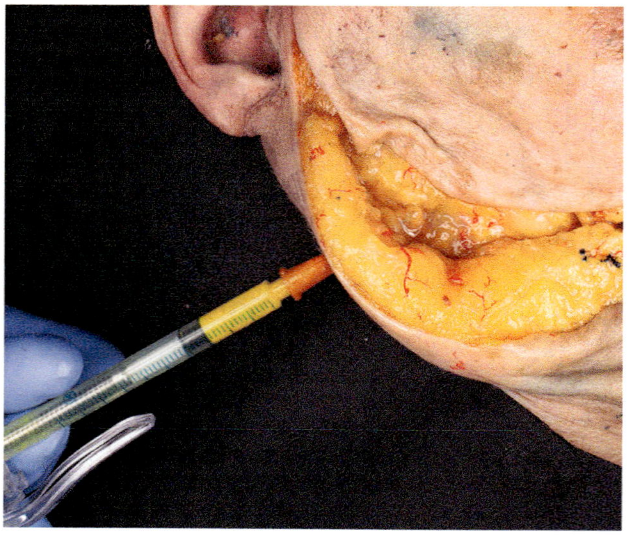

Figure 9.21 Toxin treatment of masseter showing perpendicular injection technique.

HOW I DO IT: FILLERS

- Each patient is thoroughly assessed and worked up in preassessment clinics.
- The patient's goals are carefully considered and balanced with realistic clinical outcomes.
- An aseptic field and the correct equipment are prepared.
- The injection sites are marked, and topical local anesthetic applied.
- Gentle massage is performed to enhance even distribution of filler.
- The results are evaluated at rest and in full animation per the patient's goals.
- "Less is more."
- Post-treatment, regular make-up is avoided for at least 24 hours, and a follow-up of the result for the patient is scheduled.
- Good quality pre- and post-photography is advised.

Melomental Folds/Marionette Lines

- Optimal treatment of the melomental folds requires thorough individual assessment and knowledge of regional anatomy, combined with insightful knowledge of the physical and cosmetic properties of both fillers and botulinum toxins. We prefer using a high-G′, high-viscosity HA filler, which provides the structural integrity to correct volume loss and further support the oral commissure.
- To volumize the pre-jowl sulcus, a sub-periosteal injection of dermal filler can be made perpendicular to the skin. The melomental fold and oral commissure can be volumized using a dermal filler in the deep dermal and submucosal planes. Following injection, gentle massage of the area aids even distribution and a smooth contour (Figure 9.22).

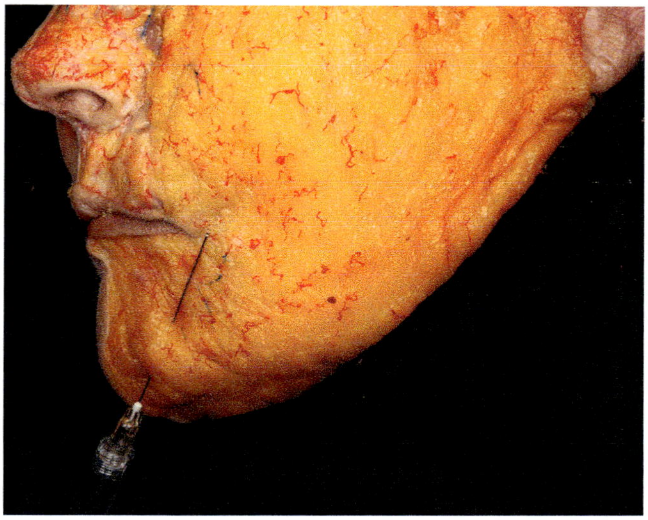

Figure 9.22 Subperiosteal perpen-dicular injection technique for filler volumization of the pre-jowl sulcus.

Jawline

- The jawline and pre-jowl sulcus are important aesthetic regions of the face. A high-G′, high-viscosity HA can be used for sub-cutaneous (sometimes sub-periosteal) injections along the border of the mandible (Figures 9.23 and 9.24). Female jawlines

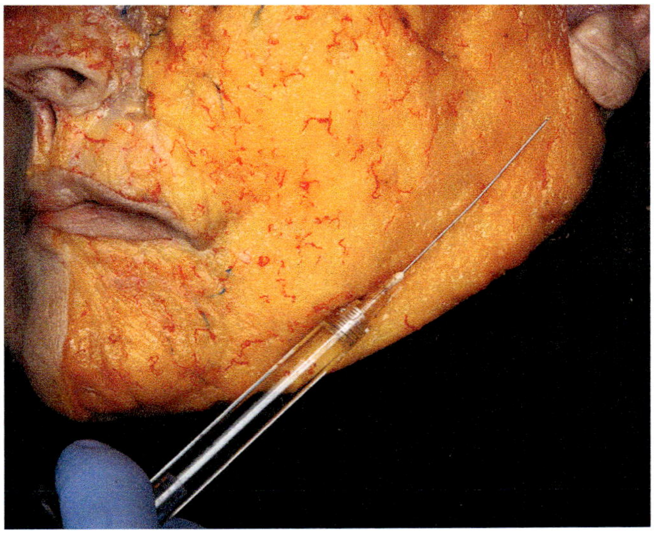

Figure 9.23 Injection technique for jawline superficial injection of high G′ filler.

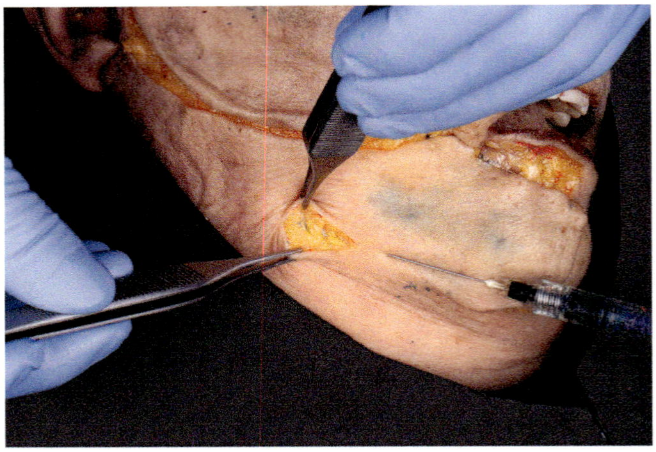

Figure 9.24 Parallel injection technique showing subcutaneous injection.

tend to be a smooth, continuous line ending at the ear, whereas male jawlines tend to be more angulated. Injecting a female jawline may therefore be done using a single entry point trough a retrograde injection, whereas a male jawline will often require two points, one for retrograde linear injection and one needed for eventual perpendicular injections.

- Injection of the pre-jowl sulcus can be made as a cutaneous injection with 25G 38 mm cannula parallel to the skin. The aesthetic aim is to smooth out and define the mandibular border, reduce the concavity of the pre- and post-jowl sulci and lift he jowl. You may also use a needle perpendicular to the bony margin.
- The decision to use needle or cannula is personal preference. Needles in this region of the face can offer improved tactile feedback and speed and are easier to glide through fibrous tissue, which can arise from previous injections or surgical procedures.

Chin

- The chin is an often a neglected area in aesthetic practice and should be viewed as the area between the mandibular ligament depressions and the oral commissure. Volumizing one area alone often leads to inadequate aesthetic results. (Figure 9.25)
- High-G′, high-viscosity HA or calcium hydroxyapatite are recommended for chin volumization.
- A 13 mm 27G needle can be used for deep subperiosteal injections, and we advise using blunt cannulas where the skin is directly adherent to the underlying bone. Special care must be taken in the vicinity of the mental foramen. A bimodal approach for filler injection can be beneficial, with deep injections to augment the mandibular fat pad, followed by injections in the subcutaneous dermal layer to improve contouring.
    - Restoring volume in the labiomental crease can support and augment the lower lip and chin interface. The ILA runs near the labial-buccal sulcus on the deep side of the lower lip and

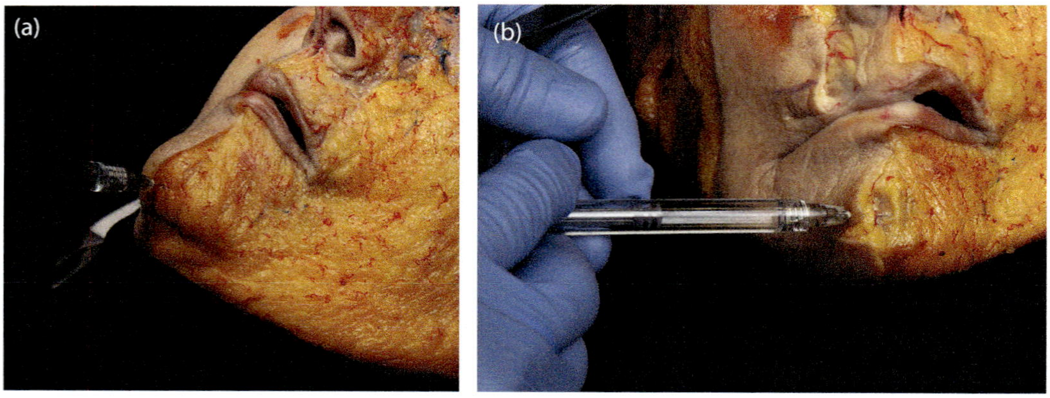

Figure 9.25 Chin injection techniques for volumization. (a) Lateral view of chin augmentation injection technique. (b) Frontal view of chin augmentation injection technique.

must be avoided. Volume can be added over the insertion of the mentalis muscle, along the posterior aspect of the orbicularis oris muscle and over the DLI. Superficial subcutaneous injections will add support and minimize complications, but fillers injected too close to the skin can be aesthetically unappealing.

- When mentalis strain is present, the mentalis fat pad can be volumized with filler. An entry point at the maximal chin convexity may be used with subcutaneous angulation off the midline until resistance is met before entering the fat pad.
- The deep lateral chin compartments are key targets for volumization. These fat pads lie deep to the DAO and facilitate muscle glide. Anterior to this fat pad is a membrane which helps protect the mental nerve. The mental nerve has a super-omedial course and often travels with the ILA, thereby posing a risk when injecting in the region. A 27G needle (Figure 9.26) or a 38 mm 25G cannula with an entry point at the paramedian inferior border of the mandible allows entry cranially into the sub-DAO plane and injection into the deep lateral chin compartments. This technique allows the injector to pass caudal to the mental foramen and over the periosteum of the mandible, medial to lateral. Volumizing here will assist in blending the jawline and camouflaging the pre-jowl.

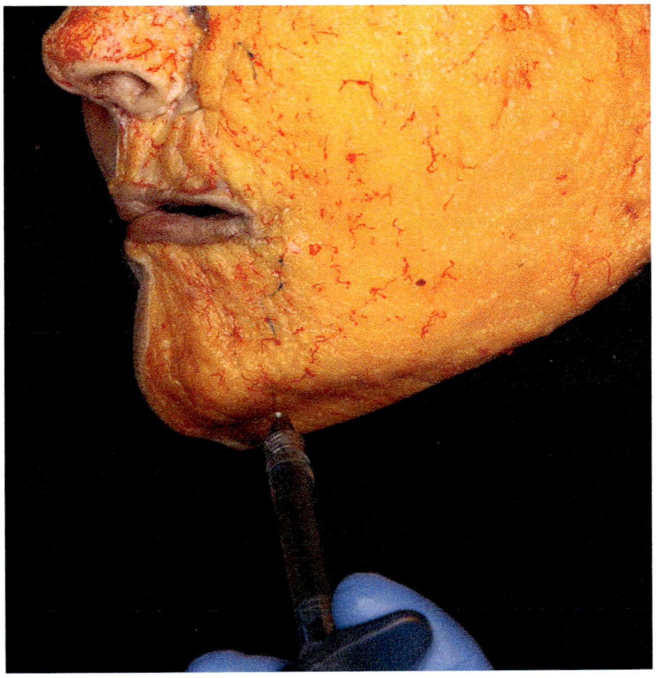

Figure 9.26 Deep lateral chin compartment augmentation with entry point at paramedian inferior border of mandible with cranial entry.

COMPLICATIONS

For general complications and the concept of "safety by depth," see Chapter G.

Seckel divided the face into seven functional danger zones [10]; in this chapter on chin and jaw injections, danger zones 3, 4, and 7 are applicable.

Toxins

- Take care with meticulous toxin placement to prevent migration into the depressor labii inferioris after either mentalis or DAO treatment.
- Take care with the dose and placement of toxin in the perioral area to prevent difficulty with phonation, whistling, and drinking.

Fillers

- Be aware of the position of the mental foramen.
- Beware of the submental artery.
- Visible contour deformity, asymmetry, and lumping may occur if placement is too superficial or when excessive volumes have been injected. Unevenness may be improved slightly with regular massage but may last for longer periods.
- Due to the mobility of the perioral area, suboptimal product placement may cause an unnatural appearance during speech.
- Large treatment volumes in the chin and the perioral area may impede natural speech in the first

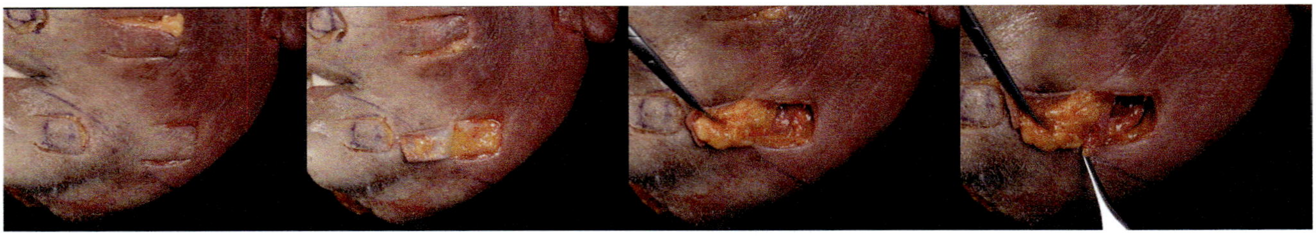

Figure 9.27 Dissection showing layer by layer location of danger zone 3 facial artery and vein.

week after treatment due to the impact on the orbicularis oris or DAO.
- The mental crease is a pain-sensitive area.
- Intraoral/bimanual massage is advised post-injection to reduce possible unevenness. Post-procedural swelling may be palpable intraorally.

Danger Zone 3

- This zone includes the marginal mandibular branch of the facial nerve at its most vulnerable point and also the facial artery and vein (Figure 9.27). This zone is located by identifying a point 2 cm posterior to the angle of the mouth and drawing a 2 cm-radius circle based on it. At this zone, the platysma-SMAS layer thins, thereby exposing the nerve and nearby facial vessels which are susceptible to injury.
- Damage to this nerve leads to significant aesthetic and functional repercussions. At rest, the tone in the normally innervated zygomaticus major muscle will be unopposed by the now denervated DAO, resulting in elevation of that corner of the mouth and the lower lip pulled up over the teeth. During grimacing or frowning, the now denervated DAO cannot depress the corner of the mouth and lower lip, meaning the lower teeth will not show on the affected side.

Danger Zone 4

- This zone includes the zygomatic and buccal branches of the facial nerve, which are superficial to the masseter muscle and Bichat's fat pad but deep to the platysma-SMAS and parotid fascia layers. These branches are no longer protected by the parotid gland and therefore more vulnerable. The danger zone is located in a triangular region bound by the body of the mandible inferiorly, the parotid gland posteriorly, and zygomaticus major anteriorly. Using surface anatomy, this can be delineated by having a point at the oral commissure, at the highest point of the malar eminence, and the posterior border of the angle of the mandible.
- Injury to these nerves can result in paralysis of the zygomaticus major, the zygomaticus minor and the LLS. This results in sagging of the upper lip during rest and a more apparent disfigurement during smiling when the contralateral unopposed zygomaticus major and minor pull the mouth toward the innervated side.
- If nerve damage occurs, the muscle paralysis is often not long-term given the multiple interconnections between branches of the buccal and zygomatic nerves.

Danger Zone 7

- This zone contains the mental nerve (Figure 9.28), which carries sensory innervation to the ipsilateral chin and the lower lip and is a branch of the mandibular branch of the trigeminal nerve. The mental nerve exits the mental foramen, which is located at the midpoint of the body of the mandible, in line with the second lower premolar. The mental foramen lies on a sagittal line drawn through the midpoint of the pupil, the supraorbital, and the infraorbital foramen.

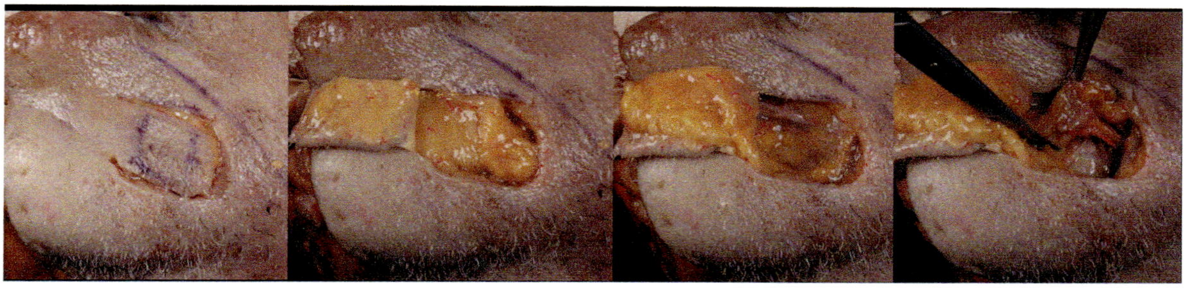

Figure 9.28 Dissection showing location of danger zone 7: Infraorbital nerve.

- Implications of nerve damage can be significant, with patients often not noticing when food is dribbling from that side of their mouth. Inadvertent lip biting may ensue while chewing.

References

1. Dallara JM et al. *J Cosmet Dermatol.* 2014;13(1): 3–14.
2. Pessa JERR. *Facial Topography, Clinical Anatomy of the Face.* Missouri: Quality Medical Publishing; 2012.
3. Carruthers A et al. *Dermatol Surg.* 2008;34(Suppl 2):S167–72.
4. Pilsl U and Anderhuber F. *Dermatologic Surg.* 2010;36(2):214–18.
5. Lamb JSC. *Facial Volumization: An Anatomic Approach.* Thieme; 2017.
6. Olszewski R et al. *Int J Comput Assist Radiol Surg.* 2009;4(4):349–52.
7. Braz AV et al. *An Bras Dermatol.* 2013;88(1): 138–40.
8. Angle EH. *Dent Cosmos.* 1899;41:248–64.
9. Mommaerts MY. *J Cranio-Maxillofacial Surg.* 2018;44(4):381–91.
10. Seckel B. *Facial Danger Zones. Avoiding Nerve Injury in Facial Plastic Surgery.* 2nd ed., Thieme; 2010.

Further Reading

Iblher N et al. *J Plast Reconstr Aesthet Surg.* 2008; 61(10):1170–6.

Penna V et al. *Plast Reconstr Surg.* 2009;124(2): 624–8.

Reece EM et al. *Plast Reconstr Surg.* 2008;121(4): 1414–20.

Rohrich RJ and Pessa JE *Plast Reconstr Surg.* 2009; 124(1):266–71.

10 NECK AND DÉCOLLETAGE

Kate Goldie, Uliana Gout, Randy B. Miller, Fernando Felice, Paraskevas Kontoes, and Izolda Heydenrych

INTRODUCTION

The neck is defined as the anatomical area that originates anteriorly from the inferior surface of the mandible and runs to the superior surface of the manubrium of the sternum.

As opposed to the face, where aesthetic treatment goals may be to both enhance beauty in younger patients and create a younger, fresher look in older patients, aesthetic treatments in the neck predominantly focus on preventing and rectifying the signs of aging.

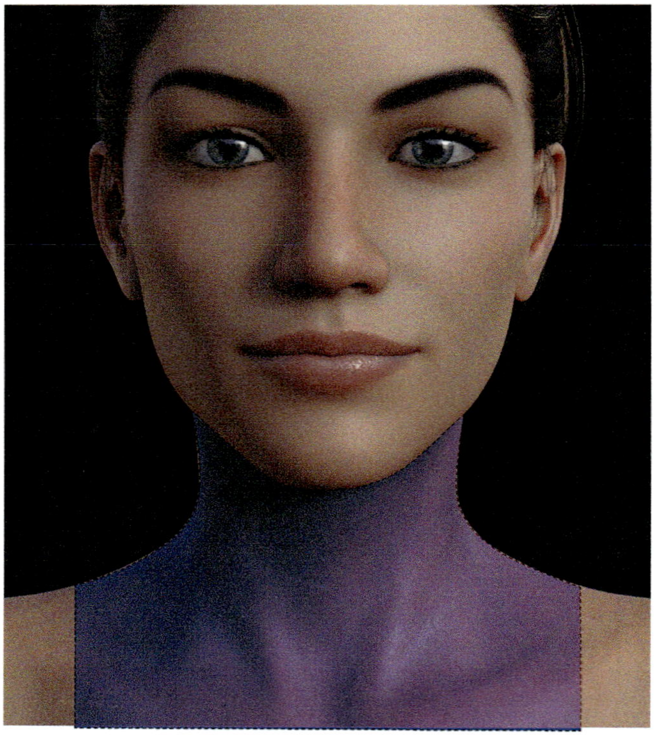

Figure 10.1 Boundaries of the neck (indicated in purple).

BOUNDARIES

The posterior neck borders are bounded superiorly by the occipital bone of the skull and inferiorly by the intervertebral disc between CVII and T1 [1] (Figure 10.1). The neck is often further divided into anterior and posterior triangles. The anterior triangle is bounded by the anterior border of the sternocleidomastoid, the midline of the neck, and the inferior border of the mandible. The posterior triangle is defined as the area of the neck bounded by the posterior border of the sternocleidomastoid (SCM), the anterior border of the trapezius and, inferiorly, the lateral third of the clavicle. The visible anterior triangle is predominately the focus of aesthetic treatments.

AGING

The aging neck is characterized by Figures 10.2 through 10.5:

- Increased soft tissue laxity
- Excess skin
- Fat accumulation
- Loss of the cervicomental angle

Considering how aging affects each of the cervical layers can help with diagnosis and selection of optimal treatment. The skin of the neck is often exposed to environmental stresses. Along with intrinsic factors of aging, cell and tissue senescence also leads to telomere shortening and Hayflick's limit. These processes result in laxity, generalized wrinkles, and horizontal necklines, along with pigmentary changes and the appearance of telangiectasia.

Histologically, the epidermis has a flattened dermo-epidermal junction. The dermis exhibits volume loss with decreased connective tissue structures and fewer fibroblasts [6].

Aesthetically, platysmal patterns impact aging. The platysma splays medially with age, loses tone, and

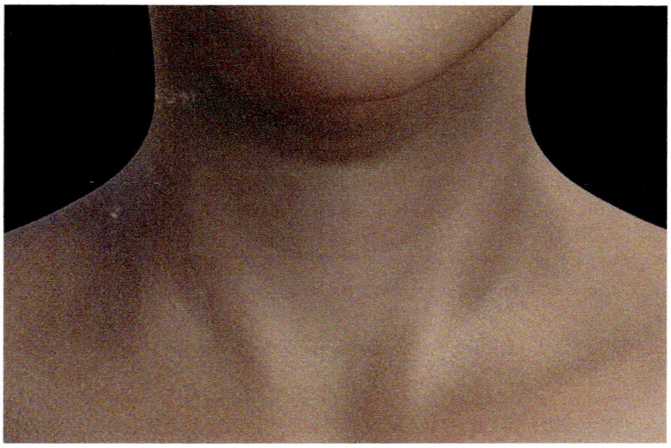

Figure 10.3 Aging neck showing excess skin, fat accumulation, and horizontal neck lines.

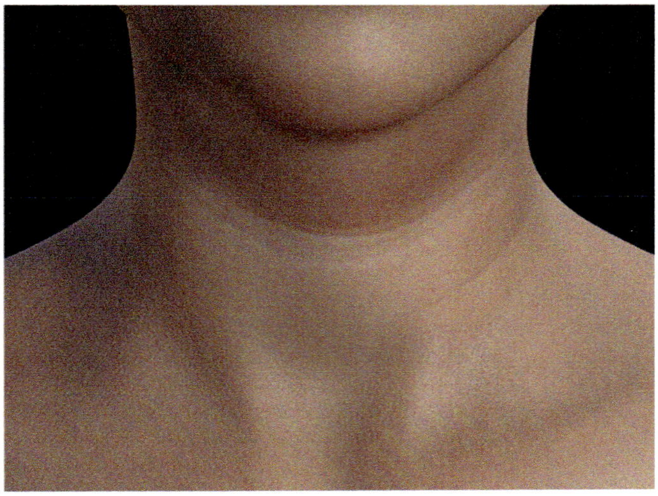

Figure 10.4 Aging neck showing horizontal neck lines.

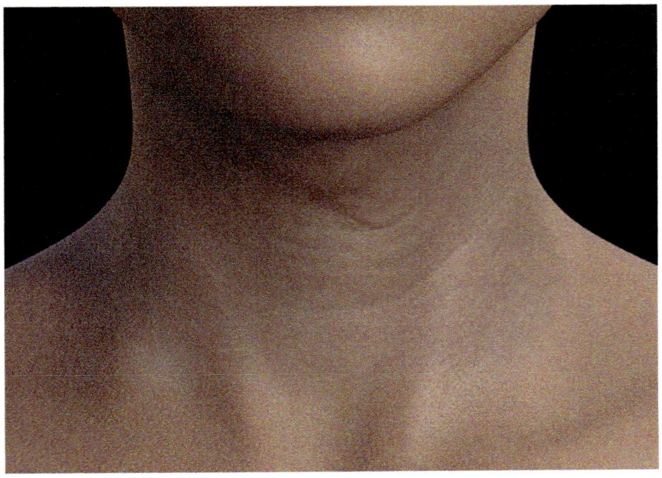

Figure 10.2 Aging neck showing horizontal and vertical neck lines.

suffers from weakened support from deep retaining ligaments. Individuals with the least decussation of platysma fibers are at increased risk of fat descent and ptosis of deep subplatysmal fat structures, thus creating poorly defined neck contours.

Deeper anatomical details, including digastric muscle length and the position of the hyoid bone, may affect neck aesthetics, and impact negatively on the cervico-mental angle (CMA). Enlarged submandibular glands can also lead to blurring of the superior neck borders (Figures 10.2 and 10.5).

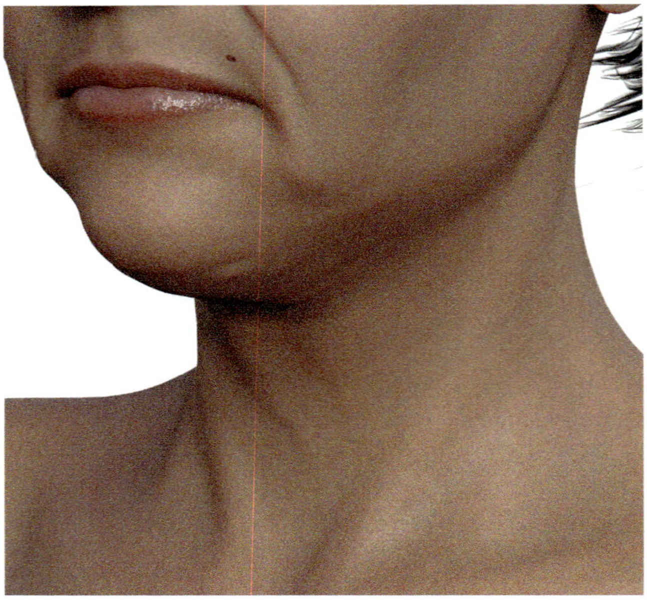

Figure 10.5 Neck skin showing horizontal neck lines and platysmal bands.

SKIN

The skin of the neck is thinner than most facial regions, but it is considerably more extensible and visco-elastic [2] as it has evolved to withstand the dynamic movement caused by the raising and turning of the head. The subdermis contains varying amounts of superficial fat, which correlate positively with increasing BMI.

FAT

Pre-platysmal fat thickness varies with age and ethnicity (Figures 10.6 through 10.8). The subplatysmal fat of the neck occurs as distinct regions that may be identified by their consistent relationship to the platysma, digastric, and mylohyoid muscles. The mylohyoid muscle comprises the posterior boundary.

There are three compartments—central, medial, and lateral (Figure 10.9)—which abut each other to form the subplatysmal fat layer. There are differences in thickness of these compartments.

Central fat is easily distinguished from medial and lateral fat due to differences in color and appearance.

MUSCLES

Aesthetically, the platysma is the single most important structure in the neck. The platysma is a wide

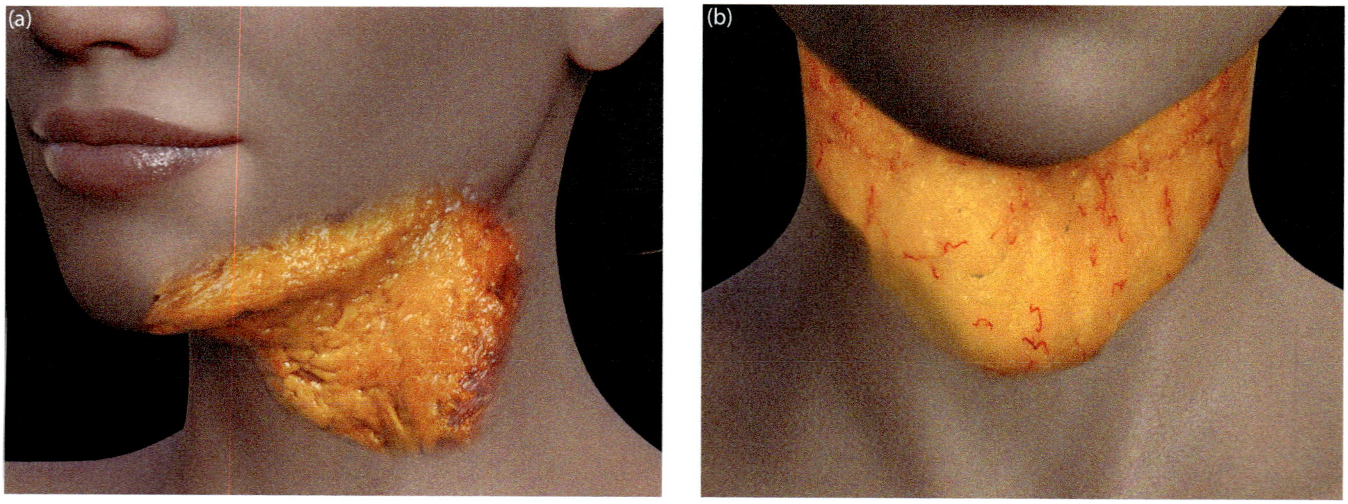

Figure 10.6 (a) Pre-platysmal fat in oblique view. (b) Pre-platysmal fat in anterior view.

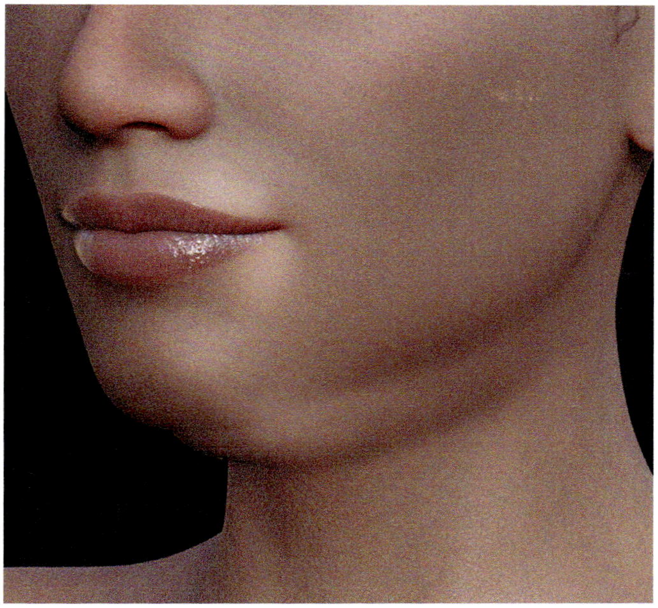

Figure 10.7 Excess fat in neck showing submental fullness.

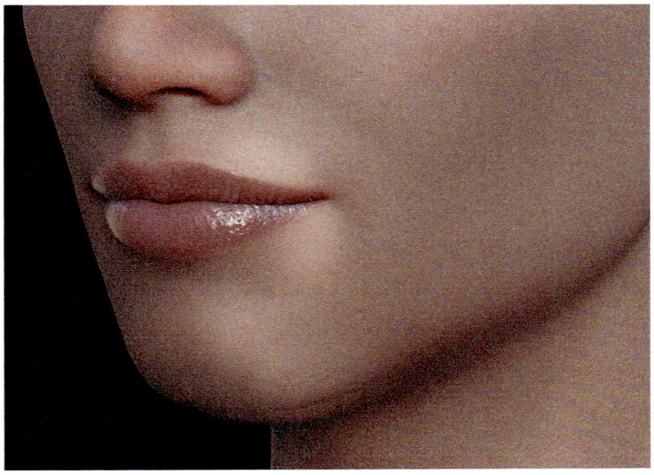

Figure 10.8 Moderate submental fat.

flat muscle that originates, in most cases, from the upper portion of the thorax anterior to the clavicle. The platysma will most commonly course superomedially; however, in almost a third of individuals, the platysma ascends almost vertically from the clavicle to the face [4].

The platysma has a variety of muscle insertion points: cheek skin (57.5%), cutaneous muscles

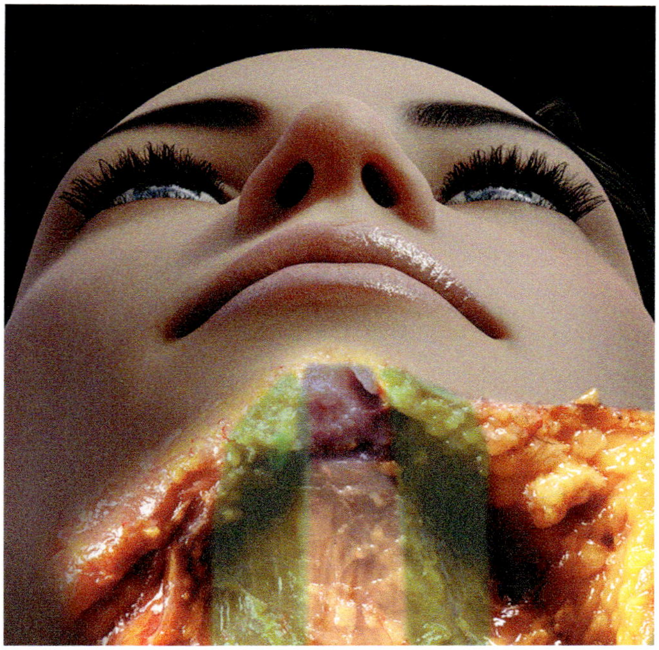

Figure 10.9 Subplatysmal fat with three fat compartments: blue (central), white (medial), and green (lateral).

around the mouth (18.6%) and the mandibular-cutaneous ligament, and zygoma [4]. In some individuals, the deep fibers attach to the periosteum of the mandible or the parotid fascia, creating a deeper anchoring point, while more superficial fibers continue superiorly.

Functionally, platysma contraction will pull the corners of the lips inferiorly, working in the concert with other key lower face depressors such as mentalis and depressor anguli oris. In addition, the platysma can help to pull the corner of the lips inferiorly and laterally. All these individual variations have potential effects on the aesthetic role the platysma plays in the lower face and neck.

The platysma has, for many years, been treated with botulinum toxin for effacing the appearance of platysmal banding. Recently the use of botulinum toxin in the neck has evolved to provide more nuanced strategies to lift and reshape the lower face, soften horizontal lines, and improve the appearance of skin, in addition to minimizing vertical banding.

Achieving lift and reshaping of the lower face while maintaining natural expression requires a deeper understanding of the anatomical interconnections between lower facial muscles and the platysma, and their joint function in the depression of the lower face. De Almeida et al. proposed that increased understanding of the functional division between the upper and lower platysma would increase aesthetic outcomes [5]. For lower face shaping, it is the upper platysma is which holds the key. The upper platysma comprises three sections (Figure 10.10):

- Platysma pars mandibularis (PPM)
- Platysma pars labialis (PPL)
- Platysma pars modiolaris (PPMo)

PPM attaches to the border of the mandible, the depressor angui oris (DAO), and the cutaneous lower face. The contraction of this platysmal section creates submandibular necklines running inferiorly and laterally from the inferior border of the DAO. Functionally, the DAO and the PPM work in conjunction. Treatment of either muscle in isolation may lead to unnatural results in patients with overly dynamic muscle combinations.

The PPL courses behind the DAO and inserts into medial lower face muscles such as the orbicularis oris and depressor labii inferioris, thus depressing the lateral third of the mouth.

Finally, there is the PPMo, which is the platysmal section lying lateral and posterior to the DAO. Predominance of this platysmal division while smiling can lead to exaggerated buccal smile lines, which corrugate the skin and disturb the aesthetic appearance of the midface.

Other superficial muscles of the neck include the sternocleidomastoid (SCM) and trapezius. These muscles are of lesser aesthetic importance. The superhyoid and infrahyiod strap muscles, situated more deeply in the anterior triangle, are important for swallowing, elevating, and depressing the hyoid bone. Consequently, excessive anterior and midline botulinum toxin should be avoided to prevent possible interference with muscle function.

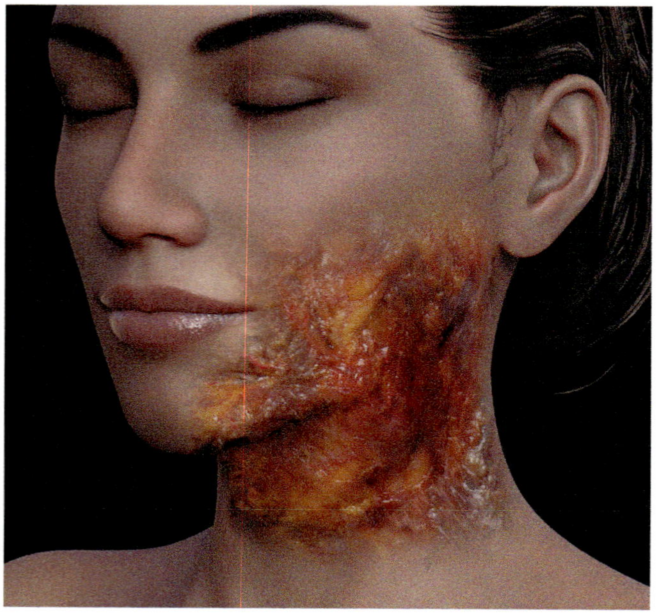

Figure 10.10 The three sections of the upper platysma: PPM, PPL and PPMo.

VASCULARIZATION

Arteries

- The main artery of the neck is the common carotid which divides at the upper border of the thyroid cartilage of the larynx (C4) to form the internal and external carotid arteries (Figure 10.11).
- The vasculature of the anterior cervical skin arises from the superior thyroid artery and the transverse cervical branch of the subclavian artery [1].
- The facial artery provides the vascular supply of platysma via the submental branch and by the subclavian artery via the suprascapular artery.

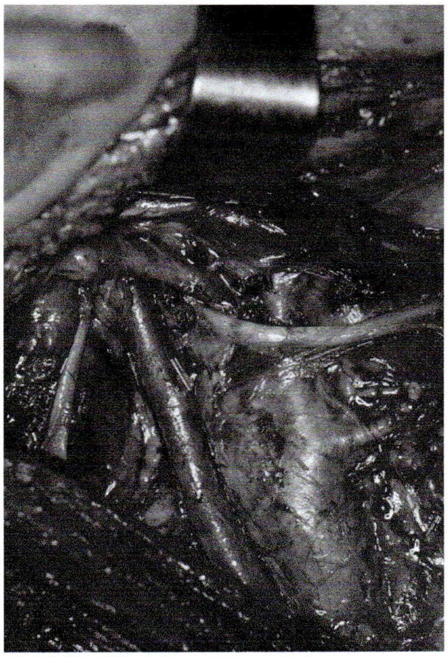

Figure 10.11 Lateral view of neck vascularization; note the common carotid artery and external jugular vein.

- Myocutaneous perforators have been described between the sternocleidomastoid, strap muscles, and trapezius to supply the dermal-subdermal plexus, which is continuous across the midline and supplied chiefly by branches of the superior thyroid artery, the facial artery, and the myocutaneous perforators of the strap muscles.

Veins

- The largest vein in the neck is the internal jugular vein, which originates at the jugular foramen and descends in the neck as part of the carotid sheath.
- The external jugular vein is located close to the angle of the mandible, near the lower auricle of the ear, and passes diagonally across the sternocleidomastoid muscle.

INNERVATION

Cervical cutaneous innervation emerges from the cervical spinal nerves.

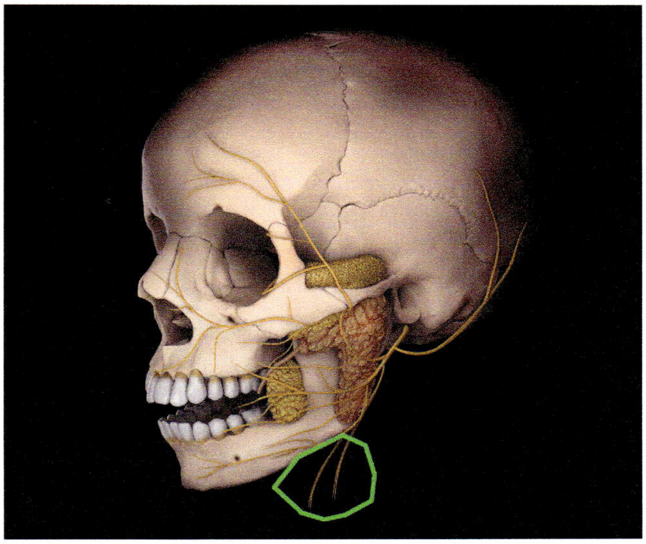

Figure 10.12 Innervation of the neck (note cervical branch of the Facial nerve).

The anterior triangle is innervated by the transverse cervical nerve, which courses medially as it emerges posteriorly to the sternocleidomastoid muscle.

Knowledge of the location of the greater auricular nerve (GAN) is of importance in preventing nerve injury in aesthetic treatments. The GAN is the largest ascending branch of the cervical plexus and sometimes runs closely under platysma. The most superficial position of the nerve is reliably found one-third of the distance between the mastoid process (or alternatively the auditory canal) and the clavicle [6].

The innervation of platysma is via the cervical branch of the facial nerve which runs deep to the platysma and is situated close to the inferior border of the mandible (Figure 10.12).

BONE

The two types of bone in the neck are the cervical vertebrae and the hyoid bones, neither of which impact aesthetic treatments. The shape, size, and conformation of the mandible, although not technically the neck, plays an integral role in the suspension of cervical soft tissue and overall neck aesthetics. One of the first steps to improving the cervicomental angle (CMA) non-surgically is to correct retrogenia with anterior submental chin augmentation, using soft tissue fillers to project the mental pogonion.

HOW I DO IT: BOTULINUM TOXIN

Treatment of the Neck

An aesthetically pleasing neck has a CMA of between 105°–120°, a defined mandibular border, a distinct subhyoid cartilage depression, and a thyroid cartilage bulge (Figure 10.13). In addition, the absence of obvious platysmal banding with minimal vertical lines and hydrated firm skin with an even tone is preferred. Depending on the diagnosis of the unique pattern of cervical aging for each patient, a variety of treatment modalities may be considered.

Botulinum toxin is ideal for vertical platysmal banding and mild-to-moderate horizontal wrinkles in patients without particularly thick skin. Botulinum toxin is also very effective at reshaping the lower face and increasing jawline sharpness in patients without excessive lower face fat. Botulinum toxin is injected with small gauge needles (30G to 35G) subdermally in small doses (Figure 10.13). Possible treatment protocols are described later in this chapter.

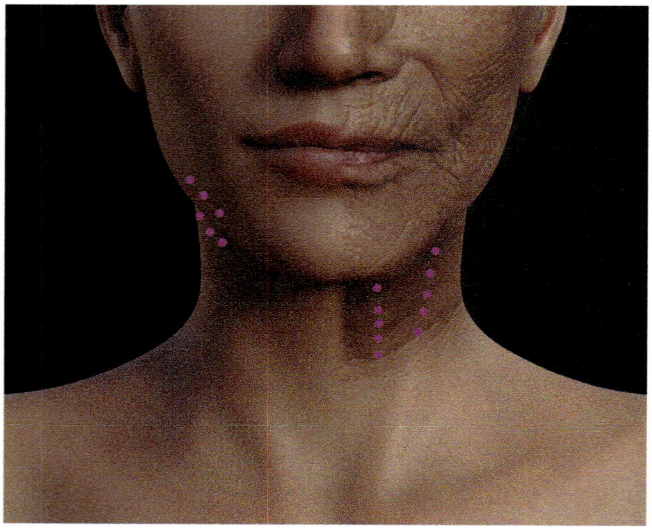

Figure 10.13 Botulinum toxin treatment areas in patient with platysmal bands and ill-defined jawline.

Precautions

- Initially, toxin doses of 30–60 U (Botox, Xeomin, Bocouture, Vistabel) in total for the entire neck is sufficient as a maximum for one treatment. More may be placed additionally after two weeks, once the effect is visible.
- Excessive neuromodulation of the platysma can lead to difficulty in lifting the head while lying down. In addition, it is important not to place excessive toxin near the midline due to the risk of migration to deep muscular structures and consequential dysphagia.
- Conversely, care should be taken to avoid neuromodulation of only the lateral neck, thus leaving the medial neck completely free of toxin. In some cases, this pattern of injection can cause recruitment and hyperactivity of the medial platysma, leading to worsening of medial banding, squaring of the face, and blunting of the CMA.
- Toxin is largely ineffective at producing satisfying aesthetic outcomes where excessive laxity and fat exist.
- As with all injections, some bruising, swelling, and redness can occur but is usually minimal.
- Hypersensitivity to toxin is possible, but extremely rare.

HOW I DO IT: FILLERS

Hyaluronic Acid

The target for HA fillers in the neck is normally direct effacement of horizontal "necklace" lines, as well

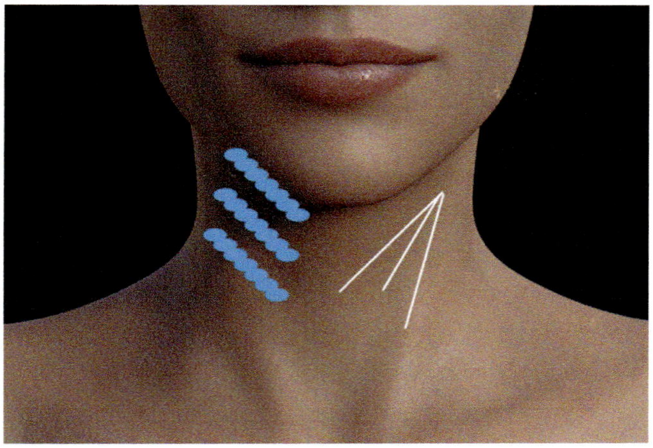

Figure 10.14 Treatment areas of the neck for hyaluronic acid filler.

as overall skin hydration, texture improvement, and easing of fine lines (Figure 10.14). The technique of delivery differs between these aesthetic goals. Ideal candidates for this treatment have mild-to-moderate horizontal lines, minimal skin laxity, and the absence of voluminous neck "rolls." HA may be effective in thicker skin patients without excessive neck volume.

Using low-viscosity, low-elasticity HA fillers is important. Identification of HAs formulated to carry minimal risk of producing the Tyndall effect is important here, as the depth of injecting is very superficial.

Direct placement of HA into horizontal necklines can be carried out with either a needle or 25G 5 cm cannula. Needles used to fill necklines are usually small gauge (~30G) or smaller. The advantage of a needle is that a very accurate intradermal depth of HA filler is possible. The delivery options include multiple slow, low volume injections, linear threading, or a continuous line of microaliquots placed at the deepest part of the wrinkle. The key here is small depots, intradermally, which appear flat immediately after injection. HA can also be injected diffusely across the neck for general hydration and skin boosting; these injection patterns do not follow lines but scatter the sites evenly across the anterior surface of the neck using either needle or cannula.

New thermally crosslinked HAs are available which are injected with a needle in fewer, higher-volume aliquots of 0.1–0.2 mL. These raised blebs of HA diffuse by osmosis across the neck over several hours, creating a firmer more hydrated skin. The longevity is about 6 months, during which a patient may have to be treated twice. Although this is not completely ideal, the ease of injection, evenness of product deposition, and skin quality changes make it a successful treatment.

The use of cannula in the neck mitigates risk of both superficial intravascular injections and inadvertently crossing into deeper, higher-risk tissues planes. Using a cannula in the neck is technically more difficult, especially in patients with previous non-surgical treatments. Using multiple injection sites where the planes of the neck are flatter, as well as using a smaller gauge cannula (25 g/50 mm), can ease this difficulty when using cannulae in the subdermis.

Precautions

- Bruising, erythema and mild edema are normal after HA in the neck. In particular, erythema and edema may last several days longer compared to what would be expected in the mid- and lower face.
- When using a needle, it is crucial that correct tissue plane is maintained with no deep placement under the thin platysma.
- The most common problem after treatment is visible product either in the depth of the vertical line or immediately adjacent to it. Small aliquots of product accurately placed can help prevent this. Some swelling and visibility after treatment is normal for the first few days, but if persistent, the product can be either completely removed or strategically shaped with hyaluronidase.

CALCIUM HYDROXYAPATITE (CAHA)

This treatment is ideal for firming and strengthening the cervical dermis and is especially effective when placed in the submandibular subdermis. Traditionally, CaHA has been used as a volumizing filler in cheeks and nasal labial folds. CaHA was originally designed not only as a filling agent but also to act through biostimulation and tissue regeneration. The gel comprises 70% carboxymethylcellulose gel and 30% calcium hydroxylapatite. Once placed under the dermis, the carrier gel resorbs over the next 3–6 six months. During this time, a matrix of collagen and elastin develops, with increased dermal thickness and angiogenesis. The collagen, although initially Type 3, is mostly converted to Type 1 over time.

In the neck it is important to dilute the products with 1:2 with sterile saline and mix thoroughly, as this allows easyapplication and decreases risk of visible product post-treatment.

Precautions

- In addition to the precautions for HA, it is important to hyperdilute CaHA before being used superficially in the neck.
- The CaHA should be deposited in multiple low-volume linear threads.

COMBINATION THERAPIES

Many treatments are commonly used in combination with botulinum toxins, HA fillers, and biostimulatory agents.

Many devices successfully treat signs of neck aging such as skin quality, tissue lifting, and fat reduction.

Skin quality improvements are achieved with intense pulsed light, fractional ablative lasers, and non-ablative fractional lasers.

Tissue lifting devices include monopolar radio frequency and microfocused ultrasound with visualization.

Effective localized fat reduction methods include cryolipolysis, chemical lipolysis, and laser lipolysis.

COMPLICATIONS

For general complications and the concept of "safety by depth," see Chapter G.

Seckel divided the face into seven functional danger zones [3]; the neck region includes danger zone 1.

Toxins

- Common complications of botulinum toxin in the neck include unintentional recruitment of the medial platysma, bruising, mild swelling, and edema.
- Excessive use of toxin in the medial platysma may lead to dysphagia.
- Excessive overall treatment of the neck risks creating mechanical issues with the raising of the head.

Fillers

- Bruising is a common side effect.
- The most common complication of dermal fillers in the neck is visible product.
- Careful technique and minute aliquots will help to prevent this.
- Prolonged and aesthetically displeasing HA placements may be dissolved with hyaluronidase.

- After treatment, the area should be cleansed again with, for example, chlorhexidine and should remain untouched and scarf free for at least 6 hours afterward.

References

1. Rohrich RJ & Pessa JE. *Plastic Reconstr Surg.* 2010;126(2):589–95.
2. Goldie K et al. *Dermatol Surg.* 2018 Nov;44 (Suppl 1):S32–41.
3. Seckel B. *Facial Danger Zones*, 2nd ed. Thieme; 2010.
4. Kim E et al. *Skin Res Technol.* 2013 Aug; 19(3):236–41.
5. Guidera AK et al. *Head Neck.* 2014;36(7): 1058–68.
6. Hwang K et al. *J Craniofac Surg.* 2017;28(2): 539–42.

Further Reading

Cardoso & de Castro C. *Plast Reconstr Surg.* 2000 Feb;105(2):764–75.

De Almeida ART et al. *Dermatol Surg.* 2017;43(8): 1042–9.

Rohrich RJ et al. *Plast Reconstr Surg.* 2011;127(2): 835–43.

Shadfar S & Perkins SW. *Facial Plast Surg Clin North Am.* 2014;22(2):161–70.

Sykes JM. *Facial Plast Surg.* 2001;17(2):99–107.

VIDEO APPENDIX: HOW I DO REGIONAL TREATMENTS

Ali Pirayesh and Dario Bertossi

1. **Forehead region**
   https://youtu.be/RuDPJn_cYYg
2. **Temporal region and lateral brow region**
   https://youtu.be/MTW0Yi0XUvA
3. **Periorbital region**
   https://youtu.be/DnhNIPQwMII
4. **Cheek region**
   https://youtu.be/FEnWrKDJbMI
5. **Nasal region**
   https://youtu.be/Kw6ZPp6LvYU
6. **Nasolabial region**
   https://youtu.be/ROrvThqY1LI
7. **Lip region**
   https://youtu.be/mxHwV-z3mjU
8. **Perioral region**
   https://youtu.be/VvfcRUCvsMA
9. **Chin region**
   https://youtu.be/efep5qEwNx8
10. **Jawline and mandibular angle region**
    https://youtu.be/rKJQX6jj8sM
11. **Neck region**
    https://youtu.be/4WjVH_Nzib4
12. **Botulinum toxin injections**
    https://youtu.be/lRAHyZCkhPM

INDEX

C

D

E

F

N

O

P